# Living with Germs

## IN HEALTH AND DISEASE

John Playfair

**OXFORD**
UNIVERSITY PRESS

# OXFORD

UNIVERSITY PRESS

Great Clarendon Street, Oxford ox2 6DP

Oxford University Press is a department of the University of Oxford.
It furthers the University's objective of excellence in research, scholarship,
and education by publishing worldwide in

Oxford New York

Auckland Cape Town Dar es Salaam Hong Kong Karachi
Kuala Lumpur Madrid Melbourne Mexico City Nairobi
New Delhi Shanghai Taipei Toronto

With offices in

Argentina Austria Brazil Chile Czech Republic France Greece
Guatemala Hungary Italy Japan Poland Portugal Singapore
South Korea Switzerland Thailand Turkey Ukraine Vietnam

Oxford is a registered trade mark of Oxford University Press
in the UK and in certain other countries

Published in the United States
by Oxford University Press Inc., New York

© John Playfair 2004

The moral rights of the author have been asserted

Database right Oxford University Press (maker)

First published 2004
First published as an Oxford University Press Paperback 2007

British Library Cataloguing in Publication Data

Data available

Library of Congress Cataloging in Publication Data

Data available

ISBN 978-0-19-280582-9

1 3 5 7 9 10 8 6 4 2

Typeset by RefineCatch Limited, Bungay, Suffolk
Printed in Great Britain by
Clays Ltd, St Ives plc

*This book is dedicated to Humphrey Kay, Leonard Cole, Ben Papermaster, and Ivan Roitt, who steered me along my way over 40 years, and to Greg Bancroft, who hauled me into the twenty-first century.*

The deviation of man from the state in which he was originally placed by nature seems to have proved to him a prolific source of diseases. From the love of splendour, from the indulgence of luxury, and from his fondness for amusement, he has familiarized himself with a great number of animals which may not originally have been intended for his associates.

Edward Jenner, 1798

An inquiry into the causes and effects of the variolae vacciniae (cow pox)

As it takes two to make a quarrel, so it takes two to make a disease, the microbe and its host.

Charles V Chapin (1856–1941)

# Foreword
by Sir Walter Bodmer FRS

Most people know that a germ is a very small living organism that causes disease. Germs are microbes, namely that part of the living world that can usually be seen only under a microscope, if at all. The world of the microbe is enormously diverse and includes viruses such as smallpox and HIV, bacteria, fungi and moulds, small worms and little animal-like organisms that cause diseases such as malaria. Most microbes are harmless to us humans, and some are beneficial not only in food such as cheeses or yoghurt, but also by playing an important role in the normal functioning of our gut.

Evolution, as Charles Darwin taught us, is driven by natural selection, and among the most adverse challenges that essentially all living organisms face is the attack from germs – those micro-organisms that do cause disease – often referred to as 'pathogens'. That is not some form of gene, but a name derived from the word 'pathology', which is the study of the essential nature of disease; so much of which, especially during most of our evolution, was due to disease-causing microbes. One of the major driving forces of natural selection has thus been to find ways of overcoming germ attacks, since survival in the face of an attack from a pathogen is clearly going to confer a significant selective advantage. A system, called the 'immune system', has evolved over many hundreds of millions of years specifically to deal with germ attacks, and its study is 'immunology'. The importance of immunology is reflected in the number of Nobel prizes given for discoveries in this field, starting from when they were first given at the very beginning of the twentieth century.

The earliest, and perhaps most primitive, immune system which we still retain mainly recognizes major classes of chemical differences which are characteristic of pathogens. This is referred to as 'innate' immunity. Subsequently, a system evolved to recognize, with exquisite sensitivity, almost any chemical difference between us and the invading pathogens. This is called the 'adaptive' immune system. Sometimes the immune system does not function properly, and itself causes disease. Sometimes the immune system can be put to good use, as in making reagents that recognize chemical differences of almost any sort, and these agents are widely used – for example by the pathologist in diagnosing what disease an individual may be suffering from. Immunity may also be put to use in attacking the differences between cancer and normal cells, forming the basis for novel treatments. Immunity may also be the basis for a form of contraception, for example by tricking the immune system into attacking sperm.

John Playfair's book deals with all these different aspects of germs and immunity in a clear and engaging way. Immunology is full of complex ideas, but here they are explained in a manner that anybody, whatever their background knowledge, should be able to understand. Concepts and organisms are clearly defined, and there is an excellent glossary at the end of the book. I could not think of a better way for the non-expert to learn about this fascinating area of science and medicine than to read John Playfair's book. Even the experts may find a few nuggets here and there, and also discover new ways to explain, in simple terms, the complexities of their field.

*Walter Bodmer*
*6 July 2004*

# Acknowledgements

As well as those mentioned in the dedication, I wish to thank my wife, Anthony Lamb, Guy Playfair, Sir Matthew Farrer, Sarah Houston, and Janice Taverne, who helped me to turn the early drafts into (I hope) a reasonably intelligible final product. I am most grateful to Michael Rodgers of Oxford University Press, who was encouraging from the first telephone call, and to Latha Menon and Marsha Filion who guided it into print.

I should add that I am alone responsible for the opinions expressed in this book, and for any factual errors that may have crept into it.

# Contents

Introduction: Living with Germs                                    1

1  Infection and immunity                                          5

2  The pathogens                                                  19

3  Defence and immunity: the old immune system                   74

4  Sharpening the focus: the new immune system                   94

5  Communication and collaboration                              121

6  The pathogens fight back                                      137

7  Getting ill                                                   160

8  Immunodeficiency                                              187

9  Controlling pathogens                                         204

10  A look ahead                                                 241

Glossary and abbreviations                                       251

Biographies                                                      264

Further reading                                                  268

Index                                                            275

# Introduction: Living with Germs

Open almost any newspaper nowadays and you will probably be greeted by a headline about the imminent arrival of mutant killer bird flu, or the ever-rising toll from AIDS or tuberculosis, the spread of West Nile virus, the reappearance of polio or SARS, an outbreak of Lassa fever, the failure of yet another malaria vaccine, or a death in hospital from a superbug resistant to all antibiotics. You could be forgiven for concluding that our planet swarms with all kinds of germs and microbes invisible to the eye and that their one aim is to wipe us all out. The first conclusion is undoubtedly true, but fortunately the second is not, and this book is an attempt to explain why.

Consider for a moment the creatures we can see. With the possible exception of ourselves, they do not seem particularly keen on mutual elimination. The dogs that half-heartedly chase our two cats if they escape into the road, or the pigeons, crows, and squirrels that forage together in our local park, may not be the best of friends, but they don't spend their time trying to kill one another. On the whole, except where you have two species directly competing for food or space, or when one of them is the other's favourite meal, 'live and let live' seems to be Nature's general rule.

Yes, but *germs*, you will object – aren't they surely the exception to this amicable arrangement? Malevolent, microscopic creatures like HIV, the TB bacillus, the malaria parasite, *do* infect and kill millions of our species every year; from time to time whole populations are decimated by the microbes of plague or flu; how can that possibly be called peaceful? How could we *live* with them? Surely what we want is to get rid of them? You would have a point, of course. It would be marvellous to get rid of HIV and flu and TB and malaria, but the fact is that these and a few others are the exception *even among microbes*. The vast majority of microbes don't infect us at all, and of those that do, only a tiny minority cause us any real trouble.

I have been using the words 'germ' and 'microbe' because everybody knows roughly what they mean, but they are not precise scientific terms. A *germ* is usually defined in dictionaries as 'a microbe that causes disease'. And when we turn to *microbe* we find it is 'a small living organism, or micro-organism, visible only under the microscope, which may or may not cause disease', or words to that effect.

Let us now be more precise. Those microbes, germs, bugs – call them what you will – that do cause disease are more correctly known as *pathogens*, and this is a scientific term. Pathogens cause *pathology* (disease), and pathology makes you ill – may even kill you. It is pathogens that are the real enemy, and they are the 'germs' this book is concerned with.

But it is not just about the pathogens themselves. There are already many excellent books about viruses, bacteria, tropical diseases, and so on (I have listed a selection of these at the end). In this book the emphasis is equally on the defence mechanisms by which we come to terms with the pathogens – eliminating them, stopping them eliminating *us*, or simply learning to live with them. This is the world of immunity and *immunology* – a subject with a reputation for being difficult. I hope I have managed to show that it is actually quite approachable. If you do find it heavy going, try re-reading Chapters 3 to 5 before continuing.

Some readers might prefer a book of this kind to carry a forceful 'take-home message' on the lines of: *if we do not immediately take such'and'such steps, disaster will follow, but if we do so-and-so all will be well.* I am afraid our topic is not that simple or sensational. Infectious disease is not one single problem and there is not one single solution. What I have tried to do is to present the known facts about infection and immunity as they appear today to the majority of experts in the field, with a sprinkling of history to explain how these facts were established, plus a few personal reminiscences to give an idea of how much has changed within living memory. You do not need to have a science degree, or even a background in science, to follow the argument, just an interest in infection – which after all affects every single one of us throughout our life. I have assumed absolutely no previous knowledge of biology, microbiology, or genetics, but I hope you will enjoy being drawn a little way into these subjects as you read. They are no more inaccessible than cooking or gardening (neither of which I have ever come anywhere near to mastering), and infinitely easier to get to grips with than the big bang, quantum theory, or relativity – which, frankly, leave even the average scientist fairly baffled. If I have a message at all, it is simply that you are bound to get infections from time to time, and you are better off knowing something about what is going on. You can then at least decide what to do on the basis of fact and not fear or fantasy.

Occasionally you will come across words or abbreviations that are new to you, in which case you can refer to the Glossary at the end. I have also listed some of the generally available books on infection and related topics, plus a few textbooks for the reader who wants to go deeper into the subject. There is of course a mass of up-to-the-minute information on the internet – most of it accurate, some of it nonsense – which I hope will be made a little more intelligible by a previous reading of the book you have in your hands.

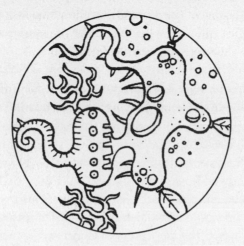

# 1  Infection and immunity

So, naturalists observe, a flea
Hath smaller fleas that on him prey;
And these have smaller fleas to bite'em,
And so proceed ad infinitum.
                    Jonathan Swift

In July 1989, just four months before the Wall was reduced to
souvenir-sized rubble, Berlin hosted the seventh International
Congress of Immunology Societies. The brand new International
Conference Centre buzzed with research students, lecturers,
professors, clinicians, specialists in biochemistry, genetics,
haematology, allergy, rheumatic disease, transplant surgery, from
fifty countries, six and a half thousand of them altogether – plus
some very nervous German security guards. It was the city's
chance to show what it could do, the World Cup of immunology.

Washington, Brighton, Sydney, Paris, Kyoto, Toronto, had already had their turn, at three-year intervals, and of course each meeting has to outshine the last one, and usually does.

I had come out of a workshop on AIDS, still a new disease then, and still the source of bad feeling between the French and the Americans, both of whom considered that it was they who had discovered the virus, HIV, six years earlier. It was just being realized how difficult it was going to be to control the disease, and opinions differed violently on how to proceed. Some rather, shall we say, unprofessional comments had been exchanged, and, feeling that a moment of calm would be welcome, I wandered into the special display room, where the laboratory of Germany's greatest biological scientist, Paul Ehrlich, had been faithfully recreated. Ehrlich flourished in the quarter-century leading up to the First World War, and he will turn up again and again in this book. If it has a hero, he is probably it.

It was a time when bearded professors in wing collars and three-piece suits sat at solid mahogany desks with a microscope and an inkstand and a pile of leather-bound journals – and in Ehrlich's case a permanent cigar – and terrorized all who came near them (not quite the lifestyle of today's professor!). There were a few of my own age group in the dim little room, but none of the younger generation. They were too busy arguing in their symposia and workshops and in any case probably didn't care too much about Ehrlich. For most of them, real science began in 1953 with Watson and Crick and the DNA double helix. Infectious diseases, which had been Ehrlich's special interest, were nowadays for GPs and hospital doctors to worry about. Immunology was concerned with ideas, theories, gene rearrangements, on/off signals, feedback, networks – not throat swabs, vaccine jabs, and temperature charts.

AIDS, of course, was to change all this, but even that year, at the small preliminary meeting held six months earlier in a magnificent Bavarian hotel, surrounded by pine forests and fields of unbroken snow, I and a few colleagues had had to push quite hard for there to be even a single workshop on vaccination at the coming conference. Vaccination – the one application of immunology from which the entire world has benefited! We got our way, I'm glad to say, but it was a near thing. Vaccines, it was felt, were somehow . . . well, *boring*. They worked, one's children had them, and that was about it. In fact, all those *microbes* were considered fairly unexciting too, the responsibility of service staff in starched white coats and masks – a far cry from the jeans, trainers, and anarchic tee-shirts of the proper lab scientist. I sat next to a brilliant molecular geneticist from Switzerland who expressed surprise, after my talk, to hear that whooping cough was a bacterial, not a viral disease. I was reminded (though I didn't say it) of the frequent newspaper articles about the 'malaria virus'. I have occasionally thought of writing in to point out that the malaria parasite was a *protozoan*, not a virus – and incidentally that the notorious 'flesh-eating virus' was in fact a *bacterium*, and that the flu virus was actually just as much a *parasite* as the malaria 'parasite' was . . . but that would be to emulate Disgusted, who writes regularly to complain of a split infinitive or a hanging participle in a news story, so I refrained. It seemed more useful to write a book.

**Parasites, pathogens, and immunity**

To return for one last time to *microbes*, it is true that most pathogens (*bacteria* and *protozoa*, for example) are indeed microscopic in size. However, some are quite visible to the naked eye (see *fungi* and *worms*, below). Others are not even properly living organisms (see *viruses* and *prions*). But one feature they do all share is of being *parasites* – that is, they live in or on the body of their host (i.e. you or me) and depend on it for some or all of their needs. Unfortunately the word 'parasite' is sometimes applied only to pathogenic protozoa and worms, especially those common in tropical countries; this use of the word is misleading and outdated. And, as already hinted, there are plenty of parasites that are not pathogens, which are not really the subject of this book, though they will get a mention now and then. If you are now thoroughly confused, have a good look at Tables 1.1 and 1.2.

From now on, I shall abandon 'microbes' and stick to the terms in the first column of Table 1.1 (bacteria, viruses, etc.), and we will look

**Table 1.1 Parasites and pathogens**

| Type of organism | Parasitic? | Pathogenic? | Examples of disease |
|---|---|---|---|
| Bacteria | Some, mostly not | A few | Tuberculosis, plague |
| Viruses | All | A few | Measles, flu, AIDS |
| Protozoa | Some, mostly not | A few | Malaria, amoebiasis |
| Fungi | Some, mostly not | A few | Ringworm, thrush |
| Worms | Some, mostly not | A few | Hookworm, tapeworm |
| Prions | All | Some (all?) | BSE, CJD |

**Table 1.2 Some characteristics of pathogens**

| Type of organism | Structure | Genetic material | Visibility |
| --- | --- | --- | --- |
| Bacteria | Single cell | DNA + RNA | Light microscope |
| Viruses | Non-cellular | DNA or RNA | Electron microscope |
| Protozoa | Single cell | DNA + RNA | Light microscope |
| Fungi | Single or many cells | DNA + RNA | Microscope/naked eye |
| Worms | Many cells | DNA + RNA | Naked eye |
| Prions | Non-cellular | Protein | Electron microscope |

at these different classes of pathogen in detail in the next chapter. But first let us pause to reflect on the second and third columns and think about the question: Why are some micro-organisms parasites or pathogens and not others?

## Parasitism is an ancient and respectable way of life

In everyday speech, the term 'parasite' is loaded with derogatory meaning. A parasite is a sponger, a lazy profiteer, a drain on society. But in the natural world parasitism is simply a consequence of the fact that some animals are large and others are very much smaller and find it convenient to live on or in the large ones. For them, your body and mine are just a part of the outside world, and one that provides them with more comfortable conditions than they would find elsewhere, a regular supply of food, a controlled temperature, free travel – a perfectly reasonable lifestyle option, though it does involve some restrictions and dangers, as the chapters on immunity will show.

Sometimes the parasite is actually useful to its host, each contributing something to the well-being of the other. This is called *symbiosis*, and we shall see many examples of this when we consider bacteria, which play an essential role in the life of both plants and animals. Some can live either on their own or as parasites, and from a comparison of closely related organisms it appears that often their evolution is from free-living to parasitic, with a progressive loss of those genes required for an independent existence (*genes* are the units of heredity in the DNA that dictate the form a bacterium – or a plant or a human – will take). One or two scientists, without bothering to hide their political agenda, have even spoken of the parasitic life in terms of 'degeneration' and 'the welfare state' – a persuasive but totally fallacious metaphor. It's all a matter of viewpoint. To us, filarial roundworms are parasites. To the roundworms, the bacterium-like *Wohlbachia* living peacefully inside it are parasites. Some bacteria are hosts to smaller parasitic bacteria called *Bdellovibrios*. And *Bdellovibrios*, like most bacteria, can in turn be parasitized by viruses known as *bacteriophages*. Substitute 'parasite' for 'flea' and Jonathan Swift was pretty well right. Anyway, from the point of view of our planet, we are all parasites and most of us are pathogens. It's a question of size.

 **Pathology is often accidental or self-inflicted**

This will perhaps be surprising news to many readers. It is human nature, when things go wrong, to blame someone or something. If we cut ourselves gardening and the wound gets infected, the painful swelling is the fault of the bacteria that got in. If we catch the flu, it is the fault of the virus – as well as the person who sneezed in our

face. Runny-nosed and miserable, it is hard to accept that all the
virus is doing is trying to make more virus, and make us sneeze it
out again and into someone else's nose, and that the shivering and
fever and pains in the muscles are the result of our own body
reacting to the invader. And if those bacteria in the garden included
the one known as *Clostridium tetani* and we were careless enough
not to have been vaccinated against it, we run the risk of dying of
tetanus, which would hardly benefit all the tetanus bacilli that
would die with us. So we must rid our minds of the idea that
pathogens *want* to hurt or kill us, like some sinister invisible 'axis
of evil'. All they want, as far as we can tell, is what all forms of life
want: to survive and reproduce themselves, and we have to live
with the fact that in doing so, they may occasionally endanger our
own survival.

 **Reproduce or perish**

The survival of any species also depends on reproduction, and in
the case of the human race this requires an absolute minimum of
about 12 years of reasonably healthy childhood. A disease that killed
all children under 10 would effectively wipe us out. On the other
hand a disease that killed everybody over 70 would in many ways be
beneficial to the race as a whole, at least in terms of consumption
versus productivity. So we might expect some process that helps to
keep children alive to be more strongly favoured during evolution
than something that kept old people going for longer. If we now
consider the commonest causes of death at various ages, it is clear
than children are most vulnerable to *infection* and *injury*, whereas
their grandparents are more likely to be carried off by *degenerative
disease* (e.g. arthritis, heart disease) or *cancer*. It follows that Nature

has put special efforts into developing mechanisms that reduce our chances of dying of infection and injury – the processes of *immunity* and *healing*, respectively. As this is a book about infection, we shall be concentrating on immunity in all its aspects – how it works, how it can go wrong, how it can (sometimes) be improved.

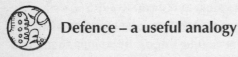 ## Defence – a useful analogy

Scientists are wisely cautious about analogies, which can so often be misleading. There will be plenty of analogies in this book and I will warn you when they are only approximate.

However, the well-used analogy between an animal protecting itself against pathogens and a country defending itself against an invading enemy is one of the better ones, because it emphasizes the fact that each side has strategies up its sleeve to outwit the other, and obliges us to look at infection from the pathogen's viewpoint as well as our own. Like a hard-fought military campaign, it is a ding-dong process of invading, repelling, eluding or destroying the defence installations, bringing in backup forces, escaping these . . . and so on until one side gives up or there is a truce. The fact that we are intelligent and pathogens are not (by our standards) did not really enter into it until very recently. Our immunological defence mechanisms are not the result of intelligence but of millions of years of evolution through selection of advantageous mutations (random genetic changes), and the same goes for the pathogen. And remember – not only have pathogens been around for millions of years longer than any higher form of animal (3 billion in the case of bacteria) but they also have an astronomically higher rate of mutation and are expert at adapting to difficult situations. So I shall

make frequent use of the 'war' analogy throughout this book, and
occasionally of the 'police-criminal' one too.

An account of the equipment at the disposal of the two sides will have
to wait until we consider them in detail in later chapters, where you
will read about the ever-shifting disguises of the flu and HIV viruses,
the biochemical trickery of bacteria and protozoa, the almost
indestructible worms, and, up against them, the built-in antiseptics
of the skin and tissues, the greedy phagocytes, the roving killer cells,
and the grasping antibodies which so unforgettably (but alas not
very accurately) grappled with a miniaturized Raquel Welch in the
wonderful 1966 film *Fantastic Voyage*. To scientists who work in this
area – microbiologists, immunologists, pathologists, epidemiologists
– it's an eternally fascinating battle, much more so than mere
human warfare, where both sides usually have more or less the
same resources and the outcome mainly depends on numbers.

 ## Friendly fire

Sadly, we are used to the concept that occasionally our armed forces
get injured by their own side. But here the analogy with infection
breaks down somewhat, because in infectious disease this is an
almost everyday event. For a substantial number of diseases the
unpleasant effects we experience – pain, fever, shortness of breath,
jaundice, skin rashes, kidney failure, even collapse and death – are
the result of our defence mechanisms responding to the invader and
going into action. To take an extreme and very rare example: a child
born without a vital part of his or her immune system who happens
to catch the measles virus will not develop the typical measles rash
but may go on to die of pneumonia; no *immune response*, no

*measles* as we know it, but no recovery either. The normal 'measles' symptoms are part of the successful outcome. Likewise with tuberculosis, hepatitis, a staphylococcal boil, and a host of fungal, protozoal, and worm diseases: the process of recovery involves a degree of damage. If that painful boil does not form, you may end up with staphylococci in the blood – the life-threatening condition of *septicaemia*. In such cases what we call the 'disease' is actually 'collateral damage', a *side-effect* of a useful immune response – a price Nature has evidently found to be worth paying for the privilege of staying alive.

In some cases the news is even worse, because the friendly fire seems to be deliberate, the immune response being actually aimed at a body component. This is known as *autoimmunity*. Autoimmunity can affect many organs – joints, heart, skin, thyroid, etc. – and trying to find out how it works has kept a lot of immunologists, myself included, busy. Later in the book (Chapter 7) I shall collect together a variety of these self-inflicted reactions, but you can already see why they are called *immunopathological*. I don't want to give the impression that it is always a question of friendly fire; in the next chapter we shall meet viruses and bacteria that are quite capable of inflicting damage entirely on their own.

 **Missing equipment**

Situations like the fatal measles described above are fortunately rare – though measles is still listed among the world's top 10 killer infections (see Table 2.1 on p. 66). However, just as in any large complex army one might expect something somewhere to be missing or not functioning, the immune system is vulnerable to a

number of defects. It is estimated that in the UK as many as 1 in
1500 individuals show an immune defect of some kind, though not
all these *immunodeficiencies* are of equal severity; perhaps 1 in 20
of them are serious or even life-threatening and the rest are so
mild as to cause no trouble under everyday conditions. Many of
them are *genetic* – that is, due to a faulty gene, and in some cases
this has been inherited, as diseases like haemophilia are. But in the
developing world a large number of other causes are superimposed
on these, of which *malnutrition* is the most important (this is the
main reason why measles is a killer in the tropics). Sometimes one
infection can itself cause immunodeficiency, leading to other
infections taking a firmer hold. HIV is by far the most serious
example of this, and will be considered in later chapters.

 **Upgrading the system**

For about half a million years, mankind has had to be content with
the immune system as Nature designed it, which in fact is very little
different from that of humbler mammals such as the mouse. Indeed
many of its components can be traced back 500 million years to the
earliest vertebrates, and a few even go back to invertebrates. So the
evolution of defence mechanisms is an extremely slow one. It is
generally assumed that our current crop of diseases were acquired
mainly from domestic animals, during the era when the hunting
lifestyle gave way to that of the farmer and human communities
grew to a size and density that allowed animal-to-human and
person-to-person spread. There must have been long periods
during which both host and pathogens made small adaptations to
each other. First encounters between human populations that had
evolved separately for thousands of years, such as Europeans and

native Americans, carrying different diseases, would have called for further rapid adaptations to each others' pathogens. There are records from the sixteenth century showing that new infections such as syphilis in Europe and smallpox in Mexico were more florid and fatal than they became in later centuries. Our 'childhood' viruses did not settle down to their present fairly benign pattern until the Middle Ages. So today's humans and their parasites are descended from those on both sides that were best fitted for survival – that is, coexistence. In the process, human behaviour was affected too. It is thought that contact with 'foreign' diseases may have been a factor in Jewish and Muslim dietary rules, the Hindu caste system, and even the decline and fall of Rome (it is said that 10 000 people were dying every day at the height of the sixth-century Roman plague outbreaks).

Then, just over 200 years ago, an enormous leap occurred. For the first time human intelligence was applied to the improvement of immunity: Edward Jenner inoculated young James Phipps with fluid from a milkmaid with cowpox and showed that he was resistant to smallpox, and the science of *vaccination* was born. I say *science*, because a hit-and-miss form of the same approach, using smallpox itself, had been in use in China and the Middle East for centuries. As with every scientific breakthrough, there is endless argument as to who should get the credit, and the question will be discussed, along with the many vaccines that have been introduced since, in the chapter on controlling infection (Chapter 9), in which we shall also look briefly at the world of *antibiotics*, that other attempt by humanity to limit the power of pathogens.

Jenner's success was all the more remarkable in that the discovery of the smallpox virus – indeed of all viruses – was still far in the future. Even bacteria, though they had been seen in the microscope, were not linked to disease until a century after Jenner, thanks to a brilliant generation of mainly German and French scientists, of whom Robert Koch and Louis Pasteur were the most outstanding. Together with Ehrlich, whom we met at the beginning of this chapter, Pasteur and Koch should certainly be considered among the top 20 benefactors of mankind, despite – or perhaps because of – the fact that they were the bitterest of enemies.

 ## Weapons of mass destruction

Having looked back a few million years, we shall end by a nervous look ahead. The last decades of the twentieth century witnessed two horrifying developments that few would have predicted in my childhood. It was always suspected that new infectious diseases would be discovered from time to time, but not that an infection from the world of the apes would jump the species barrier and within two decades be responsible for over 25 million human deaths, orphaning whole generations of children. As if the AIDS 'accident' was not bad enough, *deliberate* population decimation by any one of half a dozen pathogens has now emerged as a serious war strategy.

It is extraordinary to think that in the early days of vaccine and antibiotic development, optimistic science journalists were predicting 'human life without germs'. And not only writers made this mistake: the judgment in 1969 by William H. Stewart, the US Surgeon General, that 'it is time to close the book on infectious diseases' looks today like a classic gaffe on a level with the British Astronomer Royal's confident statement in 1956 that 'space travel is utter bilge' (the first sputnik was launched the following year). I always wonder what prompts people in the public eye to make these rash predictions which can so easily be proved wrong. Now some are saying that we have to face the possibility that it might be the other way round – the germs will finish *us* off. I hope I shall be able to convince you that this is not very likely either.

In the next chapter we shall look at today's pathogens, starting with the oldest of all life forms – the bacteria.

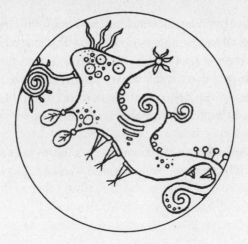

# 2 **The pathogens**

The word 'disease' ... immediately prompts the idea of a remedy.
But to begin at once searching for a cure is usually to embark on
useless labour – more or less relying on luck. Better to start by
learning the nature, the cause, and the evolution of the disease,
with the eventual hope of finding how to prevent it.

Louis Pasteur, *Pathogenic microbes and vaccines*, 1884

 **Bacteria**

Opinions still differ as to exactly how life on earth started, but there
is clear fossil evidence that about 3.5 billion years ago, only 1 billion
years after the earth itself was formed, single-celled organisms
remarkably like today's bacteria were already abundant – and
*they* were certainly not pathogens, because there was nothing

except rocks for them to parasitize! It was another 2 billion years before the appearance of the new type of cell required for the evolution of larger animals and plants. Strange and wonderful creatures have come and gone since – ammonites, trilobites, dinosaurs, the mammoth, the sabre-toothed tiger – but the bacteria are still there, so evidently the design of that single cell was a pretty good one. Before considering bacteria as parasites and pathogens, let us look closer at these two fundamental types of cell. This is not an idle detour, because as we shall see later, it has a lot to do with the difference between bacteria and other microbes *as pathogens*.

## Designs for living

### The basic plan

To make something recognizable as a living organism, you would need two basic sets of machinery: *metabolic* to generate energy, and *hereditary* to reproduce and create the next generation. Without heredity, your construction would remain a one-off, never to be replaced when it wore out. Without its own metabolism it would be inert (unless you could make it twitch with one of those lightning flashes beloved of Hollywood Frankenstein movies). For metabolism, Nature has exploited a variety of chemical chain reactions, or 'pathways', some using *oxygen* and some not, and there are bacteria that specialize in each of them. But there is only one hereditary mechanism – the one we are familiar with, using the nucleotides DNA and RNA. Some scientists believe it was RNA that came first, and in fact the resemblance between RNAs of one type (*ribosomal*) from all living creatures is one of the best pieces of evidence that life only originated once. There are organisms which have the RNA (or DNA) but no metabolic equipment of their own;

these are the *viruses* and some of them are undoubtedly pathogens, though it is hard to be sure whether they should be called living. More about them later.

Metabolically active chemicals and potentially reproductive nucleotides floating around freely still do not constitute a living organism; for this they need to be held together in some reasonably stable structure, and this happened when the first *cell membrane* evolved, to be followed later by the *cell wall*, with its increased strength and resistance to external conditions. And this is essentially the bacterial type of cell (Fig. 2.1): a cell with a wall and a membrane, containing *enzymes* to speed up the metabolic reactions, which would otherwise be painfully slow, plus DNA, its bases strung together on a *chromosome*, capable of replicating itself and arranged as *genes* that, with the help of RNA, form *proteins* able to make more walls, membranes, and enzymes – is essentially the bacterial type of cell (Fig 2.1). It is a magnificent creation, fully capable of independent existence and self-replication for billions of years, and has expanded into every possible ecological niche.

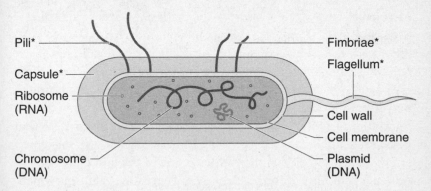

Pili*
Capsule*
Ribosome (RNA)
Chromosome (DNA)
Fimbriae*
Flagellum*
Cell wall
Cell membrane
Plasmid (DNA)

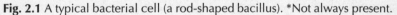

**Fig. 2.1** A typical bacterial cell (a rod-shaped bacillus). *Not always present.

Bacterial reproduction is about as simple as you can get; the cell doubles in size and splits in two. The progeny are normally identical, but do not remain so for ever because bacterial DNA is subject to change by *mutation*, and there are even mechanisms for exchanging DNA between bacteria; this can come in useful when they are under attack, for instance by antibiotics. Bacterial cells come in various shapes and sizes – spherical, rod-shaped, spiral, etc. – and are named according to their appearance under the microscope (Fig. 2.2). More precise classification depends on the pattern of staining with various dyes, analysis of surface structures, and eventually DNA sequencing.

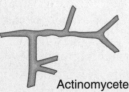

| | | |
|---|---|---|
| Coccus | Streptococci | Staphylococci |
| Bacillus | Bacillus with spore | Spirochaete |
| Actinomycete | | Vibrio |

**Fig. 2.2** Some common shapes of pathogenic bacteria. There are also hundreds of other shapes among the free-living bacteria.

*Further additions*

The bacterial type of cell is known as *prokaryotic* (sometimes spelled procaryotic), meaning 'pre-nucleated', to distinguish it from the later type of *eukaryotic* ('well-nucleated') cell of which all other creatures, from the single-celled amoeba and yeasts to large multicellular plants and animals, are built. The origin of the eukaryotic cell is still not entirely clear. Its most striking new feature was the *nucleus*, in which the majority of the DNA is packaged, now divided up into a number of different chromosomes (23 pairs in the case of humans). Prokaryotes made a contribution in the shape of bacteria which are thought to have taken up residence inside eukaryotes – a process known as *endosymbiosis* ('inside-together-living'), a good example of useful parasitism. This must have occurred at least twice: an oxygen-breathing bacterium settled down as a permanent cell component called the *mitochondrion*, providing a compact source of energy to animal cells, while a chlorophyll-containing 'green' bacterium, breathing carbon dioxide and producing oxygen, gave rise to the *chloroplast* found in all plant cells. So it was the bacteria that decided the future of the entire plant and animal kingdoms – an impressive achievement for a microscopic organism! Not so widely accepted is the theory that the first nucleus originated in a similar way as an endosymbiotic DNA virus (see later).

Several large volumes could be devoted to the activities that go on in a single eukaryotic cell, but for our present purposes there are two features with a particular bearing on infection and immunity. I will just mention them here and elaborate on them in later chapters. They are both concerned with the movement of *information*, inwards and outwards, particularly important in maintaining the stability of a complex multicellular organism. One is the process by

## 24 The pathogens

which the cell learns about its environment by using a series of
*receptors* on the outside surface of the cell membrane, which are
specialized for 'recognizing' the surfaces of other cells (including
pathogens) as well as hormones and other chemical messenger
molecules with an influence on the cell. The other is the process by
which the cell conveys information from its own interior to other
cells. One example of such information might be the important fact
that it has become infected with a virus, and the conveying is done
by specialized *MHC* molecules that transport bits of protein from
inside the cell to the surface (MHC is short for a cumbersome name
which will be explained in Chapter 4). Figure 2.3 illustrates these

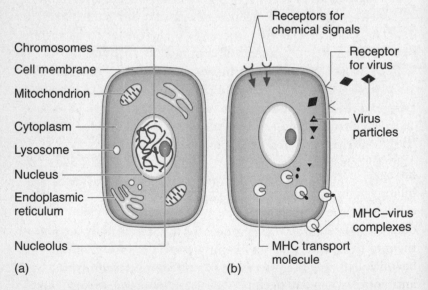

**Fig. 2.3** The eukaryotic cell. (a) Basic structure and contents. (b) Two important
pathways of information transfer, illustrated in a virus-infected cell. For
definition of terms, see text. Note, the molecules shown are not to scale;
they would be invisibly small at this magnification.

two information transfer systems for a typical eukaryotic (e.g. mammalian) cell; like all the figures in this book it is highly simplified and diagrammatic, and the various structures and molecules are not to scale.

To return to bacteria, you can see why even they cannot be considered 'primitive'. Indeed it is a mistake to call any species of creature alive today primitive, because it has been around for a great deal longer than we have, sometimes in extraordinary conditions. For example, there are bacteria that can survive freezing, boiling, enormous doses of radiation, total lack of oxygen, high salt concentrations – all of which would finish us off in no time. Living bacteria have been found frozen in Antarctic ice after 32 000 years, while one species survived temperatures of 175°C in the crash of the Columbia space shuttle. Clearly bacteria are not about to become extinct.

## Useful bacteria

In fact if bacteria *were* to disappear, life on earth would soon suffer. To take just two examples: bacteria in the root nodules of plants fix nitrogen in the soil, essential for healthy plant growth, while the billions of bacteria in the rumen of cattle are needed to digest the cellulose of the grass they eat. Even in non-ruminants like ourselves, the hundreds of species of bacteria peacefully resident in the intestine, making up over half the weight of faeces, appear to be beneficial, as judged by the effect of knocking them out with antibiotics, when pathogenic bacteria and fungi can replace them and lead to digestive problems; these 'friendly' bacteria are sometimes called *probiotic* (in favour of life) and one of them, *Lactobacillus acidopholus*, features in commercial yoghurt. And we should not forget the useful jobs we have invented for bacteria – fermenting milk into cheese, recycling waste, and synthesizing enzymes and antibiotics.

So, now that I have persuaded you to accept bacteria as remarkable and admirable little creatures and the ancestors of life on earth, let us turn to their less admirable role as pathogens.

### Ours – or theirs?

To repeat the point made in Chapter 1, only very few of the thousands of species of bacteria are pathogenic. Most are not even parasitic. Of the roughly 400 recognized *genera* (groups of species) of bacteria, less than 40 contain species that regularly cause disease in humans, although there are others that cause disease in other animals. On the whole, different species of animals have different species of pathogens, but there are some that can cross the species barrier from animal to man under conditions of close contact, such as plague from rats, brucellosis from goats, and (in the days before pasteurization of milk) TB from cattle. These so-called *zoonoses* are often particularly serious and even life-threatening to us, because the rats, cattle, etc. are the 'natural' host with which the bacteria have come to reasonably peaceful terms over the millennia, whereas we, as occasional hosts, have not had this advantage. To use a rough analogy, we are like a tribe that is accustomed to fighting with crossbows, and has evolved satisfactory defences against them (learned to *live* with them, you could say) suddenly coming up against an enemy with longbows – as the unfortunate French knights did at Agincourt in 1415. There are zoonoses among the other classes of pathogen too (viruses, protozoa, etc.) as we shall see in due course – in fact zoonoses account for just over half of all human pathogens.

## Boils and throats

Coming back to our handful of human pathogenic bacteria, let us take a look at a few of the diseases they cause, starting with some really common ones. Most people suffer a skin infection from time to time, perhaps an infected cut, which if it doesn't settle quickly may turn into a pus-filled boil or abscess, or even a dangerous infection of the bloodstream (bacteraemia). Usually the culprit is a *Staphylococcus* or, less often, a *Streptococcus*. To illustrate the way bacteria are named, *Staphylococcus* and *Streptococcus* are *genera* in the *family* of micrococci, and each genus contains numerous *species*, for example *Staphylococcus aureus*, *Streptococcus pyogenes* – often abbreviated to *S. aureus*, *S. pyogenes* – which can be further subdivided into *strains* with individual features such as capsule formation or drug resistance. This double-naming (*binomial*) system, used for all animals and plants, is also applied to bacteria and other cellular pathogens (but not viruses). However, in normal conversation among experts it is quite common to use the genus name only – *Staphylococcus*, *Mycobacterium*, *Plasmodium* – and sometimes an even more everyday term – staph, tubercle bacillus, malaria parasite – depending on the degree of precision required.

Staphylococci live normally on the skin and in the nose, and some strains are more virulent than others; people who are unlucky enough to carry a virulent strain, particularly if it is also resistant to antibiotics, are a potent source of cross-infection in crowded places such as hospitals, where staphylococci resistant to the antibiotic methicillin (MRSA) have become a common cause of infection and even death. Both 'staphs' and 'streps' do their damage by dividing rapidly – up to three times an hour – and secreting destructive molecules known as *toxins*, and the pus in the boil is a sign that defence mechanisms are at work, as we shall see later.

Streptococci are also a fairly common cause of throat infections, which may go on to tonsillitis, scarlet fever, rheumatic fever, or heart or kidney disease. In Victorian times and earlier, with dreadful housing conditions and no antibiotics, repeated streptococcal infection was a leading cause of death from heart or kidney failure; it is believed that this is what killed Mozart – although he, poor man, like Napoleon, has been retrospectively diagnosed with practically every fatal condition in the book, including deliberate poisoning. At the other end of the scale, some species of streptococci form part of the normal gut flora, and yet others are useful in fermentation and waste disposal.

## Teenage skin

Another bacterium that normally lives in the skin is *Propionibacterium acnes*, which as its name suggests, is one of the main causes of acne. *P. acnes* inhabits the tiny glands that secrete sebum and is normally harmless, but when these get blocked, as happens under the influence of sex hormones during puberty, inflammation and pus formation result – the notorious 'blackhead'.

## A poetic death; seed and soil

Another great scourge of those days was *tuberculosis* (TB, consumption, phthisis), once responsible for no less than one in seven deaths – and a good many more if novels and operas are included. We can smile as a Victorian heroine fades away, pale and coughing, from this most poetic of diseases, but she is only reflecting reality. In her day, TB killed five people in every thousand every year. The causative agent, known as *Mycobacterium tuberculosis* (and sometimes as *Koch's bacillus* in honour of its decovery by Robert Koch in 1882) is a very different proposition from the staphs and streps. 'MTB' is a tough, rod-shaped bacillus resistant in the laboratory to acid and alcohol, and in the host to most of the defence mechanisms, dividing slowly but surely, mainly in the lungs at first since it is an *aerobic* organism and prefers a good supply of oxygen. Even more than in most infections, the outcome depends critically on the state of health of the person infected, a point that is sometimes illustrated by a simple gardening metaphor – that of *seed* and *soil*, the idea being that unless the soil (the patient) is receptive the seed (the bacilli) will not grow. This is true not only of tuberculosis but of almost all infectious diseases, as we already saw with staphs and *P. acnes* (above). There is a convenient skin reaction, the Mantoux test, which can detect previous exposure to the bacillus, and in my days as a medical student (the 1950s) most of us were Mantoux positive, but healthy. So we had been exposed but had controlled the infection without being aware of it; we were literally 'living with' the bacilli. However, a breakdown of general resistance – diabetes, malnutrition, treatment with steroid drugs, or nowadays, AIDS – will lead to a flare-up, showing that some bacteria have been lurking there all along.

As a newly qualified doctor I did a six-month residency at Frimley sanatorium, near Aldershot in Surrey, where TB patients were sent to recover. Supposedly, they got their strength back by carefully graded walks round the grounds, but what really cured them was the barrage of drugs they took. Those walks were a relic of the days before drugs, and I think the patients sensed this, because they shamelessly faked their exercise record books. Today most young people in developed countries are Mantoux negative, because there is so much less tuberculosis around to infect them, and if they do get infected there are powerful drugs to cure them. However, thanks to the AIDS epidemic, TB is still the number one bacterial disease in world-wide terms, killing well over a million people a year.

## The old man's friend

Except when immunity is for some reason deficient, tuberculosis is essentially a chronic disease, with ups and downs over years, but there is another lung disease with a very different pattern: *pneumonia*. Pneumonia can be caused by many different pathogens – bacteria, viruses, and even fungi – but in pre-antibiotic days the commonest one was *Streptococcus pneumoniae*, formerly known as the *Pneumococcus* (illustrating the point that bacterial nomenclature is still not entirely cut and dried). Pneumococcal pneumonia was an acute and dramatic affair, with the patient desperately ill, blue, and gasping for breath until the *crisis*, usually occurring a week after the onset, when he or she either died or magically recovered. Jane Austen's description of Marianne Dashwood's pneumonia in *Sense and Sensibility* could not be bettered, from its beginning 'heavy and feverish, with a pain in her limbs, a cough, and a sore throat' to its height with 'hour after hour passed away in sleepless pain and delirium' and the sudden recovery with 'amendment . . . in her pulse, her breath, her skin, her lips'. When we discuss the immune response you will understand why her recovery was so rapid and complete. Penicillin has revolutionized the treatment of pneumococcal pneumonia, but it is still the commonest cause of death in the elderly and bedridden, for which many are grateful; physicians of the old school used to refer to it as 'the old man's friend'.

Other bacteria that target the respiratory system include *Bordetella pertussis*, the cause of whooping cough, *Haemophilus influenzae*, a common cause of pneumonia and meningitis in young children (named because it was once wrongly thought to be the cause of influenza), and *Legionella*, a fairly new recruit to the textbooks, only discovered in 1976, at a convention of the American Legion. Legionnaire's disease is usually acquired from contaminated water; not as its name suggests, from some oasis in the Algerian desert but, more prosaically, by aerosol inhalation from cooling and air conditioning installations.

## A medical emergency

Meningitis can also be pneumococcal, tuberculous, viral, fungal, or even protozoal, but the commonest cause is *Neisseria meningitis* (the 'meningococcus'). Up to a quarter of people carry this bacterium harmlessly in their nose and throat, and why it should occasionally get into the blood and spread to the meninges lining the brain, to the skin, and elsewhere is not really understood, but once this happens vigorous antibiotic treatment (e.g. penicillin) is the only hope. To distinguish the rash of meningococcal meningitis from all the other rashes that children are prone to is one of the doctor's most essential skills. I will return to the subject of skin rashes in Chapter 7.

## Molecules of sudden death

The toxins of staphs and streps have been mentioned; they are numerous and varied, destroying host cells and helping the bacteria to spread and avoid defence mechanisms. However, there is another group of pathogens whose toxins act more subtly, poisoning just a single biochemical pathway but with fatal consequences. Two of them belong to the genus *Clostridia* and they cause tetanus

(*C. tetani*) and botulism (*C. botulinum*). Both secrete a *neurotoxin* which prevents nerves signalling properly to muscles and leads rapidly, if untreated, to death from respiratory failure. Strangely, they work in opposite ways: tetanus toxin prevents muscles from relaxing so that they become locked in spasm ('lockjaw'), while botulinum toxin prevents them contracting, resulting in a floppy paralysis. Botulinum toxin is extremely potent, as readers of classic detective stories will know, but in minute doses it can be used to smooth out facial expression lines, which some people consider an improvement. A third organism, the *cholera* vibrio, secretes a toxin which inhibits the normal exchange of sodium and chloride in the wall of the intestine, leading to massive losses of water into the gut and, unless treated, death from dehydration. The discovery of this organism, in Egypt, was another of Robert Koch's triumphs.

Yet another toxin, secreted by the *diphtheria* bacillus, blocks a single step in the synthesis of protein, destroying cells particularly in the nose and throat, with death from suffocation or, occasionally, heart failure. Diphtheria and tetanus toxins were turned to good account when it was discovered that they could be inactivated by formalin but still retain the ability to induce immunity – the brilliantly successful *toxoid* vaccines introduced in the 1940s and still in universal use today. Before that, a doctor in a remote area had to be prepared for drastic action in a case of diphtheria: to clear the airways by opening the windpipe, if necessary with a hastily sterilized penknife – the operation of *tracheotomy*. The great doctor–novelist Mikhail Bulgakov wrote a hair-raising, but also hilarious, description of a just-qualified doctor confronted with this emergency in a rural hospital in pre-revolutionary Russia. (All the stories in his *A Country Doctor's Notebook* are well worth reading.)

Other bacteria that secrete toxins include those causing gas
gangrene, whooping cough, and many forms of food poisoning.

## Diarrhoea, vomiting, and stomach ache

In addition to cholera, gastrointestinal disease can be caused by a
variety of 'enteric' bacteria: *Shigella*, *Salmonella* (including *S. typhi*,
the typhoid bacillus), and *Escherichia coli* (*E. coli*). The latter is
interesting in that many strains are harmless members of the
'normal gut flora', while others such as O157 are extremely potent
causes of diarrhoea, dysentery, and kidney failure. There are also
viruses and protozoa that cause diarrhoea, as we shall see later. I
remember my father, who fought as a young officer in the 1914–18
war, describing the typhoid vaccine jab as his first 'war wound' – a
'three-inch needle in the stomach' (actually the abdominal muscle).
All the same, thanks to that jab there were 35 times fewer cases of
typhoid in the British than in the French or German armies.

A recent discovery that took doctors by surprise was that
*Helicobacter pylori* causes not only gastritis but the majority of
gastric and duodenal ulcers, and even cancers. A surgical colleague
of mine was dumbfounded, and even rather annoyed, that the ulcers
he had spent his life removing by operation could mostly be cured by
a week's course of three drugs. It struck me that this illustrated
particularly well the difference between clinicians and scientists.
The clinician has to obey a set of rules, mostly handed down by his
teachers, otherwise he would be paralysed with doubt in the face of
every emergency. The scientist, on the other hand, welcomes any
chance to prove that the rules are wrong (or better still 'the prof is
wrong'). Most students self-select themselves into the niche that
suits their mind-set. I was a bit slow, and it took a couple of years

of research in California to convince me I was a scientist, not a clinician – a decision that probably spared a good many lives.

## Anthrax and two great men

This fairly rare but dangerous skin disease of farm animals and their keepers is celebrated for several reasons. It was the first infectious disease convincingly proved to be caused by a microorganism. This was yet again the work of Robert Koch in Berlin, who in 1876 showed by a painstaking series of experiments carried out in the back room of his country practice, that animals with anthrax always had the bacilli in their blood while healthy ones did not, and that infected blood would transfer the disease to healthy animals, laying down the ground rules for establishing a disease – microbe association and putting an end to the theories of 'miasmas' and 'spontaneous generation' that were previously widespread. As mentioned earlier, Koch went on to discover the tubercle bacillus and the cholera vibrio, and establish the *germ theory* of disease – in a nutshell: 'one germ, one disease'. Five years later his great French contemporary, Louis Pasteur, who had already shown that micro-organisms were responsible for the contamination of wine and milk, tested the first anthrax vaccine in sheep, in the full public gaze – an incredibly risky enterprise. Fortunately his notorious good luck was with him, as it was another four years later when he successfully tried out the first rabies vaccine in a small boy. Sadly, anthrax is again in the news as a possible agent of biological warfare, thanks to its ability to survive for long periods in the form of spores and its ability to infect by the respiratory route via aerosols. Koch and Pasteur, belligerent rivals but tireless benefactors of humanity, must be turning in their graves.

The other notorious bacterial skin disease is leprosy, caused by the mycobacterium *Mycobacterium leprae* (or Hansen's bacillus, after its Norwegian discoverer) whose slow relentless growth is restricted to the skin and nerves. The resulting disfigurement was so visible and unpleasant that its victims were excluded from society in lazarettos and leprosaria from about the sixth century – a brutal but effective early attempt at disease control and the forerunner of today's isolation wards. Tuberculosis, a much more dangerous and contagious, but less obvious, disease, was not considered a candidate for isolation until the nineteenth century and the work of Koch.

## Rats, fleas, and the Black Death

It is a pity that Koch's results were not known to the populations of Europe in 1347 when the plague swept westwards across it, killing between a quarter and a third of them (about 25 million) – until AIDS the highest mortality ever recorded for any infectious disease. Had they realized it was caused by a bacillus carried by fleas from rats to humans and not a Jewish or Arab conspiracy, Saturn in the house of Jupiter, or a vengeful God, it might have been possible to plan some kind of containment strategy. As it was, the epidemic must have seemed literally a 'game with death' – as so memorably conjured up in Ingmar Bergman's film *The Seventh Seal*. The equally vivid account of the 1665 epidemic by Defoe, *A Journal of the Plague Year*, must rank as one of the first pieces of fake journalism, since he was a toddler at the time. Boccaccio, Machiavelli, and, in our own times, Albert Camus, are just a few of the other famous writers fascinated by this appalling disease. Incidentally, I have always wondered why we speak of *the* plague (and *the* measles, mumps, flu, pox) but not *the* tuberculosis, hepatitis, polio, malaria, etc. What is it about those diseases? To 'the' or not to 'the'? One for the linguists to analyse, I suspect.

The plague bacillus is unusual in being able to infect dogs, cats, goats, camels, and other mammals, as well as humans and some strains of rat. There are two classic forms of the disease, depending on the route of infection: *bubonic*, with painful swollen lymph nodes (from a flea bite), and *pneumonic* (from airborne infection) – one of the most rapidly fatal of all infectious diseases, with a typical time-course of three days or less. Fortunately the bacillus is susceptible to a wide variety of antibiotics and there is a reasonably effective vaccine, so it should be possible to nip any future epidemic in the bud. Rather like plague, but milder, is *tularemia*, named after Tulare in California, where it was first identified. Both infections are potential candidates for biological warfare (see Chapter 10).

## Fevers that come and go and a night with Venus

Fever is a common sign of bacterial infection, low and intermittent in tuberculosis, high and sudden in pneumococcal pneumonia, and though unpleasant it is part of the defence process, allowing immune processes to speed up. The old physicians prided themselves on making a diagnosis from the temperature chart alone. One pattern in particular virtually gives the game away, a series of peaks separated by a return to normal. In 'undulant fever' or brucellosis, the peaks are several weeks apart; in 'relapsing fever' about a week (peaks at two or three days' interval are more likely to be due to the protozoal disease malaria). Relapsing fever is caused by the spiral bacterium *Borrelia recurrentis*, a relative of *B. burgdorferi*, the cause of Lyme disease, another relatively recent discovery (1975).

Other spiral bacteria include the spirochaete *Treponema pallidum* of syphilis and the *Leptospira* of Weil's disease. Syphilis is a curious disease, which if untreated may proceed through all, some, or none of a series of stages, in the worst cases culminating in insanity. As a sexually transmitted disease, treated in the days before penicillin by metals such as arsenic, bismuth, and mercury, it gave rise to the cynical summary of syphilitic infection as 'one night with Venus, a lifetime with Mercury'. The drug Salvarsan, introduced by Paul Ehrlich in 1910, was the first scientifically designed antibacterial, and got him into a lot of trouble with the Catholic church and the police, both of whom disapproved of curing prostitutes of syphilis. Another extraordinary treatment for syphilis was a deliberate malaria infection, the idea being that the resulting fever helped to eliminate the spirochaetes. Two close relatives of *T. pallidum* are the causes of the tropical skin diseases yaws and pinta; however these are spread by skin, not venereal, contact.

The other sexually transmitted bacterial infection is gonorrhoea, caused by *Neisseria gonorrhoeae* (the gonococcus), a relative of the meningococcus, making the point that closely related bacteria do not necessarily cause similar diseases. In the case of the two *Neisseria* species, it is the hair-like pili on their surface that determine the site of entry and the whole pattern of infection, enabling the bacteria to attach to cells lining the genital tract (gonococcus) or the nose and throat (meningococcus). We see the other side of the same coin with tuberculosis and the fungal disease blastomycosis. Here two completely unrelated pathogens cause similar patterns of lung infection because the immune response to both, and the pathogens' strategies for avoiding it (both discussed in later chapters), are essentially the same. So in a way the opponents of Koch's germ theory, who had always maintained that it was the patient (the soil) and not the microbe (the seed) that dictated the form a disease took, did have an element of truth on their side, though not for the right reason.

## Exploiting weakness

In the previous chapter I mentioned that defects in immunity are not uncommon. As might be expected, they can make it more difficult to fight off infectious disease. Tuberculosis, staphylococcal infection, and pneumococcal pneumonia are just a few that become much more severe, depending on the type of defect. But in addition there are some normally harmless organisms that become pathogenic *only in immunodeficient individuals*. These 'opportunists', as they are called, include the bacteria *Pseudomonas aeruginosa* and *Listeria monocytogenes*, and a number of viruses, fungi, and protozoa, and even worms which have emerged from obscurity to threaten the lives of patients afflicted with AIDS, as we shall see in a later chapter.

## Exceptions to the rule

Unfortunately micro-organisms don't study medical textbooks, and some important pathogens do not fulfil all the criteria given at the beginning of this chapter, yet they remain more like bacteria than anything else. For example the *Rickettsia*, which include the causative agent of *typhus*, lack complete metabolic independence, relying on their host for certain enzymes; they are therefore obliged to live inside host cells, which makes them somewhat resemble viruses. Another group of 'obligate intracellular parasites' are the *Chlamydia*, which are even more like viruses although they have cell walls like bacteria; they are responsible for *trachoma*, the commonest cause of blindness world-wide, and the bird-derived disease *psittacosis*. Even more 'atypical' are the *Mycoplasma*, which lack a cell wall altogether; one species, *M. pneumoniae*, is a cause of pneumonia. And most bizarre of all are the enormous DNA *mimiviruses*, larger than some bacteria, whose exact place in the evolution of life is a hot topic of debate. Finally, at the other end of the scale, are the *Actinomyces*, whose filamentous branching appearance led them originally to be regarded as fungi. Later we shall meet fungi that were once considered to be protozoa, reminding us again that the classification of micro-organisms is not set in stone, but merely our attempt to make sense of Nature's experiments with the single-celled design.

## Bacteria as pathogens; an interim summary

At this point we can make some general remarks about bacteria, leaving aside all considerations of immunity, vaccines, and antibiotics, which will come in later chapters. They are by far the oldest forms of life, just large enough to be seen with a school microscope, small enough to get inside a mammalian cell, essential for the survival of 'higher' animals and plants. We harbour millions of them peacefully, on our skin, in our noses, in our intestines. Now and then they get into our tissues or deep into our lungs, setting off a battle with the defence forces. Occasionally they run riot and poison us with their toxins. From time to time a new pathogenic bacterium is discovered, even now (see Chapter 10).

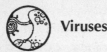 **Viruses**

If you go to the doctor with diarrhoea or a chest infection, you will quite likely be given an antibiotic 'in case it's bacterial'. Yet in many cases the antibiotic will have no effect and it will turn out to have been a *virus* infection. This similarity in symptoms is rather surprising when you consider how different viruses are from bacteria. As already mentioned, bacteria are *cells* that satisfy the criteria for 'living organisms' by possessing both *metabolic* and *hereditary* machinery. Viruses, on the other hand, are *particles* that contain the hereditary elements but not the metabolic ones. This makes them absolutely dependent on some external source of energy, which they obtain by living *inside a cell* – which could be animal, plant, or even bacterial. Now you will recall that some bacteria are already a bit like this (see *Rickettsia*, *Chlamydia*, and *Mycoplasma*, above), and some people believe that viruses are just a further step in a process of degeneration by which bacteria have become less and less independent and more and more parasitic, losing all resemblance to a cell and ending up as a few genes wrapped up in a few proteins. On this theory, the mimiviruses (see above) could be the 'missing link'. But there are problems with the 'degeneration' idea, one being that even the largest viruses possess DNA or RNA but *never both*, so a more popular theory is that viruses are really bits of DNA or RNA that have somehow learned to jump from cell to cell, taking with them instructions for making the proteins they require to form more virus particles there is in fact a precedent for this in the bacterial *plasmid*, which is a set of genes adapted for transfer to other bacteria. It is possible that both theories are right, and that different viruses originated in different ways. In either case we have an excellent analogy: viruses are *software* that can only work if inserted into the right *hardware* – a cell. No wonder the term *computer virus* caught on so rapidly; it is spot on. Richard Dawkins has carried the parallel further still with his proposal that seemingly illogical but widespread beliefs (e.g., for him, religious faiths) are examples of 'mind viruses'.

## Chemical or biological?

Though they are not cells, virus particles do have a very definite *structure*. Under the electron microscope (they are mostly too small to see with ordinary microscopes) each virus has its own characteristic geometric shape, formed by the symmetrical arrangement of a standard number of protein subunits, the whole thing looking more like a chemical crystal than a living creature. Indeed viruses can actually be crystallized. Two shapes are particularly common, rod-shaped and spherical, corresponding to *helical* or *icosahedral* (20-sided) symmetry (see Fig. 2.4). This has given rise to endless academic arguments as to whether viruses are really 'living' or not, which is like asking 'is birdsong/traffic noise/banging-on-a-saucepan, *music*?', the only answer being 'it depends what you mean by . . . ' etc. There does however seem to be general agreement that the mimivirus (see above) is sophisticated enough to be considered a living creature, and there are experts who would even deny it the name 'virus'.

Whether you accept them as living or not, viruses have their characteristic 'lifestyle'. Let us start at the point where a virus enters a cell. To do this, it must first dock with a suitable surface structure on the cell. This docking has to be extremely precise, with a molecular shape on the virus fitting exactly and sticking to another molecular shape on the wall of the cell which is referred to as

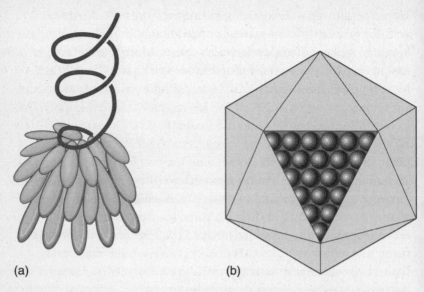

**Fig. 2.4** The two commonest types of viral structure. (a) Helical (e.g. measles); the RNA backbone is shown at the top and the surrounding protein units at the bottom. (b) Icosahedral (e.g. polio); 10 of the 20 faces are shown, and 21 of the 252 protein units.

a *receptor* – a slightly misleading term because it implies that the cell has put it there on purpose to let the virus in, whereas on the contrary it is usually some structure that the cell cannot help displaying on its surface because it is also a receptor for some essential molecule such as a hormone or growth factor (see Fig. 2.3). A receptor restricted to only some cells will confine a particular virus to infecting only those cells, which is why, for example, HIV infects certain immune (T) cells and not heart or liver cells. Once attached to their receptor, the virus particles are taken into the cell, rather as the Greek horse was by the unsuspecting Trojans. Then, almost immediately, the virus starts to *replicate*.

Here the pathways diverge, depending on what sort of nucleic acid the virus uses as its genetic core. Remember that the ultimate aim is to make more of itself, which means more nucleic acid and more protein. To make protein you must have a form of RNA known as *messenger RNA* (mRNA). So whatever it starts from, the virus must produce mRNA. A DNA virus can 'transcribe' its DNA into mRNA – a little like making a print from a photographic negative, and the normal way all cells proceed when making proteins. Many RNA viruses can simply use their own RNA directly. A small group of RNA viruses do it differently, copying their RNA 'backwards' into DNA which is then transcribed in the normal way; viruses that carry out this 'reverse transcription' are called *retroviruses* and include the dreaded HIV. Figure 2.5 may help to make this reasonably clear. Of course there is much more to it than this bare account, and the mechanisms of viral replication have been studied in great detail in order to try and design drugs to block it, as we shall see in a later chapter. The whole process is very rapid, and within a matter of hours the infected cell is full of new virus particles, ready to leave the cell and infect some others.

For a virus, there are two ways out of a cell, the brutal and the delicate. The brutal way is simply to burst the cell so that viral particles flood out, the host cell being killed in the process. You can feel the results of this in the soreness caused by the various common cold viruses, as layers of damaged membranes peel off, leaving your nose and throat raw and painful. The delicate way is by a mechanism known as *budding*, in which the virus takes with it an envelope of the cell membrane; HIV, hepatitis B, and many other viruses do this. In this case the host cell is not destroyed by the virus, but instead is liable to be killed by the immune system, because in the process of forming buds viral molecules become

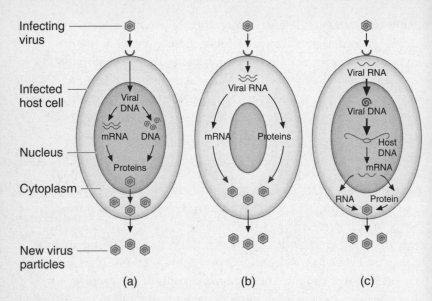

Infecting virus

Infected host cell

Nucleus

Cytoplasm

New virus particles

(a)          (b)          (c)

**Fig. 2.5** Three patterns of viral replication. (a) DNA virus (e.g. herpes); DNA → mRNA → protein. (b) RNA virus (e.g. polio); RNA → protein. (c) RNA retrovirus (e.g. HIV); the heavy arrows show the critical reverse transcription (RNA → DNA) and integration (viral DNA → host DNA) stages.

exposed on the cell surface and these are recognized as 'foreign'. But if not killed, the cell can go on shedding virus indefinitely, as happens in people who become 'carriers' of *hepatitis*. Another possibility is for the virus to simply lie quiet, flaring up at intervals, perhaps years later. This is common with the *herpesviruses* that cause cold sores and chickenpox. Finally, a few viruses can insert their DNA into cells and switch on processes that lead to *cancer*.

Now let us, as we did with bacteria, run through the main pathogenic viruses and the diseases they cause.

## Gone for ever?

We begin with a success story, one of humanity's finest. *Smallpox*, which had ravaged Europe on and off since at least the third century, was officially declared extinct by the World Health Organization in 1980, just under 200 years after Jenner's first vaccine experiment – though as long as stocks exist in locked freezers, there is unfortunately no guarantee that it will not reappear as a weapon of war. Recently the spectre of smallpox has been revived in the shape of the related *monkeypox* virus (rather a misnomer as it is carried by squirrels), which some experts fear might fill the 'niche' left by smallpox. Whether it is right to continue studying the smallpox virus is a matter of heated debate (see Germ Warfare, Chapter 10).

Smallpox was an ideal candidate for elimination: there was a good vaccine; it was restricted to humans, having mutated too far from other animal pox viruses for animals to be able to act as a reservoir of infection, and being a virus it could not survive on its own; and its 'reproductive rate' (epidemiologist's jargon for the *average* number of people infected by a single case of the disease, which can be calculated mathematically) was considerably lower than for other virus infections such as measles, mumps, German measles, and polio. Nevertheless the WHO now has these four diseases in its sights too, and in the USA, where vaccination is essentially compulsory, they are fast disappearing, as is diphtheria, the only bacterial infection with any realistic chance of being eliminated. As a young doctor I saw a teenager die of polio, unable to breathe outside his 'iron lung'; now, with two good vaccines available, this tragedy should never happen again.

## The childhood viruses

In my youth, measles, mumps, rubella, and chickenpox were a tribulation that every schoolchild was expected to endure. One caught them, recovered, and was immune to reinfection for life – which, if you think about it, means that if *everybody* was infected at the same time, the disease would die out. So for the virus to keep going in a community, there must always be a certain number of susceptible individuals; for example it has been calculated that *measles* could not survive in a closed community of less than about half a million, nor in one where 95% had been vaccinated. The resulting protection of theoretically susceptible individuals (e.g. the other 5%) is known as *herd immunity* – a reminder that to epidemiologists humans and cattle are not so different.

*Rubella* (German measles) is feared for its effects on the unborn baby, being one of the rather few infections that can get across the placenta (see Table 2.7 for some others). The herpesvirus *varicella-zoster* (chickenpox), as already mentioned, has the ability to persist for years – in this case in the spinal cord, from which it re-emerges as the painful disease *shingles*. I shall discuss the rather contentious question of vaccines against these diseases in a later chapter.

## A kissing bug

Another herpesvirus with odd properties is the *Epstein–Barr virus* (EBV), named after its discoverers. If caught by young children, as it is in the tropics, it causes a mild infection that may not even be noticed; however, the virus persists for life in certain cells and can contribute to a form of cancer known as Burkitt's lymphoma. The pattern in developed countries is different: infection occurs mainly in teenagers, and since the virus is secreted in saliva, kissing is an excellent way of spreading it. The resulting disease is the debilitating *glandular fever*, and EBV may also be responsible for some of the cases of *chronic fatigue syndrome*, that mysterious prostrating condition whose existence is still denied by some doctors but extremely real to sufferers. Other herpesviruses worth mentioning are *herpes simplex*, the cause of cold sores (type 1) and genital herpes (type 2), and *cytomegalovirus* (CMV), which has come to the fore as an opportunist in immunodeficient patients.

## Endemic, epidemic, and pandemic

These terms, which are often used rather loosely in newspapers, are rough attempts to describe the severity of a particular infection at a particular time, and they are well illustrated by *influenza*. If there is always a reasonably steady number of people with flu, as there is in most big towns, the disease is *endemic*. When there is a sudden increase and almost everyone seems to have it, we are suffering an *epidemic*. When an epidemic spreads round the world, that is a *pandemic*. Pandemics tend to occur when a highly infectious pathogen reaches a population that has no previous experience of it. This could be because it normally lives in animals (as plague does) or because it constantly changes its structure – as the flu virus does. Flu is an RNA virus put together in an unusual way, with its RNA in eight separate segments that can not only mutate but also be exchanged for segments from bird or animal flu viruses. As the RNA determines what surface molecules the virus carries, and as these are what the immune system reacts to, a new virus can appear slightly different, very different, or totally different. Imagine playing poker with cards that kept changing their appearance as well as suddenly being substituted by cards from a different pack – and trying to remember what was in your hand! The famous pandemic that followed the First World War in 1918–19 most likely originated, as later ones have been shown to, in the Chinese farmlands, where pigs, poultry, and humans live in unusually close contact. It swept round the world, infected half the entire population, and killed one in every twenty, about 40 million in all – far more than the 1914–18 war itself. The coming together of soldiers from many continents, plus the general exhaustion of war survivors, probably contributed to this exceptionally high death rate. Dreadful as it seems, it comes nowhere near the slaughter of one-third of the population of Europe in the plague of 1346–50. It remains to be seen whether history will repeat itself with the current bird flu (H5N1) that has spread from Asia to Europe but has so far killed only about 150 humans.

Tragically, we are now in the middle of what may turn out to be another record-breaking pandemic. Like flu, the *HIV* virus constantly changes its appearance, but much more rapidly, and being largely sexually transmitted it can spread even where people are thin on the ground, since they actively seek each other out. So far there have been about 25 million deaths with another 40 million infected. Every part of the world is affected, and despite numerous trials, prospects for a good vaccine are slim. The matter is made worse by the refusal of some influential people to accept that AIDS *is* a virus disease, partly because HIV causes *immunodeficiency* and its victims usually die of some other infection – bacterial, protozoal, or fungal. I shall return to AIDS and theories of its origin and how to treat it in a later chapter.

In contrast to both the above, the Asian outbreak of coronavirus

infection (SARS) in 2003, which it was feared would lead to
another pandemic, was quickly controlled, with only about 800
deaths.

## Preventable misery

I was brought up to believe that gastro-enteritis was usually caused
by bacteria. We went abroad, developed 'diarrhoea and vomiting',
and took a sulfonamide. It is no wonder this frequently didn't work,
because it is now realized that at least a quarter and perhaps a half
of all diarrhoeal infections are due to viruses – most commonly the
*rotavirus*. It is estimated that really good vaccines against bacterial
and viral diarrhoea would save 2–3 million lives a year, mostly in
the tropics and mostly in young children, but clean water and
proper sanitation would achieve the same result.

## Some yellow and bloody infections

Jaundice, a classic sign of liver disease, can be caused by a variety
of viruses. Commonest of these are the *hepatitis* viruses, of which
there are at least five. Hepatitis A is a form of 'food poisoning', from
which the sufferer normally recovers completely. Hepatitis B is
quite different, being transmitted by blood – either a transfusion, a
needle, or sexually. It is more serious because about one patient in
ten becomes a *carrier*, appearing healthy but able to infect others.
Alternatively, it may persist as a chronic infection, ultimately
leading to liver cirrhosis and sometimes cancer. Chronic infection is
even commoner with hepatitis C. Another virus disease involving
the liver as well as other organs is *yellow fever*, which is spread by
mosquitoes. Jaundice may also occur in glandular fever and in the
bacterial diseases relapsing fever and leptospirosis.

A frightening feature of yellow fever is *bleeding*, especially into the gut, due to disturbances of blood clotting. Bleeding is also prominent in *dengue* fever, another mosquito-borne disease, and in the animal-derived infections Lassa fever, Marburg disease, and Ebola fever, where it is caused by leakage from damaged blood vessels all over the body, reminiscent of the most gruesome SF movie special effects. Workers from the WHO and the US Centres for Disease Control have risked, and occasionally lost, their lives investigating these terrifying viruses; one, Ebola, nearly caused a panic in the USA, as recounted, with some artistic licence, in the 1995 film *Outbreak*. Bats are thought to be the normal reservoir of Ebola, and the virus is considered to be a serious threat to the survival of the African gorilla population.

## Mad dogs and a courageous Frenchman

To complete our summary of really unpleasant virus infections, let us have a look at *rabies*. I have already mentioned that Louis Pasteur had a stroke of luck with this disease, and if we examine its curious lifestyle we will see just how fortunate he was. The virus spreads by driving its host into a salivating frenzy – the classic 'mad dog' (foxes, wolves, bats, skunks, and racoons are some other possible victims). If you are bitten, usually on the hand or leg, virus from the saliva enters the wound and makes its way into nerves, in which it travels quite slowly upwards to the brain. This can take anything from one to three months, during which you appear perfectly well. However, soon after the virus reaches the brain, unless immunity is already in action, it triggers off convulsions, delirium, and death in coma. So there is a period of several weeks during which immunity can be induced, and this is why Pasteur's vaccine, which was given *after* the dog bite, was successful. It would not have worked with any other infection. Another bit of luck was that his vaccine was obtained from the dried spinal cord of a rabid dog, which by good fortune contained non-infective but still recognizable virus. Since viruses were not accepted as real disease agents for another 20 years, and not actually seen under the microscope for another 50 years, Pasteur had no way of being sure his preparation was safe (Koch vociferously maintained that it was not). It could have all gone dreadfully wrong, and the whole exercise would be highly illegal nowadays.

## Viruses and cancer

In the years between the two world wars, increasing evidence suggested that some animal cancers were caused by viruses. However, it was not until 1964 that a human tumour was linked to a virus – EBV and Burkitt's lymphoma, as already mentioned. Since then, four other viruses have been shown to be able to cause tumours, though by no means always; hepatitis B (liver cancer) and papilloma virus (cervical cancer) are probably the commonest. So there is clearly no such thing as a universal 'cancer virus'. Moreover, the fact that most people infected with EBV, hepatitis B, or papilloma viruses do not get cancer suggests that other contributory factors are needed, and in the case of Burkitt's lymphoma two of these have been identified: a chromosome abnormality and heavy malaria infection. People with defective immunity are more prone to Burkitt's lymphoma, so the immune system evidently plays a part in preventing it. The fact that there is a good vaccine against hepatitis B makes liver cancer the first tumour to be preventable by vaccination; cervical cancer should be the next. Unfortunately vaccines against those cancers *not* caused by viruses are still at the highly experimental stage.

## Some viruses we can live with

To end on a more cheerful note, let me remind you that some virus infections are quite mild – annoying rather than dangerous. The common cold, which can be caused by at least eight groups of viruses, each composed of dozens or hundreds of different types, is a huge cause of days off work, but not a major threat to health. In fact with today's pills that dry up the runny nose, a typical cold is no great hardship. As a boy I used to live near the Common Cold Research Unit just outside Salisbury, and I remember lurid tales of drops in the nose and walks in the freezing rain, but I am ashamed to say I never volunteered to be experimented on.

Another 'minor' affliction caused by a virus is the common wart, and I am still hoping that someone will explain how these can be 'charmed' or hypnotized away.

## Good – or at least not bad – viruses

With bacteria, we saw how the great majority were harmless and even beneficial to humans and animals. Is it the same with viruses? Certainly there are vast numbers of them that do not infect humans – viruses of other animals, plant viruses, and even a special group of viruses that infect bacteria. These *bacteriophages*, which have sophisticated syringe-like devices for literally injecting themselves into bacteria, are one of the ways in which bacteria can exchange genes, and the same idea can be used in genetic engineering and gene therapy, although bacterial *plasmids* (see Fig. 2.1) are the vectors normally used. These can be used to insert new genes into ordinary viruses, whose ability to multiply and 'home' to particular cells makes them excellent carriers for placing these genes in cells which lack them – a ray of hope for sufferers from 'single-gene' defects like cystic fibrosis or haemophilia, but still some way off as a standard treatment. Another idea is to put vaccine molecules into a 'safe' virus and use the new combination as a living vaccine. For example a molecule from hepatitis B could be inserted into cowpox to immunize against hepatitis. More about this genetic trickery when we come to discuss vaccines in Chapter 9.

Then there is the proposal that viruses have been transferring genes between animals all along, giving evolution a push, starting epidemics, even extinguishing the dinosaurs. One theory even claims an extra-terrestrial origin for viruses, and perhaps for all life on Earth. It is easy to dismiss such bizarre scenarios with a pitying smile, but that is exactly how the now widely accepted meteorite theory of the extinction of the dinosaurs was greeted at first by many palaeontologists. Napoleon famously declared that *'le mot impossible n'est pas français'*, and scientists ought to be very cautious about using that word too. Having said that, I believe that the theory that viruses came from outer space is pretty unlikely, but I doubt if it can be disproved. But *gene transfer* is another matter; there is good evidence that both viruses and bacteria can do this. We shall see (Chapter 6) an example relevant to infection when we look at how viruses interfere with immunity by sending out messages that use genes they have picked up from their hosts.

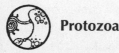 **Protozoa**

After our foray into the strange half-living world of viruses, we return now to more 'normal' pathogens, starting with the *protozoa* ('first' or 'original animals'). Like bacteria these are single cells, but with a difference: their cells are *eukaryotic*, with nuclei and a variety of specialized structures, by which they can move and attach to and ingest their prey. They are also much larger than bacteria, easily seen under the ordinary microscope. I remember studying in biology class the protozoan *Paramecium*, which wriggled across the microscope field as you watched it, like a tubby little boat with 10 000 tiny paddles (official name: cilia). *Amoeba* was another one, which preferred to slither along the glass, with its innards (cytoplasmic particles) streaming ceaselessly forward into the advancing tip. There are others with a single long paddle (flagellum), but I don't recall seeing one of those until years later.

*Paramecium* is an example of a protozoan that is quite self-sufficient and has never opted for the parasitic life. Amoebae are mostly free-living too, but one sort, *Entamoeba* is a human pathogen, as we shall see. A handful of the flagellated protozoa also cause disease – the *trypanosome* of sleeping sickness being one example. But the fourth class of protozoa, known collectively as *sporozoa*, are the really fascinating ones; they are all parasitic, with an extraordinary lifestyle of alternating *asexual* and *sexual* reproduction – that is, they switch from breeding like bacteria to breeding like higher animals, round and round for ever. This class includes by far the most important protozoan of all, one of the world's top three killers – *malaria* – and this is where our survey of protozoal disease will begin.

### Chicken and egg and a balancing act

The lifestyle of the malaria parasite *Plasmodium* is truly amazing; there is no other like it. If we start with the bite of an infected mosquito, we can follow the slender *sporozoites* from the salivary gland of the mosquito into the blood of the victim, from which they rapidly exit into the cells of the liver, where they grow for about a fortnight into *schizonts*, then briefly back into the blood with the stumpier shape of *merozoites*, to enter red blood cells, in which they multiply, to burst out and infect another red cell, at which point the patient gets the well-known shivering attack, soaking sweats, and raging temperature of malaria. Repeated two- or three-day cycles in red cells lead to anaemia and damage to many organs, sometimes including the brain.

Then the parasite turns its attention to sex. Male and female *gametocytes* form in the red cells, and if another mosquito bites at the right moment, they are sucked in, to develop into *gametes* looking remarkably like human sperm and ova, which fuse to make a fertilized egg; this works its way to the mosquito stomach where it sprouts into thousands of sporozoites, which travel to the salivary glands to start the whole cycle again (Fig 2.6). A fantastic voyage indeed! How did such a complicated process evolve? Which came first, chicken or egg? Strangely enough, parasitologists would say 'egg'. Because the sexual stage takes place in mosquitoes, they are considered the *definitive host*, and we are merely *intermediate hosts*, carrying the disease from one mosquito to another – a humbling thought.

Many tropical animals have malaria parasites of their own; we have four species, of which one, *Plasmodium falciparum*, is responsible for practically all malaria deaths – over a million a year, mostly in Africa. The other three, which are thought to have had longer to adapt to humans, cause mainly fever. Malaria kills predominantly children, so it is a very effective eliminator of genes that favour its

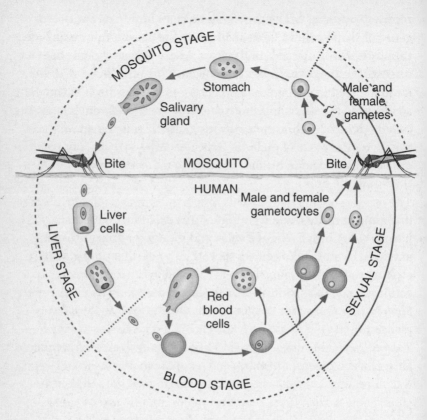

**Fig. 2.6** The life cycle of the malaria parasite is the most complex of any pathogen, with four very different stages.

growth or, to put it another way, an effective *preserver* of genes that inhibit its growth. One of these is the gene causing *sickle cell anaemia*, and though this is in itself an unpleasant disease, it gives such a strong protection against dying of malaria that the gene has become quite common in areas like West Africa where malaria is endemic – one penalty of this being that those who by bad luck receive two copies of the gene, that is, from both parents, do not generally survive long. Thus if *everyone* in the endemic areas had the sickle gene, all their children would die of severe sickle cell disease. If none of them did, many would die of malaria. So the frequency of the gene in the population maintains itself at the most advantageous level, somewhere between the two extremes. This is called *balanced polymorphism*, and a similar phenomenon, not usually so clear-cut, explains why two or more versions of many other genes persist in human populations.

The other sporozoa with a sexual stage in their cycle are primarily intestinal parasites, and were thought of as animal pathogens, fairly harmless to humans, until they began to cause severe symptoms and even deaths in immunodeficient patients (those with AIDS, etc.). These are *Toxoplasma* and *Cryptosporidium*. The latter confines itself to the intestine, causing profuse diarrhoea, but *Toxoplasma* can affect the eye and brain and can also cross the placenta to infect the unborn baby. Domestic cats mostly carry *Toxoplasma* and this has led to arguments that they should be banned altogether – surely an unthinkable prospect to any civilized person!

## Old and new world families

The *haemoflagellates* (blood-dwelling flagellated protozoa) are another fascinating group, not so much for their life cycle, which consists of repeated bacteria-like divisions with slight changes in shape and the extension, when needed, of the flagellum, but from the way they have evolved on opposite sides of the Atlantic, much as human immigrant populations do. There are two basic family names, *Trypanosoma* and *Leishmania*. In the Old World (i.e. Africa and the Middle East) there are two branches of the trypanosome family, both causing sleeping sickness, and half a dozen of the *Leishmania*, causing damage to either the skin or internal organs, but not both. In the New World (i.e. South America) we find about the same number of *Leishmania*, distinct from but causing similar diseases to the Old World ones, plus one trypanosome relative that causes a quite different condition, Chagas' disease. African trypanosomes are carried by tsetse flies, South American ones by a crawling bug; *Leishmania* everywhere are carried by sandflies. Trypanosomes in Africa live exclusively in the blood (a difficult feat from the point of view of avoiding the immune system, as we shall see later), whereas the South American ones start in the blood and then enter tissues (heart and nerves). *Leishmania* have cut the blood stage down to the minimum and make straight for the defence cells of the host in which they have learned to survive quite happily. I used to visit a beautifully equipped research institute outside Nairobi, in Kenya, which specialized mainly in trypanosomiasis, but I was surprised to find, on my first visit, that it was *cattle* trypanosomiasis that mattered most to them, since it was a major cause of meat shortages and mass under-nutrition. I was assured that far more human lives would be saved by a cure of that than of human sleeping sickness, which was an eye-opener to someone in the habit of thinking only of sick *people*.

## Tropical – or not

Malaria, trypanosomes, and *Leishmania* all depend on tropical insects for their spread and are therefore more or less restricted to the tropics, though there was, to take one example, malaria in Italy until as recently as 1935 when Mussolini, in one of his better moments, set about eliminating the marshy mosquito breeding grounds, to be followed up after the Second World War by the American-led use of DDT spraying. In theory malaria could be eliminated everywhere by eliminating mosquitoes, but this has proved to be virtually impossible in tropical areas, and malaria is actually on the increase there.

However, there are also protozoal pathogens that are spread, as the cholera and typhoid bacteria are, by sewage-contaminated food and water (charmingly known as the 'faecal – oral' route), and these can be picked up anywhere in the world. The most important one is *Entamoeba histolytica*, often harmless but sometimes the cause of amoebic dysentery (diarrhoea containing blood) and in rare cases a perforated intestine or an amoebic abscess in the liver or lung. I once had a colleague who returned from examining in Africa and developed a large mass in his liver. He looked terrible and we all thought he was dying of cancer. But a shrewd physician put in a needle and drew out a syringeful of pinkish 'amoebic pus'; he was put on an appropriate combination of antibiotics, and all was well.

Numerous other amoebae can infect the intestine, though without causing any symptoms except sometimes in immunodeficient individuals, but there are two more flagellated protozoa that deserve a mention: *Giardia lamblia*, a common cause of diarrhoea, and *Trichomonas vaginalis*, which produces the only sexually transmitted protozoal disease.

So it would only be half true to describe protozoal infections as 'tropical diseases'. The worst ones are – for the moment. But who knows what will happen if global warming and lax governments allow mosquitoes and the other insect vectors to creep back into more northern regions? This could be serious because, in general, protozoal infections are hard to cure with drugs and impossible (at present) to prevent by vaccination. We shall see why this is in a later chapter, but here is a hint: they are *eukaryotes* and so are we.

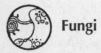 **Fungi**

If the word 'fungus' calls to mind mushrooms, toadstools, and those large colourful excrescences on the bark of trees, you may have difficulty visualizing a human fungal pathogen. However, many fungi are single-celled, or multicellular but small, and some of these (about 300) have learned to live as parasites of animals, including a few that cause important human diseases. Fungal cells are eukaryotic, like protozoa, but with special features, most notably a rigid cell wall rather like that of plants. This allows the multicellular *moulds* to grow into long filaments such as you see on 'mouldy' bread or cheese, while other fungi, the *yeasts*, remain as single cells; a third ('dimorphic') group can oscillate between the two states depending on the temperature conditions – for example whether they are outside or inside the body.

The best-known fungal diseases (official term: *mycoses*) illustrate these two extreme forms: candida (thrush) is a yeast; ringworm and athlete's foot are caused by filamentous moulds. Neither of these is life-threatening in healthy people, but some of the dimorphic fungi can get into the lungs and cause pneumonia (see below) and some yeasts and moulds can take advantage of weakened immune defences to run riot all over the body. These are therefore *opportunists*, just as *Listeria*, cytomegalovirus, and *Toxoplasma* are, and once again it is AIDS patients who are the worst sufferers. It was a cluster of lung infections with the single-celled

*Pneumocystis carinii* (which was for long believed to be a protozoan!) that first drew attention to the emergence of AIDS in 1981. In the textbooks of my student days, before AIDS, before cortisone, and before kidney transplants, pneumocystis got one line as a harmless inhabitant of the normal lung; now there are whole international meetings devoted to it (which just shows how quickly scientific and medical books can go out of date).

## Taxonomy is not a guide to symptoms

One of the dimorphic fungi mentioned above, *Histoplasma capsulatum*, can be used to make this point. You catch it, if you live in certain parts of America, by inhaling spores which settle in the lung and develop into the mature, yeast-like organisms. These are rapidly taken up by immune cells known as macrophages (more about these in the next chapter), which ought to be easily able to kill them but can't, because of the pathogen's own 'fight-back' mechanisms. The result is very like infection with *M. tuberculosis*, a bacterium that employs exactly the same strategy. The fungi *Blastomyces*, *Coccidioides*, and *Paracoccidioides* can all do likewise. So a *fungus* and a *bacterium*, worlds apart in terms of evolutionary relationship (taxonomy) and structure, cause similar diseases because of their similar location and methods of self-protection. We saw the same thing with bacterial and viral diarrhoea: it is hard to tell them apart, and we shall see countless more examples when we come to look at host and pathogen defence mechanisms in later chapters. So if we include the immune system as part of the 'soil', it can sometimes be as important to the course of disease as the 'seed' (the microbe) – just what Koch's opponents maintained (see Chapter 7 for more about seed and soil). Sometimes, though, there is no ambiguity; nothing can really be confused with ringworm.

## Occupational hazards

Allergic reactions to fungi are responsible for a number of lung diseases with exotic but self-explanatory names (cheese worker's lung; pigeon breeder's disease; thatched roof disease). However, the commonest condition of this type, farmer's lung, is caused by an actinomycete, an atypical bacterium with a filamentous, fungus-like structure.

## Useful fungi

One could argue that we would be worse rather than better off without fungi. Without the yeast *Saccharomyces cervisiae* to ferment sugars, humanity might never have invented beer or wine, and would have had to wait until the nineteenth century (when 'baking powder' came into use) for a decent loaf of bread. And without the mould *Penicillium notatum* Fleming would not have discovered penicillin and kick-started the whole antibiotic industry. Several other fungi also produce antibacterial agents, and so do bacteria themselves, presumably as part of their own defence system against other bacteria. It was a yeast cell into which a gene from the hepatitis B virus was inserted to produce the first genetically engineered vaccine. And let us not forget that some large fungi are deliciously edible – though other very similar ones are acutely fatal, which I suppose adds a certain excitement to the gourmet lifestyle.

 **Worms**

To anyone who already finds the sight of a worm wriggling in the soil fairly distasteful, the idea of the same thing in your gut or lungs must seem quite disgusting. Yet an estimated *4000 million*

people carry some form of intestinal worm and perhaps 400 million have a worm elsewhere – lung, liver, blood, or tissues. None of these are completely free of symptoms and some are chronically ill, so parasitic worms (or *helminths*, as students have to learn to call them) must rank as the heaviest infectious burden of our species. Once again it is the inhabitants of tropical countries who carry most of the load. Consider this: one can harbour up to 1000 of the roundworm *Ascaris lumbricoides* in the intestine; they can reach a foot long and a female can lay 200 000 eggs a day; the annual egg output in China alone has been estimated as 10 000 *tons*. Not all worms are as big as *Ascaris* (though there are some that are bigger); some are almost invisible. As we saw with the protozoa, some are carried by tropical insects and some (including *Ascaris*) spread by the faecal – oral route. One class has a more complex life cycle involving a water snail, and we will start our review with them.

## Don't paddle in this lake!

I remember at a meeting being very impressed when an Egyptian doctor put up a slide of hieroglyphs from the time of the pyramids (about 2500 BC) and proceeded to read off a most convincing account of *schistosomiasis* (caused by parasites in the genus *Bilharzia*), still a major health problem today in that country and the Middle East as well as parts of South America and the Far East. Schistosomes are small worms, under an inch long, which live harmlessly in blood vessels, in male-plus-female pairs, without multiplying – worms have the one redeeming feature that they don't multiply in their animal host in the way that all other pathogens do. Unfortunately, for their cycle through the water snail to be completed, their *eggs* must reach the water, and this is achieved by forcing their way across the wall of either the intestine or the bladder, depending on the species of schistosome. This would not be so bad but for the fact that some get stuck (in the bladder) or go the wrong way (into the liver), where they set up a violent inflammatory reaction. Thousands of these in the liver are sufficient to block blood flow through it, leading to dilatation of veins around the oesophagus which may rupture and bleed fatally. Likewise in the bladder there can be obstruction of the flow of urine. Some of the eggs that do reach the water find their way to a snail, in which they grow into tiny *cercariae* with a twitching tail; one can just see them shimmering in a test tube held up to the light. These now have to attach to your skin in order to infect you, so if you never paddle in water known to be infected, you are safe from schistosomiasis. You might think it would be quite easy to control the disease by vigorous public health warnings, but alas it doesn't work that way. After all, we could cut down the spread of colds and flu in our own cities by wearing masks, but they are a very rare sight in the West.

## Blindness and a yard of string

Like *Ascaris*, the *filariae* are roundworms but they are spread by mosquitoes and various flies, in which their larvae develop. Their name describes their thread-like appearance, and what disease they cause depends on where these threads end up. To take two examples: *Wuchereria* lives in lymphatics, leading to blockage and the grotesque deformities of *elephantiasis*. *Onchocerca* favours the skin and eye, where it can cause blindness, and because the blackfly that carries it breeds in running water the disease is known as 'river blindness'. In endemic areas one person in seven is blind – twice the frequency expected from trachoma (although trachoma is much more widespread). The Guinea worm, *Dracunculus*, a huge roundworm living just under the skin, is the second largest parasite of humans, growing to over three feet in length. Certainly not thread-like, it could be mistaken for a piece of white string.

The rest of the roundworms behave more like *Ascaris*, settling in the intestine after a remarkable journey through the lungs, trachea, and oesophagus. The hookworm *Ancylostoma* clings to the small intestine, drinking blood in tiny doses but with heavy infections causing quite serious anaemia. *Strongyloides* is similar, except that in immunodeficient individuals it can become disseminated – another *opportunist* to add to the list. *Trichinella* (from pork) and *Toxocara* (from dogs) complete the list of pathogenic roundworms, causing, among other symptoms, eye damage.

## Looking for the head

The third and best-known class of pathogenic worms are the *tapeworms*. I remember the excitement in the ward where I was a student when a patient came in to have his pork (or it may have been beef) tapeworm cured. In those days the treatment was a course of male fern extract, though nobody explained to us the biological basis of this weird association. It was quite interesting to examine the hundreds of flat hermaphrodite segments of *Taenia* as they came out into the bedpan (there can be up to 10 feet of them!) but less so when we realized it was our job to search for the tiny head, which if it stayed attached to the gut would grow a whole new worm; we in our youthful arrogance thought nurses did that sort of thing. Much later, visiting a village in northern Kenya, after an unforgettable flight across Lake Turkana in a tiny plane, piloted by the famous 'Flying Doctor', in which we skimmed alarmingly low over lazily basking crocodiles, I saw dozens of cases of hydatid disease, caused by another tapeworm, *Echinococcus*. This is a parasite of dogs but its eggs, if they get into humans, can grow into huge fluid-filled cysts that may need surgical removal – which was why my pilot was a regular visitor to the area.

## Useful worms?

Amazingly, even a worm infection may have its good side, by an effect on the immune system that tends to reduce the chance of allergies, and even, in one theory, multiple sclerosis.

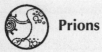 **Prions**

We come now to the last and most bizarre group of pathogens, and probably some of the most notorious, given the recent BSE epidemic and the current alarm over CJD. BSE ('mad cow disease') is short for bovine spongiform encephalopathy, which tells us what the pathology is: spongy areas of degeneration in the brain of cattle. CJD stands for Creutzfeldt–Jakob disease, named after the two doctors who first described this form of dementia 80 years ago. BSE is very much like *scrapie*, a long-established disease of sheep, while CJD is reminiscent of *kuru*, a condition restricted to New Guinea and shown to be spread by the unusual (to us) habit of eating the brains of dead relatives. Recent cases of 'new variant' CJD have been firmly linked to cattle BSE. So all these conditions have finally been brought together into the single category of 'transmissible spongiform encephalopathies'.

The question was: What is doing the transmitting? At first it seemed obvious that it was a virus of some kind, but meticulous analysis showed that it contained protein but apparently *no DNA or*

*RNA*. So unless a trace of nucleotide had been missed it couldn't be a virus. Ironically it was once thought that DNA must contain traces of protein in order to have a role in heredity. But now the boot was on the other foot! Once it was shown in 1953 that DNA was the true genetic material, nobody could imagine an infectious protein. However in 2004 the protein hypothesis was finally proved to be correct when it was shown that a fully synthetic protein could reproduce the infection. So the agent is indeed a **pro**tein which is **in**fectious, and it was baptized *prion*. There was still the question: how could it replicate? We don't know the whole answer at present, and with the current level of research I am sure this section of the book will be the first to go out of date. Infectious prions resemble but are not identical to a normal brain protein, having a shape which particularly lends itself to being deposited as masses of *fibrils*, going on to make adjacent normal proteins refold into the same shape, and so on – rather in the way that crystals grow. It is hard to think of an analogy, but you might try imagining the effect of dropping a magnet into a pile of paperclips and watching them clump together. Recently it has been suggested that there are 'good' prions with a role in normal organ development. The whole field has been one of the medical sensations of the 20th century, and its two champions, the Americans Carleton Gajdusek and Stanley Prusiner, well deserved their Nobel prizes. It remains to be seen whether, as Prusiner suspects, prions are behind Alzheimer's, Parkinson's, and other currently mysterious degenerative brain diseases, and perhaps even ageing itself.

 **Summary: pathogens, mild, severe, and fatal**

So much for the main pathogens of humans. As we have seen, they are a diverse collection, from tiny crystal-like structures to 10-foot worms, united only by the fact that when they get into our bodies, we get ill. Sometimes we recover rapidly, sometimes more slowly. Occasionally we may even die. Some are spread by personal contact; some by air, food, or water; some by an insect bite. Others are picked up from animals. Some are harmless unless our immune system is damaged. Perhaps the following tables will help to put their human impact in perspective, before we move on to examine how we defend ourselves against them.

**Table 2.1 Major killers on the world scale**

| Pathogen/disease | Type of organism | Annual deaths/comments |
| --- | --- | --- |
| HIV/AIDS | Virus | More than 3 million; mainly in the tropics |
| Tuberculosis | Bacterium | „      1.5 million;      „ |
| Malaria | Protozoan | „      1.3 million;      „ |
| Measles | Virus | 600 000; mostly children in the tropics |
| Influenza | Virus | 600 000; excluding pandemics |
| Tetanus | Bacterium | 200 000; mostly newborn children |
| Whooping cough | Bacterium | 300 000 |
| Syphilis | Bacterium | 160 000 |
| Cholera | Bacterium | 100 000 |
| Pneumonia | Viruses; bacteria | 3.5 million; mostly children |
| Diarrhoea | Viruses; bacteria | 2 million; mostly children |
| Meningitis | Viruses; bacteria | 170 000 |
| Hepatitis | Viruses | 100 000 |

**Table 2.2 Some diseases spread by the respiratory route**

| Pathogen/disease | Type of organism | Comments |
|---|---|---|
| *Streptococcus* | Bacterium | Common cause of pneumonia |
| *Haemophilus* | ,, | Common cause of pneumonia |
| Whooping cough | ,, | |
| Tuberculosis | ,, | May spread to other organs |
| Diphtheria | ,, | Laryngitis |
| Anthrax | ,, | More usually via skin |
| Plague ('pneumonic') | ,, | Also via skin ('bubonic') |
| Legionella | ,, | droplet infection |
| Common cold | Viruses | Usually self-limited |
| Influenza | Virus | May spread to lung (pneumonia) |
| Measles | ,, | Also skin rash |
| Mumps | ,, | Also salivary glands |
| Chickenpox | ,, | Rash; may recur as shingles |
| Rubella | ,, | May affect fetus |
| *Aspergillus* | Fungus | May cause allergy |
| *Histoplasma* | ,, | |

**Table 2.3 Some diseases spread by the 'faecal–oral' route**

| Pathogen/disease | Type of organism | Comments |
| --- | --- | --- |
| *Salmonella* | Bacterium | Common cause of diarrhoea |
| *Campylobacter* | ,, | Common cause of diarrhoea |
| *E. coli* | ,, | Common cause of diarrhoea |
| *Shigella* | ,, | May be dysentery (blood in stools) |
| Cholera | ,, | Mainly tropical |
| Rotavirus | Virus | Common cause of diarrhoea |
| Poliovirus | ,, | Occasional spread to brain |
| Norwalk virus | ,, | Diarrhoea and vomiting |
| Hepatitis A | ,, | 'Infectious jaundice' |
| *Entamoeba* | Protozoan | Dysentery; may cause abscesses |
| *Giardia* | ,, | Common cause of chronic diarrhoea |
| *Ascaris* | Worm | Commonest parasite of man |
| *Toxocara* | ,, | From dogs via faeces |

**Table 2.4 Some diseases transmitted by insects or other vectors**

| Pathogen/disease | Type of organism | Vector |
|---|---|---|
| Plague | Bacterium | Flea (from rats) |
| Tularaemia | ,, | Flea, tick, louse |
| Relapsing fever | ,, | Louse |
| Lyme disease | ,, | Tick |
| Typhus | Rickettsia | Flea, louse |
| Dengue | Virus | Mosquito |
| Yellow fever | ,, | ,, |
| Malaria | Protozoan | ,, |
| Leishmaniasis | ,, | Sandfly |
| Sleeping sickness | ,, | Tsetse fly |
| Chagas' disease | ,, | Reduviid bug |
| Onchocerciasis | Worm | Blackfly |
| Filariasis | ,, | Mosquito |
| Schistosomiasis | ,, | Snail |

**Table 2.5 Major diseases caught from animals (zoonoses)**

| Pathogen/disease | Type of organism | Animal reservoir/comments |
|---|---|---|
| Bovine tuberculosis | Bacterium | Cattle; rare since pasteurization |
| Brucellosis | ,, | Cattle, goat, dog |
| Leptospirosis | ,, | Horse, cattle, dog |
| Lyme disease | ,, | Deer |
| Plague | ,, | Rat |
| Tularaemia | ,, | Rat |
| Anthrax | ,, | Farm animals |
| *Salmonella* | ,, | Farm and dairy products |
| Psittacosis | Chlamydia | Birds |
| Rabies | Virus | Bat, dog, fox, racoon |
| Influenza | ,, | Birds, pig |
| Lassa fever | ,, | Rodents |
| Ebola, Marburg | ,, | Monkeys |
| HIV/AIDS | ,, | Chimpanzees; monkeys (originally, now human → human) |
| *Cryptococcus* | Fungus | Birds |
| *Toxoplasma* | Protozoan | Cat |
| *Cryptosporidium* | ,, | Birds, mammals |
| *Echinococcus* | Worm | Dog |
| Tapeworms(s) | ,, | Pig, cattle |
| *Toxocara* | ,, | Dog |

**Table 2.6 Infections mainly restricted to immunodeficient and immunosuppressed individuals**

| Pathogen/disease | Type of organism | Comments/predisposition |
| --- | --- | --- |
| Pseudomonas | Bacterium | Cystic fibrosis; burns |
| Listeria | ,, | Meningitis |
| Avian tuberculosis | ,, | AIDS |
| Klebsiella | ,, | Especially in hospitals |
| CMV | Virus | Fetus; AIDS; bone marrow transplant |
| Candida | Fungus | AIDS; antibiotic over-treatment |
| Cryptococcus | ,, | AIDS |
| Pneumocystis | ,, | AIDS |
| Toxoplasma | Protozoan | Fetus; AIDS |
| Cryptosporidium | ,, | AIDS (diarrhoea) |
| Strongyloides | Worm | AIDS |

**Table 2.7 Infections transferred from mother to fetus or newborn**

| Pathogen/disease | Type of organism | Result/comments |
| --- | --- | --- |
| Syphilis | Bacterium | Congenital syphilis |
| Leprosy | ,, | Congenital leprosy |
| Listeria | ,, | Congenital listeriosis |
| Chlamydia trachomatis | Chlamydia | Neonatal trachoma |
| Rubella | Virus | Eye, ear, brain, heart malformation |
| CMV | ,, | Ear, brain malformation |
| HSV | ,, | Neonatal infection |
| VZV | ,, | Skin, muscle, brain malformation |
| HIV* | ,, | Congenital/newborn AIDS |
| Hepatitis B* | ,, | Persistent infection |
| Toxoplasma | Protozoan | Eye, brain malformation |
| Malaria* | ,, | Rare infection of placenta |

* Also spread by blood transfusion.

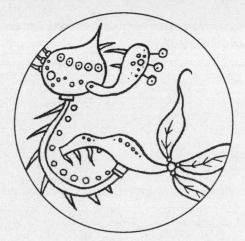

# 3 Defence and immunity: the old immune system

Qui desiderat pacem, praeparet bellum.
Let him who desires peace prepare for war.
Flavius Vegetius, fourth century

One can argue the correctness of this old Latin tag where military politics are concerned, but it is undoubtedly true for infectious disease. In the first chapter of this book I suggested that defending the body against pathogens was very much like defending a country against invasion, and now we are ready to pursue this analogy and see how far it holds good. We have met the enemy forces – viruses, bacteria, etc. – and we know that some of them, the pathogens, will cause damage, perhaps even kill us, if they get in. This is a problem that has been faced by animals of every kind right back to the earliest invertebrates, and by plants and even bacteria, which can themselves be infected by viruses. However, we will concentrate our attention mainly on the strategies adopted by ourselves and other modern mammals, except when there is something valuable to be learned from a glance backwards in time.

 ## Guarding the walls

Obviously the simplest solution to the pathogen problem is . . . keep them out – on the same principle as the massive walls, arrow slits, and vats of boiling oil that protected a medieval city. We have a tough layer of *skin* for this purpose which, as long as it is unbroken, is quite hard for many pathogens to penetrate. Unless they can get themselves established in a biting insect, as the malaria parasite does, they will have to wait for a natural break to be provided for them – a cut, wound, or burn, for example. Otherwise they must sneak round to the less fortified regions where there is a much more delicate membrane between body tissues and the outside – nose, mouth, throat, eye, lungs, intestines, bladder, sexual organs. In practice, the respiratory and alimentary routes are the entry routes chosen by the majority of pathogens (see Tables 2.2, 2.3).

Skin is more than just a barrier; it contains glands that secrete a variety of molecules with antibiotic-like activity against (mainly) bacteria and fungi. Probably these are sufficient to deal with the moderate numbers of organisms encountered on a daily basis and keep us in normal health. We know this because rare unfortunate individuals lacking one or other of them suffer endlessly repeated skin infections with staphylococci, everything else in their defence systems being absolutely normal. I say *moderate* rather than *small* numbers because the air we breathe and everything we touch contains plenty of bacteria and viruses; even without going near anyone ill, we are estimated to inhale around 10 000 micro-organisms every day.

There are more of these antimicrobial molecules in the lungs, helped by the fact that it is very hard for bacteria to penetrate to the furthest reaches of the lung because of a flow of mucus in the opposite direction (i.e. upwards) which continually washes them out again; to try and avoid this, many viruses and bacteria attach themselves firmly to the walls of the air passages. It is this mucus that is abnormally sticky and hard to cough up in the disease *cystic fibrosis*, in which lung infections are distressingly common. The flow of urine acts in the same way to flush out bacteria from the bladder, unless the bacteria can attach themselves firmly to the bladder wall, as the *gonococcus* does. The eye is another site where contact with micro-organisms is inevitable, and here we rely on the flushing effect of tears; these also contain the enzyme *lysozyme*, which kills some bacteria. There is lysozyme in the blood too, and bacteria killed by it would normally be regarded as non-pathogenic. The stomach, with its intensely acid juices, is an effective death-trap for most kinds of pathogen – but not *Helicobacter*, which neutralizes the acid by forming its own alkali (ammonia) from urea. Finally we should not forget that coughing, sneezing, vomiting, and diarrhoea are good ways to get rid of pathogens – and pass them to someone else in the process.

But already we are up against a question that is going to recur as a major theme throughout this book: Why don't these anti-pathogen weapons destroy the skin itself, and the lungs, and the stomach? This question, and others like it, go the the heart of the whole infectious disease problem – how to tell friend from foe. The Pope's generals had the same sort of problem in 13th century Provence in trying to distinguish Cathar heretics from good Catholics: their answer was simple: *kill them all; God will recognize his own.* Nature's answer is a little more subtle: to allow the evolution of only those weapons that damage pathogens and *not* human cells – like those weed-killers that are supposed not to hurt garden flowers, or like synthetic antibiotics, which are designed to kill the bacteria and not the patient. But this doesn't explain *how* they achieve this discrimination. We used to set first-year students exactly this problem to discuss during the coffee break. Perhaps you, too, would like to take 10 minutes off for a cup and think about it . . .

\* \* \* \* \* \* \* \* \* \*

We got some ingenious suggestions – and some not so ingenious. The idea that pathogens might be made of *totally different stuff* was always voted down, because every student knew that bacteria, viruses, etc., like ourselves, were made of proteins, carbohydrates, and lipids, and most had the feeling (correct) that pretty well all proteins were made from the same 20 amino acids. So that idea was evicted (somewhat prematurely, in fact). Also rejected was the proposal that human cells could spot a parasite that *intended harm*, which seemed to require almost clairvoyant powers (but was not totally crazy either, as we shall see). More plausible was the idea of a mechanism that selectively killed cells that *grew rapidly*, which ought theoretically to hit bacteria, viruses, etc. harder than body cells. However, when we pointed out that this was exactly how X-irradiation and chemotherapy for cancer worked, and that their use was restricted because of the damage they cause to the bone marrow and the intestine, where cells do divide rapidly – plus the fact that some pathogens, like the tubercle bacillus, actually grow very slowly – it was agreed that this would not be much use as a general method.

At this point, with the students beginning to think they were hopelessly stupid, we revealed the rather unsensational answer: there is no single mechanism. Nature has seized on every point at which pathogens differ from our own cells and every way in which our own cells can be protected. The lining of the stomach shields itself from gastric acid by a thick layer of mucus. It is safe to flush bacteria out of the air passages in the lung because host cells don't belong down there anyway unless they are fighting pathogens. The lysozyme enzyme in tears attacks a particular structure in bacterial cell walls that is simply absent from all eukaryotic cells (remember that bacteria are *prokaryotes* with many differences from ourselves in their structure and biochemistry). And so on. We shall be returning quite often to this absolutely fundamental question of how to make defence mechanisms safe for the host animal.

### Inside or outside

Despite these protective mechanisms, pathogens clearly do get in. Often they start by binding firmly to a cell surface, as described above and for viruses in the previous chapter. Cold and flu viruses bind to the membranes of the nose and throat, as the pertussis (whooping cough) bacterium does lower down the respiratory passages. Enteric bacteria, viruses, and intestinal protozoa and worms bind to intestinal cells. The pathogen may then either 'blast' its way in by secreting enzymes or toxins or, more subtly, trick the host cell into 'sucking' it in. Pathogens that enter the tissues are called *invasive*. If they stay in the gut or on the skin they are *non-invasive*, though they may still do damage by feeding on skin itself, as the fungus of ringworm does, or drinking blood, as hookworms do, or they may be harmless, like the estimated 100 million million 'normal' bacteria in the intestine. Non-invasive pathogens, which are technically *outside* the body, are very difficult to get rid of. Even the notorious staphylococci are normally non-invasive, living on the skin and in its glands, from which it is almost impossible to remove them even with the most vigorous wash, and from which spread to another host is quite easy. It could be argued that they have nothing to gain by getting into the deeper tissues, setting off defence mechanisms, and possibly risking the life of their host. This is 'living with germs' at its most amicable.

## Alarm bells

One of the earliest signs that something has disturbed the body's status quo, whether it is just a breach in the external defences (e.g. an injury) or whether some pathogens have got in (staphylococci perhaps, or viruses), is a resetting of various priorities. That huge protein factory, the liver, reduces its output of everyday proteins like albumin in favour of a number of proteins with useful effects in limiting tissue damage. Other cells produce messenger molecules that tell the brain to raise body temperature. Local tissue damage sets off *inflammation*, which increases local blood flow and directs the attention of defence cells and molecules to the site of invasion, as well as planning ahead for eventual healing. Unavoidably, local pressure is increased, tissues are stretched and nerves stimulated, so inflammation can be painful. The stage is being set for action.

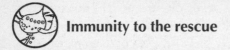 Immunity to the rescue

If pathogens have indeed entered the body, something more is needed than simply to heal the breach. To pursue our analogy of invading enemy agents, we need to call in the internal defence team, or in medical terms, the *immune system*. This is the name given to all the cells and molecules (let us lump these together for now as 'elements') scattered throughout the body whose job is to deal with pathogens – a sort of combined army and police brigade.

### A three-pronged assault

In dealing with any invasion, there are three separate tasks that have to be carried out. The invaders must be (1) *recognized*, then they must be (2) *disposed* of, and since recognition and disposal may need to be carried out by different elements, we need (3) a *communication* system to keep all elements in touch. This is exactly how the immune system works: there are recognition and disposal elements and a communication system. In lectures I used to use examples from the Second World War, when to deal with bombing raids there were (1) air spotters, (2) anti-aircraft guns and fighters and (3) a radio link between them all. Students laughed at the quaint old photos of Spitfires and Heinkels and searchlights, but I think they got the idea, which was important because *immunology* has acquired a reputation since those days for being far too complicated for the ordinary person to bother with. Since this is partly the fault of immunologists themselves, I am going to pause at this point to take a quick look at the whole subject, before getting back to the present state of knowledge of the immune system.

## A momentous decade

Many of the greatest medical scientists were immunologists in all but name. I suppose it was the country doctor Edward Jenner who started the ball rolling with his smallpox vaccine (1798). But it was in the 1880s that things really started to happen. Louis Pasteur, a chemist and microbiologist, showed that the idea of immunization could be applied to other diseases such as cholera and anthrax (1881). Soon afterwards (1890) Emil Von Behring and Shibasaburo Kitasato, in Berlin, made the vitally important discovery that a newly appearing molecule in the blood of animals that had been immunized against diphtheria and tetanus by the injection of toxins was what protected them. They called this molecule *antitoxin* and later *antibody*, but its remarkable properties were not fully explained for another 70 years and I must keep it for the next chapter.

Meanwhile, at around the same time (1882) the Russian zoologist Ilya Metchnikoff showed that cells could be protective too, by engulfing and digesting foreign material, including pathogens; he called these cells *phagocytes* ('eating cells'). Debate raged over whether antibodies or phagocytes were more important in defence, even spilling over on to the stage. George Bernard Shaw's play *The Doctor's Dilemma* (1907) is about precisely this issue; his hero, Sir Colenso Ridgeon, advocated the idea, championed by the real-life Almroth Wright at St Mary's Hospital in London, that both *opsonins* (antibodies) and cells were needed for the best results (he was correct, as we shall see). Here he is in Shaw's play, explaining his discovery to an elderly colleague:

Sir Patrick:  Opsonin? What the devil is opsonin?

RIDGEON:  Opsonin is what you butter the disease germs with to
   make your white blood corpuscles eat them.
SIR PATRICK:  That's not new. I've heard this notion that the white
   corpuscles – what is it that what's his name? – Metchnikoff – calls
   them?
RIDGEON:  Phagocytes.
SIR PATRICK:  Aye, phagocytes: yes, yes, yes. Well, I heard this
   theory that the phagocytes eat up the disease germs years ago:
   long before you came into fashion. Besides, they don't always
   eat them.
RIDGEON:  They do when you butter them with opsonin.

But already by 1897 the German chemist Paul Ehrlich (to be
honoured a century later at that Immunology congress in Berlin)
had started asking awkward questions like: How is it that these
antibodies and phagocytes can destroy foreign invaders but not the
tissues of their host?, and: How do they know what is foreign? This
question, you will notice, is closely related to the one we put to our
students, but with an extra twist, because now we have to explain
how one and the same cell (the phagocyte) can distinguish what it
should eat (a pathogen, for instance) from what it shouldn't (such as
another phagocyte or a tasty liver cell). Ehrlich's question will recur
in one form or another right through this book.

## A twentieth-century discipline

The science of immunology had begun, and eventually, after
another 50 years of sporadic discoveries, it was recognized as a
respectable academic subject; in fact when I started out in the
1960s, my department head, Ivan Roitt, was probably one of the
first people in the UK to have been appointed as an immunologist

rather than a biochemist, haematologist, or microbiologist with a side interest in immunity. Now at last there were immunology laboratories, immunology departments, immunology societies, specialist journals, local meetings, international conferences, textbooks. The subject developed its own special language. Even to this day, a slight hush falls round the medical school table when an immunologist speaks up, rather as if he or she was unlikely to say anything that normal people would understand, or contribute anything actually relevant to the problem of diagnosing and treating sick people. And it is quite true that at immunological conferences, where *everybody* is an immunologist, the talk is so littered with jargon, abbreviations, fantastic experiments, outrageous speculations, and furious arguments about detection and elimination, that you might think you had wandered into a Pentagon war game. Still, what matters is that out of all this experimentation and argument has come an understanding of the immune system which has progressed faster than developments in any other medical field except perhaps molecular biology (DNA, etc.). Immunology textbooks, to stay reasonably up to date, have to be rewritten every two or three years.

As with all branches of science, this rapid progress has been fuelled by some fairly vigorous personal and even national rivalries – carrying on the tradition of Pasteur and Koch, who fought (verbally) for France and Germany a century ago. Inevitably the centre of productivity has shifted to the USA, whose universities and biotechnology companies offer a young graduate such tempting rewards, but contributions out of proportion to population size have come from the Scandinavian countries, Israel, and Australia, and most immunologists have friends all over the world. Occasionally the thirst for priority in publication leads to a regrettable failure to give credit; most of us in Europe have heard from some overseas colleague: 'Sorry, if I'd read your paper, of course I'd have quoted it.' It must have been worse for non-English-speaking countries before they accepted the inevitable and published their national journals in English, the international language of science today. I remember WHO meetings in the 1960s where, for the benefit of one French delegate (whose English was usually perfectly adequate), every question had to be repeated by the chairman in French. This was at the insistence of President de Gaulle, and exactly doubled the length of every session, eating seriously into the lunch interval. And now, back to the immune system itself.

## Two police forces

The first point to make is that there are really two immune systems, related to each other very much as the police on the beat and the CID detectives are. Both have the three elements mentioned above (recognition, disposal, communication) but use them in different ways. The 'on-the-beat' force is the oldest, going right back to the invertebrates, and it includes all those cells and molecules that have been tried out and tested over thousands of millions of years of evolution for their usefulness in recognizing and disposing of pathogens in safety – or, in police terms, spotting a villain and locking him up. Metchnikoff's phagocytes are a good example; he actually discovered their engulfing function in an invertebrate (a starfish), but a human phagocyte engulfing a bacterium behaves almost identically. This slowly evolving immune system, as much part of our make-up as our liver, lungs, or kidneys, is known as the *innate immune system* because we are 'born with it'. As well as phagocytes, it includes some important defence molecules, such as complement and interferon.

Compare this with the second system. This is relatively new on the scene, being only found in vertebrates: the jawless fishes of 500 million years ago, the sharks, and all their successors – fishes, reptiles, birds, ourselves. Instead of, like the innate system, having gradually learned ways of recognizing pathogens, it works on a completely opposite principle, namely to start by recognizing *everything* and then learning *not* to recognize the body's own structures. This might seem a rather clumsy approach, but I shall try and show in the next chapter just how powerful it is.

Both systems, the old and the new, employ both cells and molecules; antibody is one of the 'new' molecules and the cell that makes it is called a *lymphocyte*. This amazing cell is one of Nature's marvels; there is no other like it. Unlike phagocytes, which can attack almost anything foreign (like a squad of policeman who can all spot a villain), lymphocytes and antibodies are individuals; a separate one is devoted to each foreign object, able to pick it out among millions of others, help in its disposal, and preserve a record of the fact for future use. You can see the close parallel with the way detective forces operate, putting a man on to each suspect to hound him down and keep all his details on file. Because this system is constantly updating its knowledge of the actual pathogens it has met, it is called the *adaptive immune system*. In this ability to learn from experience and retain *memory*, there is a superficial resemblance to the way the brain works, especially when you consider that adaptive immunity (like learning) is rather slow getting into action compared to innate immunity, which (like instinct) acts rapidly if it is going to act at all. However, the actual mechanisms are quite different, so the analogy between the immune system and the brain is *not* particularly useful. We shall stick to the police one, which is much better.

The above is, of course, grossly simplified. Now we shall look in more detail at innate immunity and how it contributes its quota to keeping pathogens under control.

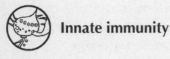 **Innate immunity**

Let us return once more to Metchnikoff's phagocytes. We last saw them engulfing a bacterium, and this is an event which occurs hundreds of times a day throughout our lives as stray bacteria wander into the tissues or a massive army of them floods in through a wound (for an idea of the relative size of phagocyte and bacterium, try imagining yourself swallowing a large bun in one piece). The process goes roughly as follows: the phagocyte moves towards the bacterium by following a trail of chemical clues and helped by the increased blood flow of local inflammation; it attaches part of its cell membrane to part of the bacterial cell membrane; a protrusion of membrane surrounds the bacterium and swallows it, so that it now lies in a hollow vesicle inside the phagocyte; other vesicles (the *lysosomes*, see Fig. 2.3) join up and squirt in their contents, which include molecules for killing and digesting the bacterium; finally, the bacterium is reduced to its constituent molecules which are recycled for the use of the host (Fig. 3.1).

So far, so good; we have dealt with *disposal*. But you may have noticed that I sidestepped that vital point – the question Ehrlich asked a century ago: How does the phagocyte know the bacterium is something it should eat? How does it know it's a pathogen? Why doesn't it eat other phagocytes? In other words, where is the *recognition*? Amazingly, the answer took almost a century to

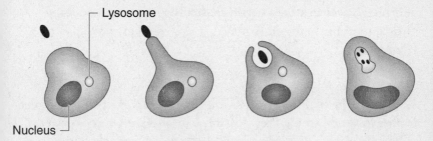

Lysosome

Nucleus

**Fig. 3.1** Four stages in the phagocytosis of a bacterium by a macrophage.

emerge, because it had to wait until the molecules on the pathogens and the molecules on the phagocytes that recognized them were fully analysed.

It was not just a question of the right 'opsonins', as Shaw's hero might have thought, because phagocytes can eat bacteria in a test tube containing no antibodies whatever. Nor was it a case of the bacterium looking completely alien because, as pointed out by our first-year students, bacteria are made of the same kinds of chemicals – proteins, carbohydrates, and lipids – as phagocytes are. However, it turns out that there *are* certain molecular patterns that are found in some pathogens and not at all in mammalian cells – in somewhat the same way that jerseys knitted from the same wool can still feel different because of their different patterns. Microbial examples are (a) lipopolysaccharide (usually abbreviated to LPS), a carbohydrate–lipid structure only present in the walls of some bacteria; (b) particular sugars restricted to the cell wall of bacteria, fungi, and some protozoa; (c) double-stranded RNA in some viruses (mammalian RNA is always single-stranded), etc. – all are undoubted signs of *foreignness*. Once again, Nature has ferreted out those few features that do distinguish pathogens, and it is safe for phagocytes to attack anything that displays them. So there was something in the students' idea of a cell that could 'scent danger'.

To recognize these 'pathogen-associated molecular patterns' – known in the trade as PAMPs (immunologists, like text messagers, abbreviate everything they possibly can) – Nature has endowed phagocytes with a set of special *receptors*. An example of the immense time-span over which innate immunity has evolved is the fact that insects and humans use closely similar receptors to recognize PAMPs – in fact one set was first discovered in flies and subsequently found in humans! Phagocytes can also recognize patterns that are exposed when host cells or molecules become damaged, which allows them to carry out their other useful function of clearing away worn-out body components. They can also recognize utterly foreign objects like carbon particles, which is fortunate for smokers and people living in smoky areas, whose lungs would otherwise become silted up with carbon. In short, without phagocytes our lives would be impossible.

The pathogen-recognizing skills of phagocytes do unfortunately have their limitations. They are pretty good at dealing with many bacteria and fungi, but not those that are coated with *capsules* and, most importantly, not bacterial *toxins*. Toxins are small proteins which for the most part lack any of the PAMPs mentioned above; not only that, but some of them are also capable of killing phagocytes (you may recall that the pus in a staphylococcal abscess is mainly dead phagocytes). Many believe that it was largely in order to cope with bacterial capsules and toxins that the antibody molecule evolved, as described in the next chapter – though there is a limit to how far one can look back in time and say precisely *why* something occurred. After all, we don't really know for certain why our ancestors came out of the forest, lost their fur, and evolved speech – and that happened only a few million years ago.

## Large and small phagocytes

The duties of *phagocytosis* are split between two sets of cells. The larger of the two, the *macrophages* ('large eating cells') reside mainly in the tissues and organs, where they live for months or years, eating, killing, and digesting their prey day after day. The smaller phagocytes, known as *polymorphs* or *neutrophils* (PMNs for short) because of their shape and colour under the microscope, travel round in the blood, waiting to be summoned to an inflammatory site where pathogens have made an appearance; if not used, they quickly die. The number of PMNs in the blood is one of the things the doctor wants to know when he asks for a 'white cell count', because too few PMNs could spell trouble from bacterial or fungal infection. There should be about 5000 million per litre, or five times that in all (about 10 times the human world population), and they are replaced daily from the bone marrow.

Another white blood cell, present in much lower numbers, is the *eosinophil*, whose role has been hotly debated. Eosinophils contain a number of powerful molecules with the curious effect of damaging worms, which may have been their original function in prehistoric days when worm infections were a major human health hazard – as in the tropics they still are. They owe their name to the fact that their granules stain with the dye eosin – another contribution by our hero Paul Ehrlich, who was the first to exploit fully the value of staining in pathology and bacteriology.

## Complementary molecules

In 1893, 10 years after the discovery of antibody, a clever but simple experiment revealed a new element of innate immunity. It was already known that the serum (clotted blood minus cells) of an animal that had been injected with a particular type of bacteria would agglutinate (clump together) the bacteria it had been injected with (but not others), even if the serum had been heated; this clumping substance was antibody and agglutination became a standard method of demonstrating its presence. Now it was shown that the addition of unheated serum, *even from a normal animal*, would cause the agglutinated bacteria to be *lysed* – that is, made leaky and destroyed. A cloudy suspension of bacteria in a test tube would go clear as the bacteria literally disappeared (see Fig. 3.2). The unavoidable conclusion was that something in normal serum helps antibody to destroy bacteria, but is knocked out by mild heating (in fact, about 56°C).

This new substance was called *complement*, and we now know it is actually a set of about 30 proteins which interact with antibody and then with each other in a sort of chain reaction, or 'cascade', one of whose effects is to punch tiny holes in the walls of bacteria so that the contents leak out. (Cascades are an effective way of generating a large and rapid biological effect from a small starting signal; the *clotting* system works in a similar way to generate a blood clot as soon as a blood vessel is damaged.) It was later found that some pathogens can set off the complement cascade without antibody being involved. So, rather like phagocytic cells, complement represents both a *recognition* and a *disposal* system for at least some pathogens – again, predominantly bacteria and fungi. In fact complement can not only lyse them but 'butter' them for

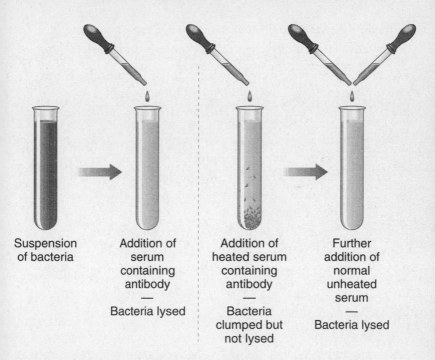

| | | | |
| --- | --- | --- | --- |
| Suspension of bacteria | Addition of serum containing antibody — Bacteria lysed | Addition of heated serum containing antibody — Bacteria clumped but not lysed | Further addition of normal unheated serum — Bacteria lysed |

**Fig. 3.2** An experiment to show that antibody can clump bacteria, but complement is required to destroy them by lysis.

phagocytosis too, so it is also an *opsonin* – altogether a most useful element in defence.

## Togetherness

The effect of complement is not confined to helping antibody and helping phagocytes; it can help both at once. A bacterium with antibody bound to its surface will be eaten by phagocytes more rapidly than one without, and if there is complement bound to it as well, the process will be speeded up even more. This is an example of the theme that runs through almost all immune functions, namely *collaboration* between two or more (in this case three) different elements of the immune system.

We shall encounter many other examples of collaboration when we come to look at adaptive immunity and lymphocytes, which collaborate with phagocytes as well as among themselves. Note that collaboration is not quite the same as communication. One could liken the collaboration between phagocytes, antibody, and complement to the combination of soldier, gun, and vehicle; each of them has its own function but they are most potent when working together. *Communication* implies one element sending information to another, and the best examples of this are when the innate and adaptive immune systems communicate with and among each other, as we shall see in Chapter 5.

### Nature's antiviral drugs

In discussing viruses (Chapter 2), I mentioned that it was possible, though not easy, to design drugs that interfered with their replication. As so often happens, Nature was there first. Bacteria have enzymes that cut up viral DNA – the same *restriction endonucleases* that are so indispensable to the molecular biologist today. In higher animals, the *interferon* molecule (actually a set of 14 slightly different molecules) has the ability to flood out from a virus-infected cell to its neighbours and protect them from the virus. It is made in response to a signal that only viruses provide (RNA in its double-stranded form) and it acts only against viral RNA and viral protein formation.

Thus Nature has discovered another pathogen weak spot, and

interferon passes the 'Ehrlich' safety test of killing the pathogen without killing host cells; it has now been made commercially and is used to treat certain persistent virus infections such as hepatitis as well as some tumours. However, it has the drawback of making the patient feel quite ill, in fact the 'flu-like' symptoms of many virus infections (fever, muscle pains, etc.) are actually caused by raised levels of interferon – some compensation, perhaps, for feeling so rotten. The picture is also complicated by the fact that the interferons have indirect effects too, stimulating various other types of cells to exert their own activities against not only viruses but also other pathogens as well. This takes us into the realm of communication and introduces the fascinating molecules known as *cytokines*. More about them in a later chapter. First we need to take a closer look at adaptive immunity and the lymphocyte.

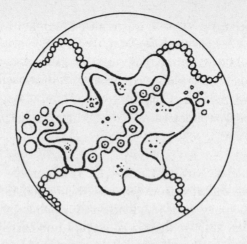

# 4 Sharpening the focus: the new immune system

Lymphocytes, like wasps, are genetically programmed for exploration, but each of them seems to be permitted a different, solitary idea. They roam through the tissues, sensing and monitoring. Since there are so many of them, they can make collective guesses at almost anything antigenic on the surface of the earth, but they must do their work one notion at a time. They carry specific information in their surface receptors, presented in the form of a question: is there, anywhere out there, my particular molecular configuration?

Lewis Thomas, 1974

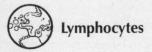 **Lymphocytes**

As we have seen, antibody formation, immunological memory, and the success of vaccines were well known before 1900, yet it was another half century before it was realized that they were all due to the properties of *lymphocytes*. Up to then the favourite theory was that lymphocytes were the 'stem' cells that gave rise to all the other blood cells – one of the classic wrong ideas of the twentieth century. It was not until the elegant experiments of James Gowans in Oxford (1959) that the lymphocyte took its rightful place as *the* cell of adaptive immunity.

Lymphocytes make up about a third of the white cells in blood and they are utterly different from the other major population of white blood cells, the phagocytic polymorph/neutrophils (PMNs). To begin with, they are very long-lived – years, and perhaps decades. Unlike PMNs, they do not just enter the blood, leave it when they are needed, and die; they *recirculate* from blood to tissues and back again, each endlessly searching for its unique quarry, because when a particular pathogen appears somewhere in the body, only a few out of millions of lymphocytes will be able to recognize it. Remember the analogy with the detective and think of Javert and Jean Valjean, Holmes and Moriarty, Father Brown and Flambeau, each in single-minded pursuit of his one and only 'familiar face'.

To increase the chances of a 'sighting', there are special locations where pathogens and lymphocytes are more likely to meet; these are the lymphoid organs, of which *lymph nodes* (or glands) are the most important. When these glands are swollen or painful, for example during a sore throat, there is a lot of activity going on inside them, lymphocytes recognizing the invading viruses or bacteria having homed in from all over the body to do battle. Unless it takes extraordinary precautions, a pathogen cannot avoid, sooner or later, coming in contact with the 'right' lymphocyte and that, for the pathogen, is the beginning of the end. One way or another, via antibody or various killing devices, the lymphocytes will do all they can to finish it off.

This scenario raises a number of intriguing new questions, such as: What is meant by the 'right' lymphocyte? How does a lymphocyte get to be 'right'? How many sorts of lymphocytes do we need? I shall tackle these one by one.

## Specificity

What do I mean by 'right'? Once again, it is a question of *receptors*. On their surface, lymphocytes carry protein molecules that can fit and bind tightly to other suitably shaped molecules, rather as a glove fits a hand – the 'glove' in this case being the receptor and the 'hand' some tiny portion of a pathogen. You will recall that I said much the same about phagocytes, but there is a fundamental difference between the two types of cell, because whereas all phagocytes carry the same set of 15 or more types of receptor (to recognize those pathogen-associated molecular patterns, or PAMPs, we discussed in the last chapter), each lymphocyte carries thousands of copies of just *one single* type, so that it can recognize only one single shape, unique to that lymphocyte (see Fig. 4.1), rather like the glass slipper that fitted only Cinderella's foot.

This idea of unique receptors on cells, so unexpected but so fundamental to the whole of immunology, was put forward as long ago as 1890, and you will not be surprised to know that its author, once again, was Paul Ehrlich. He arrived at it by thinking about why different dyes stained different cells and different microbes – another favourite topic of his which also led him to the concept of chemotherapy. It was 70 years before the techniques were available

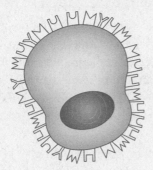

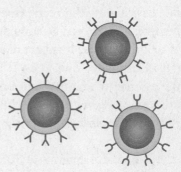

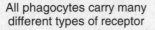

All phagocytes carry many
different types of receptor

Each lymphocyte carries
one type of receptor only

**Fig. 4.1** The cells of innate immunity (e.g. phagocytes, *left*) and those of adaptive immunity (lymphocytes, *right*) use completely different approaches to the recognition of pathogens.

to demonstrate receptors on lymphocytes and provide confirmation of his amazing insight. Ehrlich's one mistake was to assume that receptor 'gloves' bound to their microbial 'hands' by a *chemical* bond – the type of union he, as a chemist, was most familiar with. In fact the bond is *physical* (just as the hand–glove one is), and quite capable of coming undone – in scientific terms, it is *reversible*. But every great scientist is surely allowed an error or two; Koch and Pasteur were not always right either.

Immunologists employ the term *specificity* to make the distinction between the lymphocyte and the phagocyte type of recognition: lymphocytes are described as 'highly specific' in their recognition, phagocytes as 'less specific'. At one time, innate immunity in general was referred to as 'non-specific immunity', but this is a bit unfair to phagocytes, which as we saw can distinguish perfectly well between most pathogens and normal body cells. In fact this is more than lymphocytes can do, because when they recognize 'their own' particular molecular shape, they have no way of telling whether it is part of a pathogen, or a harmless parasite, or one of the body's own cells. It is just a *shape*. And here we come to the essence of adaptive immunity: it is based on the recognition of millions of shapes through the possession of millions of receptors. Rather than *pathogen-directed*, it is *shape-directed*.

Where do these millions of different types of shape-detecting receptors come from, and how does each lymphocyte manage to end up carrying only one type? This question bothered immunologists for years and many strange theories were proposed. However, we now know the answer which, as one might expect, shows perfect logic on the part of Nature, though it, too, may seem strange at first sight.

## Receptor diversity

Let us imagine there are about 100 million different varieties of lymphocyte receptor – enough to recognize every conceivable molecular shape. The actual number is impossible to calculate, and is different for the two types of lymphocyte, T and B (a complication to be introduced shortly) but 100 million different varieties is probably not far off. We can rule out straight away the notion of 100 million separate genes in our DNA, because this is vastly more than the total number of human genes (a mere 25,000).

Instead, we have a combination of three things. (1) Receptors are composed of two protein *chains*, each different; this saves genes because, for example, 100 genes for each (= 200) will give $100 \times 100$ combinations (= 10 000). (2) Each of the chains is built of three *segments*, each coded for by a separate gene, and as a result of duplications and mutations accumulated over millions of years, each of these genes exists in anywhere from 5 to 200 slightly different versions, and they can be shuffled in any combination to make a new composite gene for each of the two protein chains. The shuffle will be different for each lymphocyte and once it has occurred it can't be unshuffled, so the lymphocyte is 'locked in' to that one shape-recognizing configuration – or *combining site* as it is known. (3) However, the six areas of the genes that code for the parts of the receptor that actually do the recognizing are susceptible to further small changes due to mutations occurring within individual lymphocytes. Multiplying up all these possibilities, we arrive at a figure of at least 100 million different possible receptor 'specificities' – a fairly awe-inspiring number.

This means that each one of 100 million lymphocytes carries a receptor (or to be precise, many copies of it), similar in *general* structure to those on other lymphocytes but different in the *recognizing* part. The closest analogy might be a hand of six cards dealt from a pack of thousands, with further changes occurring spontaneously in the cards after the deal. Perhaps you will recall that this is the same analogy as I used in Chapter 2 for the way the influenza virus varies its appearance, and if you bear in mind all the other pathogens that the immune system needs to recognize, you can see how the two sides in the battle are using a similar strategy – generation of as many variations as possible and selection of the most successful and useful variants. In other words, both are using the basic ingredients of Darwinian evolution – *mutation* and *natural selection*.

We have about 10 000 million lymphocytes, quite enough to recognize every possible molecular shape, and therefore every possible pathogen, *even though they may never encounter most of them*. This was the part of the theory that upset many early immunologists (see below), their argument being: Why carry around millions of lymphocytes you may never need? The answer, which seems obvious now, is that *we never know which ones we are going to need*. Pathogens are mutating and evolving the whole time; the immune system must do the same if it wants to keep up. In a sense, then, 'living with germs' involves your genes keeping pace with their genes.

## Clonal selection

Still thinking about numbers, you might object that it is all very well to have all these millions of lymphocytes with different receptors, but doesn't that mean that there will be only a small number to deal with any one particular pathogen? In police terms, is *one* detective per criminal enough? This is not really a problem because a pathogen, even the smallest virus, offers not one but dozens of shapes (antigens) to be recognized by different lymphocytes, and anyway, once a lymphocyte has recognized its pathogen, one of the things that happen is that the lymphocyte *proliferates* – dividing into two identical cells, then four, and so on – ending up with a *clone* of identical lymphocytes, all ready to do battle (see Fig. 4.2). Here I am afraid our police analogy breaks down, unless you can imagine the triumphant detective rapidly cloning himself, like some warrior from *The Matrix*!

As a result of all this, the numbers look more manageable, because about 1 in 10 000 to 1 in 1 000 000 lymphocytes will recognize *some part* of any one pathogen. With a population of

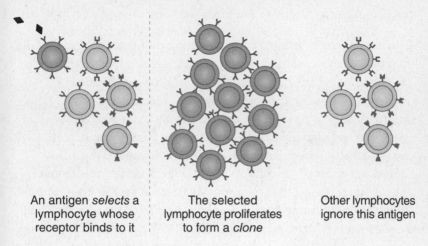

| An antigen *selects* a lymphocyte whose receptor binds to it | The selected lymphocyte proliferates to form a *clone* | Other lymphocytes ignore this antigen |

**Fig. 4.2** Clonal selection, the basis of the adaptive immune response.

10 000 000 000 lymphocytes, we are in the range where there might be as many as a million lymphocytes per pathogen, *even before they start to proliferate*. So there is no real shortage. Because the 'right' lymphocytes are selected by contact with the pathogen, and grow into clones, which gradually come to dominate the lymphocyte population of the individual concerned, the whole process is called *clonal selection*. It allows the person to *adapt* to the world of pathogens he or she actually inhabits – whence the name, adaptive immunity. Someone who has been exposed to measles will have more anti-measles lymphocytes than someone who hasn't. The clonal selection theory of 1959, the whole basis of adaptive immunity, was the brainchild of a brilliantly clear-sighted Australian virologist, Macfarlane Burnet, doing for immunology what Darwin did for zoology, and nothing has happened since to question its essential rightness.

## A wrong turning

The clonal selection theory was not universally accepted at first. As mentioned above, some immunologists, including double Nobel laureate Linus Pauling, had difficulty swallowing the idea of millions of unused lymphocytes. A rival idea, known as the *instructive* theory, proposed that all lymphocytes started out the same and individually somehow fashioned their receptor to fit the antigens they were exposed to – rather analogous to the anti-Darwinian theory of evolution by 'intelligent design' and popular for the same reason: it is easier to understand for the non-scientist. As far as the immune system was concerned, once it was realized how proteins were actually made (DNA to RNA to protein), this theory became impossible to sustain – in addition to which it failed to explain various other results to be described later. It was soon obvious that on this point Burnet was right and Pauling wrong (both were wrong on other occasions, as we shall see).

## T and B lymphocytes

This does not mean that nothing has changed since Burnet's day. Only a few years after clonal selection, there occurred another breakthrough in understanding what lymphocytes actually did. It had been known for some time that while many infections and toxins were evidently dealt with by antibody (plus complement and phagocytes in many cases, as described in the previous chapter), others appeared not to involve antibody at all, yet they all still obeyed the 'adaptive' rules of high specificity, memory, effective vaccination, etc., and all seemed to be mediated by lymphocytes. Tuberculosis was a leading example, and the rejection of tissue grafts was another. The terms humoral (for the antibody-type) and cellular immunity (for the tuberculosis/graft-rejection type) came into use. It was generally accepted that antibody was made by lymphocytes, but not at all clear how cellular immunity worked.

Then people started noticing that the thymus (a lymphoid organ in the neck, especially prominent in children and young animals) seemed to play a key role in immunity; if it was removed from mice very early in life, cellular immunity did not develop, while humoral immunity remained fairly normal. I remember in 1961 hearing a brilliant seminar in which a young French-Australian, Jacques Miller, at that time working in London, described these pioneer experiments. Not long after, I heard him give exactly the same talk in California, and I wonder how many times he was invited to present his sensational results. He soon acquired 'star' status, to the annoyance of a group in Minneapolis headed by Robert Good, who had come to the same conclusion at around the same time but had not publicized it with the same panache. Such things are unfortunately quite common in science, where priority in an important discovery is one of the most treasured rewards for years of not very well-paid work.

Not everybody was immediately bowled over by Miller's and Good's results. Peter Medawar, who had shared the Nobel Prize with Burnet the previous year, is said to have remarked that the presence of lymphocytes in the thymus was 'an evolutionary accident of no very great significance'. Burnet himself was quicker to see their importance, but went to the other extreme and assumed that *all* lymphocytes originated in the thymus. The truth emerged from an unexpected quarter when it was discovered that in birds another organ, the bursa, produced the antibody-forming lymphocytes. In mammals, however, they come, like other blood cells, from the bone marrow.

Finally in 1966 it was accepted that there were two distinct kinds
of lymphocytes, those that came from the Thymus and those that
came from the Bone marrow (or the Bursa), looking alike but with
different functions. They were baptized T and B, respectively, and
suddenly a lot of other observations began to make sense. I will
spare you the details of five decades of research, during which
dozens of laboratories took up the challenge, and skip to the present.

## Indoor and outdoor detectives

The division of labour between B and T lymphocytes turns out to
correspond to two fundamentally different groups of pathogens,
inhabiting two compartments of the body – extracellular and
intracellular. *Extracellular* means free in the body fluids or tissues
and extracellular pathogens would include staphs and streps,
viruses on their way from one cell to another, trypanosomes in the
blood, worms, and – though they are molecules rather than
organisms – toxins such as those from tetanus and diphtheria.
*Intracellular* pathogens are those living inside body cells, including
viruses during most of their life and – a most important group –
bacteria, fungi, and protozoa that can survive inside phagocytes,
such as tuberculosis bacilli and *Leishmania*.

In a nutshell, B lymphocytes deal with the extracellular
compartment by secreting antibodies; T cells deal with the
intracellular compartment in a variety of ways *not* involving
antibody. For a police analogy, you would have to imagine two kinds
of detective, one monitoring the outdoor world, and the other
trained to spot villains lurking indoors – a bit like plain clothes
officers versus the fraud squad. B lymphocytes are the easiest to
understand, so we will consider them first.

## Extracellular pathogens, B lymphocytes, and antibody

### A (fairly) recent development

In the previous chapter I mentioned that adaptive immunity appears to have evolved with the first vertebrates some 550 million years ago, possibly to give better protection against bacteria, armed with their anti-phagocytic capsules and toxins. This emerged from a search in primitive animals (or, strictly speaking, their modern descendants) for signs of lymphocytes or antibody. One of the most unforgettable episodes of my two-year spell at the University of California at Berkeley was struggling to hold a 10-foot-long anaesthetized shark at the San Francisco zoo while my supervisor, Ben Papermaster, injected an antigen through a six-inch needle. At weekly intervals we returned to take blood samples and – yes, there were undoubtedly antibodies there, not quite like those of contemporary mammals but clearly molecules of the same basic design. Similar experiments in invertebrates have failed to find antibodies or lymphocytes, which seem to have first appeared in jawless fishes like the hagfish, the earliest vertebrates still surviving today and even more ancient than the sharks.

Exactly why adaptive immunity and the backbone should have evolved at the same time is not obvious, but it makes an excellent topic for speculation. Perhaps another 10-minute coffee break would be appropriate here for you to think about it . . .

\* \* \* \* \* \* \* \* \* \*

Here are some of the 'usual suspects'. In general, vertebrates are larger, live longer, inhabit land areas, breathe air, have a higher body temperature – all of which might favour more serious infections and therefore call for an improved immune system. But none of these features by any means distinguishes *all* invertebrates from *all* vertebrates (think of fish, spiders). The backbone also brought with it a much more comlex nervous system – another 'recognition' element. I rather liked the impromptu suggestion by palaeontologist Professor Richard Fortey that it might have had to do with feeding habits; today's hagfish are notorious for feasting on rotting flesh – a rich source of bacteria. Perhaps it was just a coincidence. At any rate, vertebrates certainly do need their lymphocytes, as we shall see when we examine the problems of patients with lymphocyte defects.

## Antibody

In simple terms, a B lymphocyte is a little antibody factory, able to switch on the formation of antibody and export it at the rate of some 100 000 molecules a minute, which flood out into the blood and reach all parts of the body. But the B lymphocyte does need to be switched on, and in its 'resting' state it makes only enough antibody to display on its surface as a receptor and a sample of what it can produce. So its product is to all intents and purposes *the same as its receptor*. B cells develop in the bone marrow, circulate through blood and tissues to find 'their' pathogen, and move to lymph nodes or other lymphoid organs to settle down as *plasma cells* to producing antibody, usually for a matter of a few days, after which they either die or survive as *memory* cells.

The antibody molecule is a tiny masterpiece of design, a flexible Y-shaped molecule with two recognition areas or *combining sites* at the tips of the Y (Fig 4.3). These two combining sites are identical (because each B lymphocyte is 'locked in' to making only make one type of combining site), and two sites bind much more strongly than one, so when antibodies do bind they bind extremely strongly to their small portion of pathogen, or *antigen* as it is termed. And because the antibody B lymphocytes secrete is the same as the receptor on their surface, it will bind to the same antigen that was recognized by the cell and switched it on in the first place. A measles virus will switch on only B lymphocytes carrying receptors for one or other of the measles virus antigens, and only antibodies against measles will be made. Tetanus toxin will stimulate a completely different set of B lymphocytes, leading to the production of completely different antibodies. Measles antibody will not bind to tetanus toxin and vice versa. This is what is meant by antibodies being 'highly specific'.

## Class distinctions

Now the *other* end of the Y enters the fray. It may bind to both complement and phagocytes; if so, the pathogen is headed for

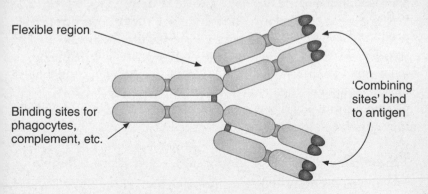

**Fig. 4.3** The four-chain structure of the antibody molecule (IgG).

destruction. Adaptive and innate immunity have collaborated in a perfect outcome. Nature has experimented with slightly different structures for this end of the antibody molecule too; they are called *classes* and given the names IgA, IgD, IgE, IgG, and IgM. Each has a distinct role in immunity, as we shall see (IgG is the phagocyte-binding one). There are classes of antibody for crossing the placenta to protect the fetus (IgG again), for protecting the lung and intestine where enzymes would destroy normal antibody molecules (IgA), and for triggering inflammation (IgE). Individual B cells tend to start by making IgM antibodies and moving on to IgG, IgA, etc. as the need arises – without, of course, changing the specificity of the combining-site end of the molecule, which is locked in to that B lymphocyte.

Most of the really effective vaccines work mainly by boosting the numbers of B lymphocytes – that is, expanding their clones – so that when the real live pathogen comes along there are more B lymphocytes to go into action, and more antibody (especially IgG) is made in less time. It is as if the system remembers the pathogen. This is immunological *memory*. The same thing happens with T lymphocytes (see below), and it happens after recovery from a normal infection, which explains why we do not get measles, mumps, etc. twice. We may not remember whether we had mumps as a child, but our lymphocytes do. In a later chapter we shall see why this immunity following recovery unfortunately doesn't happen with every disease.

### The time factor

The only slight problem in all this is that antibody production, and the lymphocyte proliferation that goes with it, take time, so it is usually several days before enough antibody is made to be effective. This is why in a disease like measles or pneumonia you can be quite ill for a week or so, until enough antibody has been made to knock out the pathogen (as far as I can calculate, Jane Austen's Marianne Dashwood recovered on the sixth day of her illness). In the case of toxins or viruses, there is usually no need for complement or phagocytosis – simply blocking their binding to cells is enough to neutralize the danger. So a good antibody response can be life-saving in toxic diseases like tetanus, diphtheria, and cholera, and in virus diseases like measles and polio.

Note that the need for antibody to collaborate with phagocytes and complement in staphylococcal and streptococcal infections, particularly pneumonia, does not add to the time delay, because the phagocytes and complement *were there already*. Innate immune elements had to wait for adaptive immunity to get going (or if you like, the policemen were on the beat but didn't know who to arrest until the detectives had tagged them for disposal). In this case, *recognition* and *disposal* are carried out by separate immune elements.

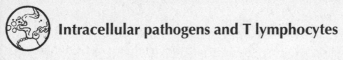 **Intracellular pathogens and T lymphocytes**

The antibody response is simplicity itself compared to the task faced by T lymphocytes – the ones that recognize and dispose of *intracellular* infections. How can a cell monitor the *interior* of another cell? In the case of viruses it was originally assumed that the T lymphocyte was simply recognizing virus antigens as the particles budded or burst out of the infected cell. But this convenient explanation could not account for the fact that T lymphocytes could sometimes be shown to be recognizing proteins associated with the viral RNA – antigens which were never exposed on the surface of the infected cell! As you can probably guess, there were some wrong theories and one right one. One of the most bizarre wrong ones was that T lymphocytes could put out a sort of 'finger' and 'feel around' inside the infected cell, and electron microscope photographs were even produced that seemed to show this (you can find an electron micrograph to support most theories).

Incidentally, on the subject of what T cells do, a very popular theory at one time was that they were responsible for preventing cancer. This idea is not absolutely wrong, but it was dealt a nasty blow when it was discovered that a well-known mutation that made mice hairless also knocked out the development of their thymus. Thus these poor little pink skinny creatures had no T lymphocytes. Everyone expected them to develop all sorts of tumours but scientists in Denmark, who followed thousands of them from birth to death, reported that they got *fewer* tumours than normal! We now know that T lymphocytes do play a part in tumour control, but other cells and molecules are equally important.

To return to virus-killing, the correct solution came from experiments in the 1970s by Rolf Zinkernagel and Peter Doherty in Australia, in which they showed that mouse T lymphocytes able to recognize cells infected with a certain virus would only do so if they came from the same *strain* of mice (mouse strains are genetically different, just as individual humans are, but within a strain the mice are all identical, like identical twins). This was the first hint of any connection between the genes that determined strain and those that determined virus recognition. To cut a long story short, it turned out that bits of virus were continuously being carried from inside the infected cell to its surface, and that the molecules doing the carrying were the same ones that defined the strain of mouse – the so-called *major histocompatibility complex* or MHC molecules. You may recall that I mentioned these in an earlier chapter as an important part of the cell's information-transfer system (see Fig. 2.3).

## Molecular haulage

Nobody really likes the name MHC, which makes one think, if anything, of graft rejection (histocompatibility means tissue compatibility, which is what grafted organs need in order not to be rejected, and 'tissue typing' really means 'MHC typing'). So at the risk of outraging my professional colleagues, I would like to propose a new definition, purely for the purposes of this book, namely *molecular haulage contractor*, which highlights the role of MHC molecules in transporting molecules within the cell, from the interior to the surface. Whenever you see the letters MHC from now on, think of a fleet of tiny lorries (12 different sorts per cell, in fact) permanently ferrying molecules from inside the cell to the surface.

This was a wonderful solution to the problem of intracellular monitoring, because not only did it explain how T cells 'saw' what was inside an infected cell, but it also revealed the real role of MHC molecules – since obviously grafting of organs was not part of Nature's plan. The picture was completed by showing that the receptor on the T lymphocyte, which is not antibody but a somewhat similar two-chain protein molecule, was recognizing the *combination* of MHC molecule and a tiny bit of virus – as it were, the lorry and its contents. We now know that MHC molecules are moving to the cell surface all the time (see Fig. 2.3), carrying with them tiny pieces, only a few amino acids long, of whatever proteins are inside the cell – not just viral proteins but normal cell proteins too, which the T lymphocytes have to learn to ignore. So in their different way, the T lymphocytes are like the B lymphocytes in that they recognize *shapes*, not pathogenicity.

## Divisions of labour

All T lymphocytes recognize their target in this way, but they vary in what they do to it. One approach is to bind to the virus-infected cell, punch holes in it, and inject a lethal dose of enzymes. The cell dies and the T lymphocyte moves on. T lymphocytes that do this are called *cytotoxic* ('cell-killing'). This is an example where *recognition* and *disposal* are carried out by the same cell. Cytotoxicity is especially valuable against viruses that do not themselves destroy the cells they infect, such as herpes, hepatitis B, and influenza (Fig. 4.4).

Other T lymphocytes act quite differently, binding to phagocytes or B lymphocytes and releasing proteins called *cytokines* to stimulate them into action; these are known as *helper T lymphocytes* and the cytokines they secrete play a decisive role in pushing adaptive responses in the right direction – either towards a macrophage or an antibody-dominated response, depending on which is most appropriate for the pathogen in question. We shall look more closely at these collaborative T lymphocyte functions in the next chapter.

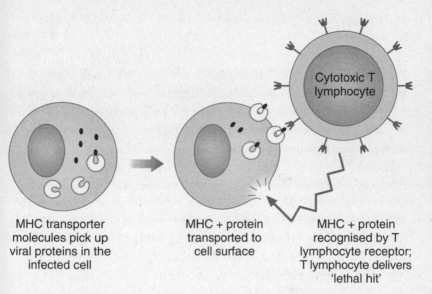

MHC transporter
molecules pick up
viral proteins in the
infected cell

MHC + protein
transported to
cell surface

MHC + protein
recognised by T
lymphocyte receptor;
T lymphocyte delivers
'lethal hit'

**Fig. 4.4** Killing of a virus-infected cell by a cytotoxic T lymphocyte.

## Self and not-self; Ehrlich again

It is easy to say that T lymphocytes must 'ignore' normal cell
components, but not so easy to see just how this is actually
achieved. In fact this is Ehrlich's question all over again: how to
distinguish your own proteins, etc. (let us call them 'self') from
foreign ones ('non-self'). As we saw, phagocytes manage this by
having receptors for a few common features (PAMPs) only found
on pathogens. But the problem is far more acute for B and
T lymphocytes because they are designed quite differently, with
receptors that recognize every conceivable molecular shape,
*millions* of them, some of which are bound to turn up on our own
cells and molecules. It would be absolutely fatal if antibodies

and cytotoxicity were unleashed on these – we would literally self-destruct.

We don't self-destruct, obviously, except to a very small extent in certain *autoimmune* diseases which, again, will have to wait until a later chapter. So here is yet another discussion topic: How do we avoid self-destruction by our own lymphocytes? In general we tolerate the presence of our self components while reacting vigorously to the non-self components of pathogens. In fact immunologists use the word *tolerance* to describe this lack of reaction to self. So Ehrlich's question can be restated once more as follows: *How does our adaptive immune system maintain self-tolerance?* Wherever two immunologists get together, this question is sure to be discussed. It is the Big One. The asterisks below are intended to give you a pause to consider it.

\* \* \* \* \* \* \* \* \* \*

If you haven't come up with a solution, you may be relieved to hear that once again there is not one all-embracing answer, but a whole list of little adjustments during T and B lymphocyte development and function that give an overall satisfactory result. It would take us far away from the theme of this book to go into them all, but let me just mention three: deletion, help, and presentation.

### Deletion

Firstly, T and (probably) B lymphocytes whose receptors bind strongly to a self component are *deleted* (that is, killed) before they leave the thymus or bone marrow. In the thymus, as many as 90% of all T lymphocytes are killed in this way. You can see how Burnet's clonal selection theory always accounted for this much better than the instructive one, because according to clonal selection, lymphocytes display their receptor *before* contacting antigen, which means that their 'intention' to react against 'self' is already evident from the start and they can be picked out for deletion. The instructive theory, according to which all lymphocytes start out the same, could not explain the deletion of only the self-reactive lymphocytes, and its adherents were obliged to deny that it happened. Even scientists can sometimes overlook awkward facts.

*Help*

Secondly, most B lymphocytes will not make a large amount of antibody, or switch from IgM to the more potent IgG etc. unless *helped* (see above) by a T lymphocyte. So as long as T lymphocytes are tolerant to 'self', B lymphocytes can at worst make some anti-self IgM antibodies (which do little harm).

*Presentation*

Thirdly, T lymphocytes are only activated by antigens they meet in special sites such as lymph nodes, and these are more likely to be from pathogens brought in by special *antigen-presenting cells* (APCs) than from self components that don't normally travel to these sites. These APCs are related to phagocytes, except that they retain antigens on their surface instead of taking them in, so they represent a collaboration between the innate and adaptive systems (a theme that will reappear in the next chapter). The term 'presentation' always struck me as rather grandiose for the process of two cells slithering over each other; it seemed more suited to the ecstatic moment in Strauss's *Der Rosenkavalier* when the handsome prince Octavian presents the silver rose to young Sophie and their eyes meet . . . but who knows? Perhaps that's how it is for a lymphocyte when it finally encounters that one-in-a-million antigen.

So in fact the whole recognition system is something of a compromise, which is just as well, because if every receptor that recognized, *however weakly*, every possible molecule that *in any way* resembled a self molecule was deleted, there would be very few left to recognize pathogens. So the set of lymphocyte receptors we end up with are the ones that have proved, during evolution, to give the most balanced result – enough recognition of non-self, not too much of self. A rough analogy would be the issue of police 'stop and search'. Too little lets criminals get away; too much leads to social breakdown.

### The Persian chessboard

We have seen how lymphocytes, starting from a tiny minority with the right recognition receptors, can proliferate up into clones large enough to mount a life-saving response – antibody or cytotoxic as the case may be. This raises one last problem: how to *stop* the cloning process. The Persian legend of the grateful ruler and the gift of rice – one grain on the first square of a chessboard, two on the second, four on the next and so on, doubling each time and ending up on the last square with a pile of rice weighing 100 000 000 000 tons – gives an idea of what could happen if clonal expansion of one B or T lymphocyte was allowed to carry on unchecked. Obviously the body would run out of space and nourishment long before this, but Nature has devised more subtle ways of keeping lymphocyte clones to a suitable size. Many of the cells die, having discharged their duty. Others are designed to *suppress* proliferation. And of course if the antigen is completely eliminated, the stimulus for proliferation has gone too, and what is left is a population of *memory* lymphocytes, both B and T, ready to mount a larger and more rapid response if the same antigen turns up again. It is these memory cells that stop you going down with measles, mumps, etc. a second time, by secreting antibody and becoming cytotoxic and eliminating the virus before it has had time to cause any symptoms. You are *immune*, thanks to the extraordinary properties of the lymphocyte – something the innate system could never have achieved by itself.

## Natural born killers

Like the infamous pair in Oliver Stone's movie, the *natural killer* (NK) cell does not quite fit in anywhere. In appearance NK cells are lymphocytes, and they kill virus-infected cells in exactly the same way as cytotoxic T lymphocytes do. However, they do not use the same receptor as T lymphocytes, they do not show memory, and they do not recognize MHC molecules – just the opposite in fact; they only kill their target when MHC molecules are *absent*. They refuse to accept any molecules brought by the haulage contractor. This is extremely useful in certain circumstances, because some viruses, such as herpes, have evolved ways of preventing MHC molecules reaching the cell surface, which protects them against T lymphocytes but invites killing by NK cells. NK cells can also release the antiviral antibiotic *interferon* – a second line of attack against viruses. They react rapidly, like phagocytes, rather than slowly like lymphocytes, so they are poised somewhere between the innate and adaptive camps – emphasizing that our attempts to put immune mechanisms into neat categories are always an oversimplification.

## Innate and adaptive immunity compared

Summing up this and the preceding chapter, we can say that higher animals have, and need to have, two immune systems that act side by side and very often in collaboration. Their main differences are illustrated in Table 4.1.

**Table 4.1 Innate and adaptive immunity compared**

|  | Innate immunity | Adaptive immunity |
| --- | --- | --- |
| Evolutionary origin | Earliest animals | Vertebrates only |
|  | All invertebrates |  |
|  | Vertebrates |  |
| Principal cells | Phagocytes | Lymphocytes |
|  |   Macrophage | B |
|  |   PMN | T |
|  | Natural killer cells . . . . . . . . . . . | Natural Killer cells |
| Important molecules | Complement | Antibody (B) |
|  | Interferon |  |
|  | Cytokines . . . . . . . . . . . . . . . . . | Cytokines (T) |
| Recognition units | Receptors for PAMPs | Antibody |
|  |  | T-cell receptor |
| Specificity of recognition | Many pathogens | Antigenic shapes (B) |
|  |  | Antigens + MHC (T) |
| Speed of action | Rapid (minutes/hours) | Slow (days/weeks) |
| Development of memory | No | Yes |

PAMP: pathogen-associated molecular pattern; PMN: polymorphonuclear neutrophil; MHC: major histocompatibility complex.

## Adaptive immunity – our sixth sense?

In the previous chapter I was rather dismissive of the analogy between immunity and the brain, which really only have the phenomenon of *long-term memory* in common, and achieve it by quite different means. The brain relies on networks of fixed, non-dividing, interconnecting neurons; the adaptive immune system uses mobile, dividing lymphocytes. There was a vogue a few decades ago for interpreting immune responses in terms of networks of lymphocytes whose receptors recognized and regulated each other, but it has still not achieved wide acceptance as a major element in immunity (which doesn't, or course make it wrong).

However, there is a curious resemblance between recognition of antigens by lymphocytes and that of *smell* by the millions of receptor cells in the nose which are responsible for detecting more than 10 000 distinct odours. To do this they employ about 1000 different types of receptor, each able to recognize several but by no means all odours, and distributed unequally between the receptor cells. So while the system does not have a separate cell for each detectable odour, as the lymphocyte system does for antigens, we can see the principle of *selection* at work in the use of a variety of cells and receptors. A further parallel with immunity is the continuous turnover and replacement of odour-receptor cells, and there is even a hint of *self-tolerance* in the way we are more sensitive to other people's odours than to our own – though this probably occurs at a brain rather than a receptor level. Dogs, as we shall see in a later chapter, actually distinguish individuals by recognizing their MHC molecules.

The hair cells in the cochlea of the ear work on a similar principle, in this case using different cells for different pitches of sound. The other senses (vision, taste, touch) discriminate using a much smaller number of distinct receptors plus a good deal of subsequent processing by the brain, but the element of cell-specialization is still there. So it may not be entirely fanciful to regard the whole lymphocyte system as a super-discriminatory, unconscious, mobile sixth sense (or seventh, if you happen to be a believer in telepathy).

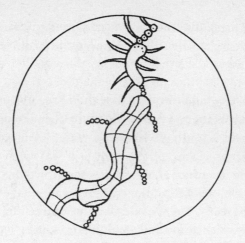

# 5 Communication and collaboration

Corpora non agunt nisi fixata.
Things do not interact unless they make contact.

Paul Ehrlich

Like an anti-aircraft battery, immune defences could not function
without collaboration and communication. In Chapter 3 I described
the collaboration of phagocytes, antibody, and complement in
dealing with a typical bacterium. In Chapter 4 I mentioned that
helper T lymphocytes collaborated with B lymphocytes to make a
larger antibody response, and T lymphocytes with macrophages to
improve their handling of intracellular pathogens, while in the
reverse direction, antigen-presenting cells were needed to start the
process of lymphocyte activation. I listed all these interactions as if

they were simple and self-evident truths. In fact, however, it was not always so easy to prove that immunity really did work in this collaborative way.

One obvious experiment we can do is to put together, for example, phagocytes, antibody, and complement, in various combinations, with some bacteria and see what happens. This can easily be done in a test tube in the laboratory, exactly as it was when complement was discovered a century ago. But does this prove that the same thing happens in real life, in the body of an animal with a bacterial infection? Not really. There could be some quite different mechanism at work in the body and the test-tube effect could be just that: a test-tube effect or *in vitro artefact* ('in-glass unnatural effect') – a very common event in the laboratory. Obviously we need a more critical test, and perhaps a homely analogy will help.

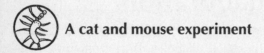 **A cat and mouse experiment**

Let me introduce you to our two cats: Louis, a large black male named after Louis Armstrong, one of my musical heroes, and Josephine, a dainty female named after the wife of Napoleon, my wife's most famous compatriot. Between them they keep the house free of mice, leaving the corpses proudly displayed at the foot of the stairs. But which is the killer? It always happens while we are asleep. We could do a scaled-up version of the laboratory experiment, putting one or the other of the cats, or both, in a locked room with a mouse, but that would only prove whether they *could* kill a trapped mouse. A better experiment would be to lock one or the other alone in the room every night and see what happens to the mouse population. If locking up Louis puts a stop to the appearance of corpses, then he is the killer, and ditto for Josephine. But if locking up *either* him *or* Josephine stops the killing, we have to conclude that it needs both of them. Perhaps he does the catching (*recognition*) and she delivers the fatal bite (*disposal*), or vice versa. At any rate, *they are in it together*.

Now, to apply the same approach to our bacterial infection, we need to *remove* phagocytes, antibody, and complement, in all possible combinations, and see which combination knocks out the killing of the bacteria. This sounds rather brutal, but fortunately (for us) there are people with inborn defects of phagocytosis, others with missing complement, and others who cannot make antibody (they are all described in detail in Chapter 8). And what we observe is that *all* of them have difficulty eliminating many bacterial and fungal infections. So, just as with our cats, we can conclude that these three elements do work hand-in-hand *in real life*. Almroth Wright was right. I have laboured this point because it establishes an important general rule, namely that you only learn the real function of some organ, cell, or molecule by removing it. Exactly the same approach was used, in 1889, to prove that the pancreas was needed to control blood sugar; when it was removed from a dog, the animal developed diabetes – the first essential step towards the discovery of insulin. Likewise the importance of the thymus in immunity was only proved in 1961 by removing it, as described in the previous chapter.

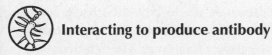 **Interacting to produce antibody**

The collaboration between T helper and B lymphocytes was the subject of another long-running dispute in immunological circles.

Let us backtrack in time to the 1960s. The starting observation was that mice made better antibody responses if they had both T and B lymphocytes. This could be shown by injecting purified T and/or B lymphocytes into mice that lacked both, and with most antigens the results were clear cut. Next it was proved that the B, but not the T, lymphocytes were actually making the antibody. Though this was at first an *in vitro* finding, it seemed most unlikely that it would be any different *in vivo*, and so it was later proved. So what were the T lymphocytes doing? One idea was that the T lymphocyte somehow 'told' the B lymphocyte what antibody to make by transferring some kind of genetic information, but this had to be abandoned when it was realized that B lymphocytes already had their own unique antibody on their surface even before antigen came along, as we saw in the previous chapter. Some experiments (*in vitro* again) suggested that a 'soluble factor' from T lymphocytes could substitute for the T lymphocytes themselves, which implied the existence of some kind of 'communication' molecule. But communicating what?

Opinions formed up in two camps: one favoured the idea of a sort of T lymphocyte-derived 'antibody', different for every antigen. The other camp maintained that the soluble factor was the same for all antigens – a general purpose B lymphocyte stimulant. T and B lymphocytes were patiently and laboriously cultured in tiny plastic chambers, separated or not separated by membranes allowing different-sized molecules to pass through. Chamber shape, source of plastic, membrane pore size, culture fluid, batch of serum (phase of the moon too, we onlookers used to joke) all had to be just right or one got the wrong answer – or no answer. A few years later exactly the same controversy arose over the T lymphocytes which, in certain circumstances, could *suppress* antibody formation by

B lymphocytes. Antigen-specific and antigen-non-specific factors battled it out in the journals and at meetings. The controversy became ever more furious. Pasteur and Koch would have felt quite at home. I remember being rather glad I was working on something else.

Then a third camp emerged with a new story. According to this, just as in the T cell cytotoxicity experiments described earlier, the interaction worked best if T and B lymphocytes were from the same strain of mice. This implied some sort of cell contact and focussed attention on the MHC molecules and their 'molecular haulage' function. Further confusion reigned, and several more years of work were required to establish the true sequence of events, as follows.

 ## Two of the three camps were right

We can look at the antibody response in three stages (Fig. 5.1). The first two stages are quite similar to the procedure for killing virus-infected cells already described. On the B lymphocyte side, the surface antibody molecules recognize an antigen and drag it into the cell. Here small portions of it are picked up by MHC (think 'molecular haulage contractor') molecules and sent back to the surface, where they are recognized by any T lymphocyte with the right receptor, which will, as always, have to 'see' both antigen and MHC (or lorry plus cargo). The chances of the right B and T lymphocytes meeting are facilitated by the tendency of both types of cell to circulate through lymph nodes (this is reminiscent of the claim that if you sit long enough in St Mark's Square in Venice, you will meet everybody you have ever known).

The third stage, however, is quite different, because obviously there would be no point in the T lymphocyte killing the B lymphocyte. That would defeat the whole purpose of the interaction, which is to stimulate antibody production. Instead it releases a variety of communication molecules which bind to receptors (again!) on the B lymphocyte and stimulate it to do various things: to enlarge, to divide, to release antibody, to switch from making IgM to IgG, etc. (Fig. 5.1). Each of these molecules has a different function; there are at least 30 of them and they are collectively known as *cytokines*. They are the 'soluble factors' that were hinted at in earlier experiments, but their usefulness extends far beyond antibody production, with effects on all types of immunological cell, bone marrow, blood vessels, and even the brain. Most are stimulatory, a few are suppressive. But there is one thing they *cannot* do, and that is recognize antigens. They are completely *non-specific*, just as interferons are (remember that interferons recognize the presence of a virus but not what virus it is). In fact the interferons are regarded as members of the family of cytokines. So the only people who were altogether wrong were the supporters of antigen-specific T lymphocyte factors, though I believe there are still those who cling to the notion and probably always will. This is not too serious because, as I've mentioned, an otherwise respected scientist is generally permitted one completely wrong idea without being written off as a crank; Ehrlich, Metchnikoff, and Medawar had theirs and Pauling, with his two Nobel prizes, was allowed two: the instructive theory and megadose vitamin C therapy.

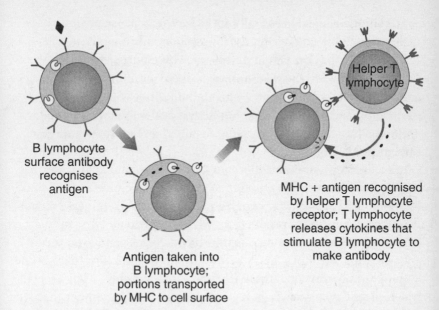

**Fig. 5.1** B lymphocyte–T lymphocyte interaction in the stimulation of an antibody response.

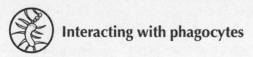 **Interacting with phagocytes**

A very similar process to the above operates between
T lymphocytes and macrophages. Imagine a macrophage that has
engulfed some bacteria. If they were, let us say, streptococci, there
is a good chance that they would be killed and digested and that
would be the end of the story. But now suppose they were tubercle
bacilli. As you may recall, these are extremely tough and hard to
kill. So in a normal quiescent macrophage some of them will
survive and may even multiply. This is where the T lymphocyte

comes in. By recognizing small bits of bacterial antigens on the surface (hauled there by MHC molecules, of course!), the T lymphocyte gets the signal to release cytokines which increase the killing power of the macrophage – or in immunological jargon, *activate* it (Fig. 5.2). The cytokines that do this are partly the same, partly different from the ones that activate B lymphocytes to make antibody. This overlap in functions is one of the many fascinating things about cytokines.

## Helper and cytotoxic T lymphocytes compared

One rather critical thing arises from all this; perhaps you have already spotted it. How does the T lymphocyte, having interacted with its 'target' cell, know whether it has to activate it or kill it? The tiny portion of antigen on the surface will give no clue of what sort of pathogen it came from – it is just a strip of a dozen or so amino acids. You might like to take a pause now to invent a way in which the system could be made safe: to provide *help* for B lymphocytes and macrophage, *death* for virus-infected cells . . .

\* \* \* \* \* \* \* \* \* \*

Perhaps this is an unfair task, because with the receptors and non-specific cytokines so far described, it simply cannot be done. We need one more receptor, which can detect the difference between two kinds of 'target' cell – a virus-infected cell (to be killed) and a B lymphocyte or macrophage (to be activated). In fact Nature has designed a pair of receptors, known by the not-very-exciting names of CD4 and CD8 (all surface molecules on cells have a CD number as a sort of identity card). Helper T lymphocytes carry CD4, cytotoxic ones CD8. You may have guessed that CD4 molecules only

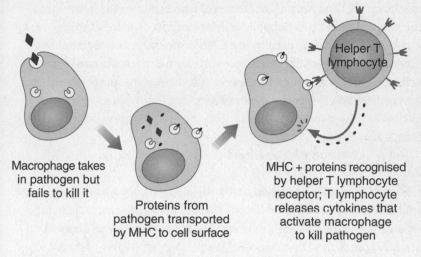

Macrophage takes in pathogen but fails to kill it

Proteins from pathogen transported by MHC to cell surface

MHC + proteins recognised by helper T lymphocyte receptor; T lymphocyte releases cytokines that activate macrophage to kill pathogen

**Fig. 5.2** Macrophage–T lymphocyte interaction in the killing of a pathogen surviving in the macrophage.

recognize B lymphocytes and macrophages, but that CD8 molecules must recognize *all* types of cell – since any type of cell could be infected with a virus and may need to be killed.

But even this is not enough; we still need something on the receiving end of the CD4 and CD8 receptors. Nature could possibly have come up with two completely new molecules, but instead, with a beautiful display of economy, it is the *MHC molecules themselves* that are used. All that was needed was for different target cells to use different sorts of MHC (different haulage contractors or, if you like, lorries of two different colours). Antigens that have been *taken in* (as they are in B lymphocytes and macrophages) are loaded into one kind of MHC; those that are *growing* in the cell (as viruses do) on to another. CD4 molecules bind to the first sort, CD8 to the others. It is a virtually foolproof system. The only drawback, which is hardly Nature's fault, is that the AIDS virus happens to use CD4 molecules as one of its receptors for getting into cells, with the unfortunate consequence that it infects and destroys helper T lymphocytes – knocking the very heart out of the immune system.

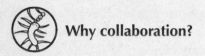 **Why collaboration?**

The collaboration between antibody, complement, and phagocytes is not hard to understand. Like the Three Musketeers, each can function alone but together they are more potent ('all for one, one for all', as Athos, Porthos, and Aramis used to boast). But the collaboration between T helper and B lymphocytes in antibody formation is of a different kind. B lymphocytes on their own can make some IgM antibody but no IgG; T lymphocytes can make neither. Why did Nature not leave it all to the B lymphocytes?

One way to think of it is as an order to attack that has to be signed and counter-signed. The B lymphocyte, having seized a pathogen by one of its antigens, offers up other portions of it (duly bound to an MHC molecule) to the T lymphocytes, as if requesting permission to proceed. If both are satisfied, the intruder is stamped as doubly foreign, the attack gets the go-ahead, and the cytokines are released. But if the 'intruder' is in fact 'one of ours' which the B lymphocyte has recognized (as can happen), the request will be turned down, because T lymphocytes, as we saw in the last chapter, are quite rigorously screened against self-recognition. So T–B collaboration is a vital part of preventing *autoimmunity* – or in Ehrlich's vivid phrase: *Horror Autotoxicus*. Using a similar argument for the collaboration between T lymphocytes and macrophages, we could say that activation of macrophages should only be allowed to occur when it is really essential, because large numbers of permanently activated macrophages would amount to a constant state of chronic inflammation. So the T lymphocyte has to check on the foreignness of the antigen before releasing its cytokines and giving the macrophage its licence to go into 'overkill'. In both cases the T helper lymphocyte is acting as a kind of higher authority whose approval is needed. Some rare situations where this ingenious system breaks down are reviewed in Chapter 7.

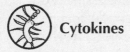 Cytokines

### Terminology gone mad

The only less-than-fascinating thing about cytokines is their names. Who would guess that four molecules called *tumour necrosis factor alpha*, *transforming growth factor beta*, *interferon gamma*, and *interleukin-1* (abbreviated, immunology-style, to TNFα, TGFβ, IFNγ, and IL-1, respectively) had anything in common? Yet all of them, and many others, are simply 'communication' molecules which cells use to send instructions to other cells. You may have noticed that in this they are a little like the *hormones* by which endocrine glands (pancreas, thyroid, pituitary, etc.) regulate metabolic processes all over the body. But this analogy is not all that good, because unlike most hormones cytokines are made by more than one type of cell and have more than one effect. Also, rather than flooding out into the blood from fixed organs like the pancreas and thyroid, they tend to be produced in the tissues close to where they are needed, by mobile cells such as T lymphocytes and phagocytes, which therefore have to be in contact, or almost, with the cells that are responding. So Ehrlich's dictum at the top of this chapter was essentially right as far as cytokines are concerned.

As for those strange names, the reason for them is that when a cytokine is first discovered, it is usually only one of its functions that is identified; the others emerge later. TNFα provoked great excitement when it was shown to cause certain tumours in mice to shrivel up, but unfortunately its anti-tumour effect is quite limited and it is mainly a mediator of *inflammatory* responses (to be described in a later chapter). TGFβ, on the other hand, is an *anti-inflammatory* molecule. IFNγ is antiviral but also has powerful activating effects on many cells, including macrophages, as described above. IL-1 is the only one of the four with a sensible name; *interleukin* simply means 'between white cells', indicating that it acts as a cell-to-cell messenger (in fact its effects overlap considerably with TNF). There are nearly 30 other interleukins and the list keeps growing. If only we had the chance to start all over again, they could all be called interleukins. (At one of the early meetings on cytokines, in a Bavarian hotel, it was suggested that they should be called 'Heidikines', in honour of a pretty barmaid, but unfortunately the proposal was turned down in the cold light of the next morning.)

Like the interferons, some of the cytokines are being tried out in the treatment of diseases, though the results are rather unpredictable. Because some of them (like TNFα) play a role in inflammation, there is also an interest in *inhibiting* them; a recent successful example is the use of TNF inhibitors in rheumatoid arthritis and a similar idea has been tried in severe malaria. Pharmaceutical companies distribute enormous multi-coloured charts, which we dutifully put up on our office walls and laboratory corridors, listing the properties of cytokines (especially the ones they manufacture and sell!) criss-crossed with arrows showing stimulatory and inhibitory pathways, complete with lists and molecular structures of the receptors through which they act. It is far too much for most immunologists to memorize, and when contemplating them I used to feel that if only I had the mind of a Gary Kasparov or a Stephen Hawking the 'whole picture' might emerge, but it never quite happened.

Nevertheless, we can stand back and review the main forces at our disposal in the fight against pathogens, as heads of state in warlike countries do: the phagocytic *macrophages* and *PMNs*, with their faithful assistants *complement* and *antibody* for keeping the body fluids and tissues free of pathogens; the *B lymphocytes* to make the antibody; *interferon* and the *NK cells* and *cytotoxic T lymphocytes* for knocking out viruses; the *helper T lymphocytes* keeping everyone in order; the special worm brigade of *eosinophils*; and flitting around everywhere the busy *cytokines* and a host of *inflammatory* molecules. Table 5.1 sums this up; it is an impressive army and any invader will obviously have to work hard if he wants to survive for long against it.

### Gene wars

At this point you are probably beginning to understand why immunology is regarded as rather complicated! However, there is a way of cutting through the mass of detail, and that is to temporarily forget all those receptors and antigens and antibodies and cytokines and just think of the *genes*. On one side are the pathogens' genes; on the other side we have the human immune genes. Each set of

**Table 5.1 The principal defence elements of the immune system**

| Cells/molecules | | Main recognition/activity |
| --- | --- | --- |
| **(1) Recognition** | | |
| Phagocytic cells | | Bacteria, fungi, protozoa |
| Complement | | Bacteria, some viruses, fungi, protozoa |
| NK cells | | Intracellular viruses (without MHC) |
| Lymphocytes | (B/antibody) | Protein/carbohydrate antigens |
| | (cytotoxic T) | Intracellular viruses (+ MHC molecules) |
| | (helper T) | Intracellular antigens on B lymphocytes and macrophages (+ MHC molecules) |
| | | |
| **(2) Disposal** | | |
| Phagocytic cells | | Kill bacteria, fungi, protozoa |
| Eosinophils | | Kill worms |
| Complement | | Lysis: helps phagocytosis |
| Interferon | | Kills intracellular viruses |
| NK cells | | Kill virus-infected cells |
| Lymphocytes (cytotoxic T) | | Kill virus-infected cells |
| Antibody | | Blocks toxins, viruses |
| | | Helps phagocytosis |
| | | |
| **(3) Communication** | | |
| Cytokines | | T lymphocyte–phagocyte |
| | | T lymphocyte–B lymphocyte |
| | | T lymphocyte–T lymphocyte |
| Inflammatory molecules | | Inflammation |

genes is evolving to keep pace with the other. Today's sets represent the successful survivors on both sides. Over millions of years pathogen species and the immune system have settled down to their basic patterns, while at the short end of the time scale the flu virus is still trying out new variants from year to year, and HIV from week to week, to which the immune system does its best to respond from its own huge gene bank. As we shall see in the next chapters, failure to control an infection is usually due to either pathogen fight-back strategies or an immune defect, and almost never to a failure of the normal immune system to *respond*.

### Are we still evolving?

Until recently it was assumed that human evolution has been fairly stationary for the last 1–200 000 years or so, but with the unravelling of the human genome it has emerged that some genes are still changing surprisingly rapidly – 'rapidly' in this case meaning a time-scale of thousands of years. Attention is mainly focused on the brain, reopening old controversies about intelligence. But infectious diseases are the most powerful selective influence of all on survival; for instance as long as malaria and AIDS continue to be major childhood killers, we should expect the frequency of the sickle cell gene and the mutant HIV-receptor gene to go on rising, and the same might apply to many other genes not yet identified. Within the immune system itself, complement, interferon and other cytokines, phagocyte receptors, and the pack of genes from which the antibody and the T lymphocyte receptor are shuffled every time a lymphocyte is born, could still probably benefit from small changes, and perhaps are even now doing so. On the negative side, the improved survival of immunodeficient individuals (see Chapter 8) will inevitably tend to preserve genes generally considered undesirable, which might otherwise tend to die out. So the immune system, over the long term, could theoretically evolve in either direction.

Nevertheless the fact that nowadays many people live into their seventies and beyond without ever suffering a serious infectious disease, shows that the present combination of innate and adpative defences is a pretty effective one. At the same time the continued existence of persistent infections and epidemics shows that the pathogens, on their side, are fairly resourceful too. So we will now turn to the question of how they manage to keep on 'living with us'.

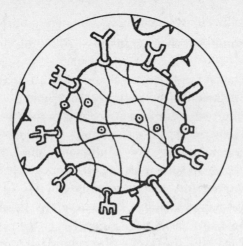

# 6 The pathogens fight back

Cet animal est très méchant,
Quand on l'attaque il se defend.
P.K., *La menagerie*, 1868

This cynical couplet could have been written with pathogens in mind. When attacked they defend themselves – not very *sportif* of them! But a pathogen with an efficient defence mechanism for survival is obviously more likely to cause disease than one without. It may be one of those pathogens that goes on to injure cells directly, or it may set off self-damaging responses by the host. All these properties of the pathogen that increase the chance of disease are often lumped together as *virulence factors*. In the next chapter we shall look at the virulence factors that actually cause damage, but first we shall consider the ones that allow survival.

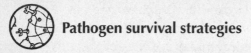 **Pathogen survival strategies**

They are up against pretty powerful opposition. The army/police force of immune mechanisms we have just reviewed – phagocytes, lymphocytes, antibody and the rest – would probably have been capable of keeping higher animals virtually pathogen-free if the pathogens had not evolved ways round them. Clearly they have. Some do it by living outside the body, where they are generally left in peace. But others live – from their point of view – deep in enemy territory, in our tissues, inside our cells, even free in our blood. How do they manage it? Let us put ourselves in the position of a pathogen and see what the options are, taking the immune obstacles cell by cell and molecule by molecule, starting with the innate ('old') system.

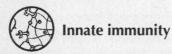 **Innate immunity**

**Defence against phagocytes**

Imagine you are a bacterium, let us say a staphylococcus, and you have found your way into the body – intentionally or not. Within minutes, along come the phagocytes – macrophages or PMNs – ready to engulf and kill you. You are in the position of a cornered criminal with a police posse closing in. What is to be done? (Just ten seconds for a quick break to consider your options.)

\*    \*    \*    \*    \*    \*    \*    \*    \*    \*

For the criminal there are essentially four strategies, with fairly close parallels for the pathogen. You can (1) bring them to a halt (inhibit phagocyte movement); (2) shoot it out (kill the phagocytes);

(3) resist arrest (avoid being engulfed by the phagocyte); (4) go quietly but stay alive (survive by resisting the phagocyte's killing mechanisms). The staphylococcus makes use of all of these.

1.  There are bacterial *toxins* that prevent the movement of phagocytes through the tissues, and even reduce the production of new PMN in the bone marrow.
2.  Other toxins induce the phagocyte to *self-destruct*; in fact the yellowish pus in a boil or abscess consists mostly of dead PMNs.
3.  The most virulent strains of staphylococcus have a sugar coating (official name: 'polysaccharide *capsule*') which covers up the molecules that phagocytes normally recognize. Staphylococci also make a molecule that blocks the attachment of antibody to the phagocyte, thus knocking out both recognition and collaboration.
4.  One of the strongest intracellular killing mechanisms makes use of *hydrogen peroxide* (the same substance as the antiseptic that chemists sell). Virulent staphylococci produce the enzyme *catalase* which destroys this – a chemical neutralization reaction occurring inside the phagocyte. The yellow pigment of *Staph. aureus* is another defence against killing.

Other pathogenic bacteria, fungi, and protozoa employ some or all of these strategies, plus other ingenious tricks such as getting out of the vesicles in which killing occurs and into the cytoplasm of the phagocyte, where any attempt to kill the pathogen would also endanger the phagocyte itself, or preventing the movement of vesicles within the phagocyte (see Fig. 3.1). The exact balance of forces determines whether there is a quick victory for one side or the other, or a long drawn-out battle.

In terms of peaceful coexistence, probably the most successful outcome for the pathogen is number 4: to resist killing and take up long-term residence in the phagocyte – to live, so to speak, in jail, like some privileged aristocrat. Only macrophages are suitable for this, as PMNs are too short-lived. This will result in a *chronic infection*, which may be relatively symptom-free unless the pathogens break out again; some examples are tuberculosis, herpesviruses, the protozoa *Leishmania* and *Toxoplasma*, and the fungus *Cryptococcus*. Here the adaptive immune system can help to turn the tide against the pathogen, because helper T lymphocytes, spotting that there is a pathogen in the macrophage (using the MHC haulage pathway described in the last chapter), can secrete cytokines such as IFNγ and stimulate the macrophage into greater efforts at killing the pathogen, or at least controlling its growth. This is why tuberculosis, *Leishmania*, etc. flare up when T lymphocytes are defective, as they are in HIV infection.

### Defence against complement and interferon

Pathogens have also evolved answers to these molecular challenges. In the case of the *complement* cascade, much the same strategies apply as to phagocytes – bacterial capsules to block recognition, destruction of complement components by enzymes. The protozoan *Leishmania*, as soon as complement molecules have been assembled to induce a leak in its membrane, simply expels the whole assembly, like a punctured tyre spitting out the offending nail and re-sealing itself. Many herpesviruses have learned how to prevent the production of *interferon*, while the hepatitis B virus can block its antiviral pathway.

An extraordinarily subtle device used mainly by viruses is the *decoy molecule.* Some herpesviruses make proteins that *imitate* certain complement molecules, bringing the cascade to a halt. Poxviruses make decoy proteins similar to the receptor on host cells to which interferon binds. These proteins then bind to the interferon molecules and stop them reaching the proper receptor on cells – so, no protective interferon effect (Fig. 6.1)! This is not too serious since the disappearance of smallpox, because cowpox (vaccinia) is well controlled by cytotoxic T lymphocytes, but it illustrates the ingenuity of viruses. The same approach is used against other *cytokines*, as we shall see later.

 ## Adaptive immunity

### Defence against lymphocytes

With lymphocytes, the problem facing pathogens is even more acute. Apart from the cytotoxic T variety, lymphocytes do not get involved in *disposing* of pathogens, leaving that task to the phagocytes of the innate system. But lymphocytes are phenomenally good at *recognizing* anything foreign ('non-self'), thanks to their millions of different shape-detecting receptor molecules. They are the *detectives* of the defence system. And once they have recognized something, they set off dramatic events – clonal proliferation, antibody and cytokine secretion, memory, etc, as we saw in the last two chapters, making disposal by the innate system vastly quicker and more effective. So for the pathogen up against lymphocytes the crucial thing is to avoid being *recognized*.

Here there is another quite helpful analogy. Imagine you are an agent obliged to survive incognito in enemy territory. Once you are

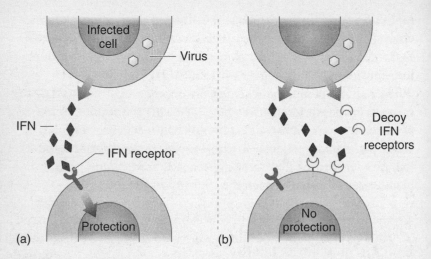

**Fig. 6.1** (a) Normally a virus-infected cell (*top*) releases interferon (IFN) which switches on antiviral protective mechanisms in neighbouring cells (*bottom*). (b) Pox viruses release 'decoy' IFN receptors that bind IFN without triggering protection.

spotted, you are effectively done for, because a spy in jail or shooting off bullets in the street may still be alive but he is no longer much good as a spy. The detectives (lymphocytes) are out there and *they know what you look like*. What to do? As usual, Nature has unerringly identified the various ways to proceed: concealment, mimicry, variation, suppression, and misdirection.

*Concealment*

Obviously, you can stay indoors, becoming an *intracellular parasite*. This is fine, as long as you are not betrayed by someone living in the same block with a habit of going out and passing around your details. Unfortunately for you this is exactly what the MHC haulage pathway does. You might try preventing MHC molecules travelling to the surface (as herpes- and adenoviruses do), but now their absence will itself attract attention (by NK cells). You could emulate the malaria parasite, which hides in liver cells just long enough to multiply up its numbers, then leaves for a different habitat – the red blood cell, which has no MHC. You could come to terms with the police: they know where you are but you promise to keep quiet, as the chickenpox virus does in nerve cells – for many years anyway. Or you might settle down peacefully and give up the thought of occupying enemy territory altogether, like the harmless bacteria on the skin and in the intestine.

A more aggressive approach to concealment is to barricade yourself in, which is essentially what those worms do that survive in *cysts*, in the liver (e.g. *Echinococcus*), or muscle (e.g. *Trichinella*). There may be antibody around, but it doesn't penetrate the thick cyst wall, so the entombed worms are safe, though they have lost their chance to spread to another host – one of the penalties of this form of escape from the immune system.

## Mimicry

It may still be possible to go out if you can persuade the detectives that you are a local inhabitant. You might try dressing in clothes bought locally – like the blood stage of the schistosome worm, which covers its surface in molecules picked up from the blood of its host and ends up completely camouflaged, despite living inside a vein, attached to the wall. A lymphocyte would take it for a large 'self' object. Hidden from the immune system, these centimetre-long worms can survive for up to 30 years.

If you are a good actor you might even try making your own face look a bit more 'local', though this is unlikely to fool a good detective (nor did it when streptococci evolved surface molecules that resembled those on human heart cells; rather than escaping immunity, they trigger off *autoimmunity* against heart muscle, causing rheumatic carditis).

## Variation

A more practical solution than mimicry would be to keep changing your appearance, preventing the detectives from building up a proper *memory* file on you. Each time you go out you will be recognized as a foreigner, but not the *same* foreigner – the one they have been warned about. Applied to pathogens, this is called *antigenic variation*, and it is extremely effective (remember, *antigens* are the molecules which induce antibody and which antibody binds to). Many viruses, bacteria, and protozoa use antigenic variation, and it illustrates the battle between host and pathogen genes in its most dramatic and accelerated form. We will examine two pathogens that illustrate two quite different approaches.

## Influenza

If it were not for antigenic variation, flu would probably be a childhood disease like measles or mumps: catch it once and you are immune for life. But as we know, flu is not like that; you can have it over and over again, each new attack, and each *epidemic* or *pandemic*, being due to a new antigenic variant. As mentioned in Chapter 2, the influenza virus has its genetic material (RNA) in eight separate segments, which can be shuffled between viruses, almost like chromosomes in higher animals with a sexual stage. This RNA codes for the two main proteins exposed on the surface of the virus, haemagglutinin (H) and neuraminidase (N). Each can exist in several forms, numbered 1, 2, 3, etc. The last three major pandemics were caused by the strains H1N1 (1918), H2N2 (1957), and H3N2 (1968), but there are many other possible combinations. A new strain that emerged in China in 1997, H5N1, was mainly restricted to birds and only killed 18 humans; however, it has recently reappeared in 2003 in what may be a more pathogenic form and has travelled to Europe, killing huge numbers of birds and (so far) some 150 humans (see Chapter 10). Each strain can undergo small changes by *mutation*, producing viruses with a slightly different surface appearance. The memory T and B lymphocyte clones built up from the last round of infection will not recognize the new strain as well as they should, so there is only a feeble memory response and we all get flu again. This is referred to as *antigenic drift*. Every decade or so a much more radical change occurs, due to exchange of whole segments of RNA between human and bird viruses, resulting in a totally new flu virus. This is *antigenic shift* and it is what gives rise to epidemics and pandemics, because nobody will have encountered such a virus before (Fig. 6.2). Worst of all, if a pure animal strain mutates to be able to infect humans and to spread between them, this would threaten a major pandemic; this is what probably happened with the 'Spanish flu' after the First World War, and what is feared might happen with the current H5N1 strain. Whether a vaccine is the answer or not is discussed in Chapter 9.

Variation is commoner in RNA than DNA viruses, because DNA can 'self-repair' errors that occur when the virus replicates. The fact that smallpox was a DNA virus and did not show variation was a great help in the success of the vaccine. Other RNA viruses that undergo antigenic variation include *HIV*, which does it extremely rapidly, during the course of disease in a single individual, *polio*, *dengue*, and some of the *common cold* viruses, which have done it so slowly and so long ago that their variants have all become established in the

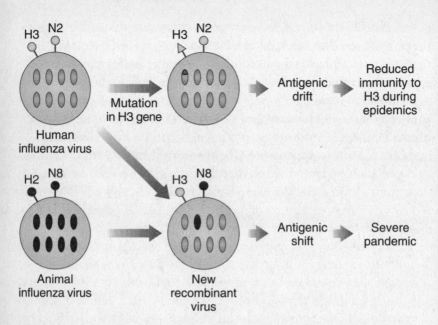

**Fig. 6.2** Antigenic variation by the influenza virus, showing 'drift' (*top*) and 'shift' (*bottom*).

community as different stable *types* of virus. With polio there are only three types, but with the various cold viruses there are hundreds, so each cold you catch is almost certainly different from the last – which is why we never seem to become immune.

*Sleeping sickness*

The African trypanosome, a flagellated protozoan that spends its entire life free in the blood, adopts a quite different approach to antigenic variation. In this case the whole surface is coated with thousands of copies of a single type of molecule, which cannot help inducing antibody since the trypanosome is exposed to lymphocytes in the blood all the time. A few days later, with antibody all over them, the trypanosomes begin to be removed by phagocytes. Then, just in time, a new population appears, with a *completely different* surface coat. A new antibody response starts, with no benefit of memory, and again the surface coat changes – and again and again. If the patient survived that long, the pathogen could keep this up through no less than *a thousand* variants, because it has a thousand different genes in its DNA, each coding for a different surface coat (Fig. 6.3).

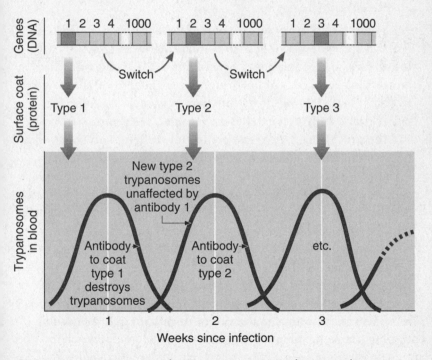

**Fig. 6.3** Antigen variation in African trypanosomiasis (sleeping sickness), showing three waves of antigenically different trypanosomes within the same patient.

It is interesting to compare the strategies of two pathogens that have chosen to live in the inhospitable habitat of the bloodstream – equivalent to an enemy agent standing permanently in the middle of the main street. The *schistosome* worm is slow-growing and non-dividing, so keeping its surface coated with molecules from the blood is not too difficult. For the rapidly dividing *trypanosome* this would be an impossible race against time; much better to have their own changes of coat ready and waiting.

## The vaccine problem

Antigenic variation is a feature of many other infections, including malaria and the bacterial diseases relapsing fever, Lyme disease, brucellosis, and gonorrhoea – where it is the hair-like *pili* which attach the gonococcus to the urethra that undergo variation. Apart from the effect in prolonging infection, antigenic variation is a major problem in trying to design vaccines. A sleeping sickness vaccine containing a thousand completely different antigens would be a commercial nightmare. But with a smaller number of stable variants it is not impossible to make an effective vaccine; the polio vaccine contains all three different antigens, and the vaccine against *Streptococcus pneumoniae* no less than 35 – although this is under half the total possible variants. Surprisingly the vaccine against yellow fever, another RNA virus, has remained effective since 1937, despite changes in the virus. However, with flu, a new vaccine is needed for each epidemic. In the case of viruses like flu and HIV, tremendous efforts are being made to identify parts of their surface molecules that do not show variation and that might be used in vaccines or as the target of drugs.

## Immunosuppression and AIDS

Just as there was the possibility of escaping innate immunity by killing the phagocyte, a pathogen may opt to knock out some part of the adaptive immune system. In a small way this probably happens frequently, because if the immune system of patients with diseases like measles, mumps, or glandular fever is examined carefully, it is found that immune responses to quite unrelated infections are reduced during the illness, and even for some time afterwards. Sometimes this can be of real importance; for example vaccines against meningitis or pneumonia given to people with quite mild *malaria* have been shown to work less well than they should. This is no doubt part of the reason why some diseases that are considered minor in temperate countries (like measles) can be much more serious in the tropics; however, malnutrition is another and even stronger reason for this (see Chapter 8).

All these *immunosuppressive* infections were put in the shade with the arrival on the scene, in 1981, of HIV and the beginning of the AIDS epidemic. HIV is the most immunosuppressive pathogen known. The virus infects mainly macrophages and helper T lymphocytes – the very heart of the immune system – leading to a progressive loss of helper T lymphocyte numbers (see Chapter 5); this results in a series of opportunistic infections – tuberculosis, *Pneumocystis*, cytomegalovirus, toxoplasmosis, *Strongyloides*, to name just a few – that almost invariably kill the patient. The danger level is considered to be 200 helper T lymphocytes per cubic millimetre of blood (the normal level is about 1000). Clearly the virus is doing more than just facilitating its own survival, and it probably makes more sense to think of HIV in humans as an infection so new that it has had no chance to establish any kind of equilibrium.

Indeed some workers claim that it has already started to reduce its virulence. But there are considerable variations on the host side too, ranging from a small population with a mutation in one of the essential receptors for HIV, who are completely resistant, to others whose genetic make-up allows the disease to progress unusually rapidly.

By contrast the chimpanzee virus SIV, from which HIV probably originated by 'jumping species' about 70 years ago, has had tens of thousands of years to 'settle down' in chimpanzees, which tolerate the virus without developing AIDS. You might expect that this is because they mount more vigorous immune responses, but on the contrary they appear to react against SIV-infected T helper cells with a *weaker* cytotoxic T lymphocyte response than humans do against HIV. It is as though the chimps ignore the virus and simply replace their T lymphocytes as they are destroyed. They seem genuinely to be 'living with their germs'. But new data on HIV come out almost every month and I am sure there are many more surprises in store.

Regrettably, a few scientists have argued that AIDS is not caused by HIV at all, but by drugs, malnutrition, and other 'lifestyle' factors. In the face of all the evidence these views could be dismissed as merely eccentric, but for the fact that they have been taken up by politicians, particularly in parts of Africa, as an excuse not to embark on demanding and expensive campaigns of treatment: a recipe for disaster. Current therapy, and the prospects of a vaccine, are discussed in Chapter 9.

*Misdirecting immunity*

To return to some less sensational examples of pathogens interfering with adaptive immunity, let us look at a few cases where immune responses are induced but seem to be the wrong sort. Some bacteria have the curious habit of triggering not just the tiny number of lymphocytes that specifically recognize them but also a substantial proportion of the whole population. Because many clones are switched on this is called 'polyclonal activation', and it can affect either B or T lymphocytes. With B lymphocytes the result is a lot of apparently useless antibody being made, which is probably not too serious, but with T lymphocytes, polyclonal activation by staphylococci or streptococcal molecules called *superantigens* (see Chapter 7) can lead to excessively high levels of cytokines and severe toxic symptoms. The *toxic shock syndrome* (formerly known as 'tampon disease') is one example.


Even less dramatic, but still important, are those situations where the helper T lymphocytes seem to have made the wrong choice in dictating the direction in which the immune response should go – towards antibody production ('humoral') or towards macrophage activation ('cellular'). A classic example is *leprosy*. This bacterial disease can take three different forms. Some patients appear to develop normal immunity and are never ill. Others eliminate the bacilli but in the process become severely scarred, with nerve damage leading to loss of feeling, mainly caused by over-vigorous *cellular* immunity. In a third group the skin is swollen and teeming with bacilli so that they are highly infectious; these patients make a predominantly *antibody* response which, while it fails to eliminate the bacilli, does not damage nerves in the same way. Clearly the second and (especially) third groups have both responded less appropriately than the first. Many other bacterial, protozoal, and worm diseases show this 'spectrum' of response.

## Avoiding natural killer cells

We saw in the previous chapter how NK cells specialize in recognizing and killing cells infected with viruses like herpes that have blocked the normal movement of MHC molecules to the cell surface (which would otherwise expose them to being killed by cytotoxic T lymphocytes). You might think that in this case the score was 2–0 to the host. But yet again the viruses have an answer; they export decoy molecules that look like MHC, giving the NK cells the signal 'don't kill'.

## Avoiding antibody

I have already mentioned the staphylococcal protein that blocks the binding of antibody molecules to phagocytes. The *Neisseria* (gonococcus and meningococcus) produce an enzyme that cuts some antibody molecules (the IgA class) in half, rendering them useless. Some bacteria liberate large enough amounts of their surface antigens to 'mop up' the specific antibodies that would otherwise home in and bind to the bacteria. Once again, the message seems to be: 'you name it, some pathogen has thought of it'.

## Avoiding cytokines

Viruses treat cytokines with the same disdain as they treat complement, by making decoy molecules that imitate the cytokine or its receptor. Once again it is *herpesviruses* that excel in this, and you can begin to see why they are so good at persisting for long periods, and often indefinitely. Perhaps surprisingly, these cytokine-like molecules have no DNA sequences in common with their human equivalent, so they must have been evolved independently. In contrast, *poxviruses* have genes for cytokine receptors (see Fig. 6.1) that are very close to the human equivalents, so they may have been acquired from humans. One useful spin-off of the study of all this molecular mimicry is that it helps us to identify which immune molecules are actually a threat to viruses. One new cytokine was even discovered *after* the viral version.

### Togetherness (again)

We saw how immune cells generally operate best when collaborating, and surprisingly this turns out to be true for some pathogens as well. Large colonies of bacteria, often containing several different species, growing on surfaces such as teeth or surgical implants surround themselves with a sugary coating ('polysaccharide matrix') – a sort of communal capsule, which protects them against immune attack, and unfortunately also against antibiotics. These colonies are called *biofilms* and within them bacteria appear to communicate and to regulate the size of the colony; they call to mind, given a little imagination, the highly organized world of wasps or ants. Keeping down the size of the biofilm is probably the most useful result of a vigorous tooth-brushing.

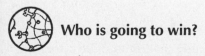 **Who is going to win?**

We have now seen what the two sides – pathogens and the immune system – are capable of in the struggle for survival. Evidently both sides are extremely well endowed. The immune system has at its disposal devices to hit pathogens inside or outside the body's cells; pathogens seem to have devices for evading every one of these (see Table 6.1). It looks almost like a case of the 'irresistible force meeting the immovable object'.

However, from the safety of our War Room, we can envisage three possible outcomes. (1) One side will completely overwhelm and wipe out the other; (2) the battle will go on for ever, with one or

**Table 6.1** The main pathogen escape mechanisms

| Escape/mechanism | Organism/disease |
| --- | --- |
| From phagocytes | |
| Inhibit phagocyte movement | Streps, staphs, gas gangrene |
| Destroy phagocytes | Staphs, streps, *Chlamydia, Entamoeba* |
| Resist phagocytosis | Streps, *Haemophilus, Pneumococcus* |
| Pneumococcus | |
| Resist intracellular killing | Tuberculosis; Toxoplasma |
| Escape into cytoplasm | Leishmania |
| From complement and interferon | |
| Decoy molecules | Pox-, herpesviruses |
| From lymphocytes | |
| Concealment | Intracellular viruses, bacteria, etc. |
| Mimicry | Schistosomes |
| Antigenic variation | Flu, HIV, trypanosomes, malaria |
| Immunosuppression | HIV, measles, malaria |
| Misdirection | Leprosy |
| From antibody | |
| Inactivate antibody molecule | Staphs (IgG), gonococci (IgA) |

both sides suffering continuous damage; (3) a treaty will be drawn up and both sides will agree to live in peace.

Infectious diseases offer examples of all three scenarios.

## Victory and defeat?

A healthy schoolboy catches measles and recovers, becoming immune to reinfection and no longer infectious. He has won his battle against *his* measles virus. But he probably infected someone else while ill, so the population of measles viruses as a whole has not suffered. Still, it is a *personal* victory. He at least does not have to live with the measles virus. But only when the virus population has nowhere to go can we really speak of complete victory, and this has only happened once so far – in the case of smallpox. And *that* would never have happened without the vaccine. Vaccines have certainly tipped the scales in our favour. We may see total victory against measles, mumps, and rubella, and conceivably polio, in the next quarter century – provided the level of vaccination does not drop because of scares, apathy, or ill-informed propaganda. We shall see.

At the opposite extreme, influenza and plague have occasionally come a little closer at times to 'winning', with very efficient transmission and mortality rates during the worst pandemics of 5% and 30%, respectively, but this is still a long way short of total victory. Smallpox had a high mortality (40%) but less efficient transmission. HIV, with an estimated long-term mortality in infected and untreated cases of perhaps 98%, could theoretically come very close, except that it is intrinsically an *avoidable* disease (if it was spread by aerosol, like flu and tuberculosis, that would be another matter). In fact it is highly unlikely that any pathogen will wipe out the entire human race, simply because humans are so different from each other in their patterns of susceptibility and resistance. Even the 'killer' myxomatosis virus, deliberately introduced into Australia to get rid of rabbits, failed to do so and merely selected a more resistant strain of rabbit. There are people who cannot be infected with HIV (see above), and if a cure is never found, their frequency in the population will presumably increase.

## A running battle

A gardener cuts himself while digging and picks up tetanus. His vaccination was over 40 years ago and protection has waned. He ignores the injury and in a week, his respiratory muscles paralysed, he is dead. He has undoubtedly lost his personal battle, but the impact on the tetanus population is negligible, since although *his* bacilli died with him, there are billions more where they came from, in the soil, and always will be. Tetanus is fairly easily avoided, and kills mainly newborn babies in unhygienic conditions, so the total impact on population numbers is not very significant either. So tetanus bacilli and the human race will continue to coexist for the foreseeable future. The same, I am afraid, is true for almost all bacteria – staphs, streps, tubercle bacilli, and the rest.

Or consider malaria. In a tropical village, children are exposed every time the wet season comes round. Some will be unlucky and die in a coma. The rest will just go on getting it, resigning themselves to a level of anaemia, tiredness, occasional bouts of prostrating fever, and perhaps eventually damaged kidneys. From time to time they are infectious to others. There are plenty of mosquitoes about, despite strenuous attempts to get rid of them. Nobody in the village is completely immune, though the adults suffer less serious malaria than the children, suggesting that a degree of immunity can develop with time. However, if they leave the village – perhaps to come to university in Europe – they are likely to get severe malaria on return, showing that their immunity needs constant 'boosting'. There is no effective vaccine yet, and as fast as new drugs appear the malaria parasite becomes resistant. The best protection is still by bed-nets. Clearly neither side is going to win this battle either, although at present malaria seems to have the upper hand. The same could be said of most of the protozoal and worm infections, which for the moment look like continuing to cause their sufferers lifelong misery, and to feature gruesomely in textbooks of pathology.

## Peaceful coexistence

Given all I have said, this would seem the least likely outcome, but it is commoner than one might at first think. Remember that seething mass of bacteria in your intestine, that layer of staphylococci on your skin, those herpesviruses sleeping in your nervous system, even the few tuberculosis bacilli walled up somewhere in your lung – just some of the potential pathogens that are currently doing you no harm. You seem, *for the time being*, to be in control. But this can soon change if you puncture your intestine, burn yourself, or become seriously run down or even just very elderly. Then – watch out for peritonitis, a wound infection, shingles, or a flare-up of TB.

Ironically, the upsurge in *opportunistic* infection by organisms that are only pathogenic in the presence of an inadequate immune system (the subject of a later chapter) has drawn attention to a category of micro-organisms which in normal individuals are evidently held in control without difficulty. *Toxoplasma* is a good example; nearly half of the population have antibodies to this protozoan, but are unaware that they have ever been infected. Remove T lymphocytes and it can become a killer. Obviously toxoplasma and humans *can* live peacefully together. Some more examples of 'normally non-pathogenic pathogens' are listed in Table 2.6, and from them we have learned that you can indeed live permanently with many 'germs' provided your immune system is healthy. Whether their numbers are kept down by a steady rate of killing or by a block on their multiplication (or a bit of both) is not clear at present.

Some pathogens have a different approach to peaceful coexistence. Without causing you any further symptoms after you have 'recovered', they retain the ability to infect others. You are a *carrier*. Two diseases where healthy carriers can be responsible for epidemics are typhoid and hepatitis B. The famous 'Typhoid Mary' was a New York cook who infected hundreds of people and twice had to be imprisoned, because she refused to have her gall bladder removed (this is where the bacilli were lurking) or to give up cooking. Years after recovery from hepatitis B, more than 1 person in 10 still has the virus in their blood (the original hepatitis B vaccine was actually made from the blood of carriers). In this case living with germs is more of a truce than a permanent peace treaty.

So the question 'Who is going to win?' seldom has a clear-cut answer. We *should* manage to get rid of a few virus diseases, and one or two virus diseases *might* come rather near to getting rid of us. However, as far as most viruses and bacteria, and all protozoa, fungi, and worms go, we are going to have to live with the pathogens we have now, plus any new ones that we acquire – for example from animals or from deliberate human mischief. In the last chapter of this book I shall indulge in a little more 'future gazing', but first we need to look more closely at how the existing ones actually earn their title of *pathogens* – in other words, how they make us ill.

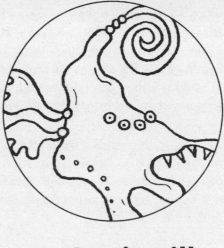

# 7 Getting ill

> Diseases are neither self-subsistent, circumscribed, autonomous organisms, nor entities which have forced their way into the body . . . but the course of physiological phenomena under altered conditions.
>
> Rudolf Virchow

Up to this point the emphasis has been on *pathogens* – what they are like, how we try to combat them, the mechanisms by which they fight back. Not much has been said about *pathology* itself, although when we have an infection this is what we notice. Some people might think of pathology purely in terms of post-mortems and the coroner's inquest, but in reality it covers everything that makes you feel ill. Illness implies *symptoms*, which mean *tissue damage* or at least some loss of normal function somewhere, and that is pathology. A pathogen is by definition a parasite that induces pathology – makes you ill. The question is, how?

The answer is: in all sorts of ways. To begin with, we must look at the very earliest symptoms, as the body realizes something is amiss. Next, assuming that the problem is the arrival of pathogens, we have to distinguish between diseases where the pathogen damages tissues *directly* and those where the damage is done by the *immune system* (the 'friendly fire' scenario). We can then divide the immune group into *innate* and *adaptive*. The adaptive group can be further subdivided into *humoral* and *cellular* damaging mechanisms. And then there is the special situation of *autoimmunity*. So let us have a look at some representative diseases in each of these categories and the pathogen's *virulence factors* that induce them.

 **Inflammation**

Often the first symptom of infection is simply the feeling of being *ill* – a sort of lethargic overall glow. Perhaps you already have a temperature. If so, it is a sign of increased cytokine production, mainly TNFα, IL-1, and IL-6 – an *acute inflammatory response* involving the whole body. Probably this will soon be followed by some clue as to where the trouble is localized – runny nose, sore throat, cough, diarrhoea, painful urination, stiff neck, jaundice. But there are infections where fever is the only sign for weeks on end. If it lasts longer than three weeks without a diagnosis it is known as PUO (pyrexia of unknown origin), and about half such cases are due to infection. I remember as a student looking after a Greek lady who ran a high swinging fever with no localizing signs for over a month. Cultures of sputum, urine, faeces, and blood were negative. She was very beautiful, and students (male) lined up to listen to her chest every day. Finally, the third blood culture showed bacterial

growth; it was a not-quite-typical case of *brucellosis*, to the surprise
of everyone from the consultant down. She was treated with
tetracycline – at home, somewhat to our regret.

Sometimes inflammation is clearly visible from the start. A cut
finger becomes infected – with staphylococci, most likely. In a few
hours it is red, swollen, and painful. These are classic signs that
blood flow to the site has increased, enabling the cells and
molecules of the *immune system* to flood into the area. The
stimulus for this consists of chemical signals from the bacteria as
well as from damaged cells (including *prostaglandins*, the target of
the anti-inflammatory effect of aspirin). If the invaders are wiped
out, inflammation dies down in a matter of days, and even sooner if
you helped with a quick dab of iodine on the wound to kill off most
of the bacteria. But it may also go on to become *chronic*, as we shall
see later in this chapter.

If pathogens have gained entry to the body, the next symptoms may
be entirely due to them.

 **Direct tissue damage**

This is the easiest type of pathology to understand in terms of cause
and effect. There are two main groups of pathogens that damage
cells directly: the *cytopathic* ones (mainly viruses) and the *toxin-
producers* (mainly bacteria).

### Cytopathic infections

In Chapter 2 I described how some viruses can leave the cells they
infect either brutally (by lysis) or delicately (by budding). Here we

are concerned with the brutal kind, which kill their host cell before moving on to infect others. Polio, influenza, hepatitis A, rotavirus, and many of the common cold viruses behave in this way. Killing the cells that line the throat or the intestine may cause discomfort, but it is only a temporary problem since they can quickly regenerate. But neurons in the nervous system cannot, so the damage caused by polio is permanent.

Cytopathic effects are not entirely restricted to viruses; they are also seen with other intracellular organisms such as *Rickettsia*, *Chlamydia*, and mycoplasma. Bacteria that survive in macrophages, such as the tuberculosis bacillus, may cause them to rupture, but macrophages are easily replaced. The malaria parasite destroys a small number of liver cells, followed by a significant number of red blood cells, sufficient to cause quite serious anaemia.

## Toxins

The direct-acting toxins of tetanus, botulism, diphtheria, cholera, staphylococci, and streptococci have already been mentioned in Chapter 2, and a more complete list is given in Table 7.1. Because they are actively secreted by the bacteria, they are called *exotoxins* ('outside toxins') to distinguish them from the *endotoxins* ('inside toxins') built into the wall of some other bacteria, to be discussed later.

Exotoxins are responsible for some of the most acute and dangerous effects of bacterial infection, but it is not always obvious what their usefulness is to the pathogen. With staphylococci and streptococci they are part of the defence against phagocytes; with

**Table 7.1 Some important bacterial exotoxins and their actions**

| Bacterium/disease | Toxin | Action |
|---|---|---|
| Staphylococcus | Leucocidin | Kills phagocytes |
| | Enterotoxin | Causes diarrhoea |
| | 'Toxic shock' toxin | Causes shock |
| Streptococcus | Streptolysin | Kills phagocytes |
| | Streptokinase, hyalase | Help spread through tissues |
| Diphtheria | Protein synthesis inhibitor | Destroys cells in throat, heart |
| Whooping cough | Adenylate cyclase | Prevents bronchial ciliary beating |
| Tetanus | Nerve–muscle stimulation | Spastic paralysis |
| Botulism | Nerve–muscle block | Flaccid paralysis |
| Gas gangrene | Phospholipase | Kills cells in deep wounds |
| Cholera; Escherichia coli | Cell permeability altered | Fluid lost into gut |
| Anthrax | Cytotoxin | Kills phagocytes; damages blood vessels |

cholera, the diarrhoea they cause helps to spread the infection. But the nerve paralysis of tetanus and botulism and the respiratory obstruction of diphtheria seem to be examples of bacterial 'overkill' or perhaps one should say 'unfortunate accident' – tragic for the individual host but of no consequence to long-term host–pathogen relations.

The filamentous fungus *Aspergillus flavus* produces an exotoxin ('aflatoxin') which can contaminate food sources such as grain and ground nuts, and has been incriminated in the development of liver cancer. Another non-bacterial exotoxin is the one used by the protozoan *Entamoeba histolytica* to penetrate the intestinal wall.

**A cytokine storm**

*Endotoxins*, despite their similar-sounding name, act in a quite different way from the exotoxins just described. Bacterial endotoxin (chemical name 'lipopolysaccharide', or LPS) is part of the cell wall of some bacteria and is only released when they die. It can then stimulate an extraordinary range of biological pathways, including the complement and clotting systems and, most significantly, excessive release of the inflammatory cytokines TNFα, IL-1, and IL-6 by macrophages – an over-response by the whole innate immune system. This 'cytokine storm' as it has been dubbed can have drastic effects on blood vessels, leading to a massive drop in blood pressure and the life-threatening condition of *septic shock*, which requires immediate transfer to intensive care. Other bacterial products that behave similarly include lipoarabinomannan of tuberculosis, which may be released during drug treatment of the disease, and the staphylococcal exotoxin TSST-1, trigger of the toxic shock syndrome – although in this case it is T lymphocytes, not macrophages, that are mainly guilty of over-responding. It has recently been found that viruses, too, can trigger excessive cytokine release, and this may be the cause of the sudden worsening in such diseases as flu and SARS.

Attempts to treat these dangerous conditions with drugs or antibodies that inhibit cytokines (e.g. TNF) have had some success, but an antibody against LPS itself failed to block the development of septic shock, causing the share price of the company that made it to collapse spectacularly. The problem was that the *lipid* portion of the lipopolysaccharide does not stimulate antibody, whereas the *polysaccharide* (sugar) portion, which does, is highly variable. So you would need a different antibody for each patient – a hopelessly impractical and uncommercial prospect.

A miniature version of the endotoxin effect used to be experienced following the old typhoid/paratyphoid vaccine, which consisted of killed bacteria with their endotoxin intact. I can remember the feeling, the evening after being vaccinated, of having gone down with something at least as bad as typhoid. Nor was it much consolation to learn afterwards that the vaccine was not regarded as very effective.

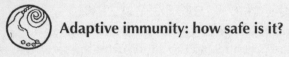 **Adaptive immunity: how safe is it?**

According to the description in Chapter 4 of how lymphocytes are purged of any tendency to react to 'self' antigens, their recognition should be restricted to foreign material, and one would expect the resulting damage to be restricted in the same way. In the majority of cases this is true. Antibodies block toxins and viruses from entering cells. Or they coat viruses, bacteria, etc. which are then disposed of by phagocytes or complement. Cytotoxic T lymphocytes kill virus-infected cells, many of which were probably doomed anyway. It all sounds neat, tidy, and safe.

Unfortunately there are exceptions to the rule, and a lymphocyte response can itself cause damage. So Rudolf Virchow was quite right, in the quotation at the head of this chapter, to say that disease could be due to 'altered physiological phenomena' – which include what we today would call 'immune responses'. Considering that he was writing in the 1880s, when cell function was only just beginning to be understood and almost nothing was known about immunity, his insight was remarkable. Nowadays we refer to all tissue damage caused by an immune response as *immunopathology*, and it can happen in a variety of ways. Some antibodies, having bound to their antigen, trigger off violent inflammation; this is the basis of *allergies*. Sometimes the antibody, bound to its antigen (official name, 'antigen – antibody *complex*') sticks to a blood vessel where the activity of phagocytes and complement is *not* wanted. Sometimes the stimulation of macrophages by T lymphocytes reaches a point where normal tissues are significantly damaged. And most unexpected of all, sometimes B and T lymphocytes *do* react against 'self' antigens. This is called *autoimmunity*, and ever since Ehrlich, immunologists have puzzled over exactly what has gone wrong.

You may be rather shocked to discover how often the unpleasant symptoms of a disease are due to one or other of these immune responses. Many people's reaction is: if this is the case, surely we need *less* immunity, not more? All I can say is that whenever some part of the immune system is defective or damaged, the result is usually more dangerous and sometimes more fatal infection (the following chapter spells this out in more detail). So we have to accept that the strength of our various immune mechanisms is set at the level which Nature has found to give the best overall results, in terms of survival in the face of our major pathogens. Now and then there will be freak situations (worm allergies are one and Ebola fever is another) where a less vigorous immune response probably would be to our advantage, but Ebola is an animal disease with no significant evolutionary impact on the human race as a whole.

*Allergy*

Most allergies are nothing to do with infection. They are inappropriate reactions to pollens, house-dust mites, etc., which would be harmless if they did not trigger off a particular class of antibody (IgE) that binds to inflammatory cells, called *mast cells*, in the skin and elsewhere; these discharge their contents, including *histamine*, as soon as they meet the antigen. The result is hay fever, urticaria, asthma, or even shock, depending on where the inflammation occurs. There is a connection with infection, however, because it is thought that this rather pointless-seeming response may have evolved to help expel *worms* from the intestine. Certainly worm infections are one of the most powerful stimuli for the production of IgE antibodies, which normally make up only a tiny fraction of antibodies in the blood. One striking example of the worm–allergy link was drawn to my attention during that visit to the hydatid-infested villages of northern Kenya. When removing a hydatid cyst, the surgeon had to be extremely careful not to rupture it, because worm antigens, flooding out into a body full of IgE antibodies, can precipitate *anaphylactic shock*, a massive allergic reaction occurring everywhere at once which is frequently fatal.

Recently a more subtle link between infection and allergy has been proposed, namely that exposure to repeated infection in childhood *protects* you against allergies, perhaps by altering the balance of those all-important T helper lymphocytes. According to this *hygiene* theory, allergies are the price we pay for controlling infection too well. But allergy tends to run in families, so there are probably 'allergy genes' involved as well.

While on the subject of allergy I cannot resist mentioning *homoeopathy*, that strange form of treatment lying somewhere between medicine and religion, and supposedly dependent on memory in water molecules. Allergies are among the diseases for which homoeopathic practitioners claim their biggest successes, and the experiments of Jacques Benveniste in 1988 with mast cells seemed, to him at least, to support the idea that pure water could retain the 'image' of an allergic substance shaken up with it and subsequently diluted away to nothing. The English-speaking world poured heavy scorn on the work and some of the French press responded with the traditional charge of Francophobia. This is one of those disputes where neither side is ever likely to yield. Science really needs a new word that means '*impossible to disprove totally but so improbable that almost any other explanation is preferable*'.

## Complex diseases

No pun intended, but the way an *immune complex* (antibody bound to antigen) can end up damaging blood vessels is quite a complicated story. Let us follow the course of an infection with a particularly vicious streptococcus (full title: Group A beta-haemolytic *Streptococcus pyogenes*). This starts with a typical 'strep throat'. Antibodies are made against various streptococcal antigens, and if they bind to the whole bacteria they rapidly cause them to be removed by phagocytes – a large and tasty meal for a PMN or a macrophage. But some streptococcal antigens will be shed as small molecules, and antibodies against these will result in small complexes which are not only removed more slowly but also have an unfortunate tendency to stick to the walls of blood vessels in the kidney, at exactly the place (the *glomerulus*) where waste products are filtered out of the blood into the urine. These complexes still have the ability to bind to phagocytes and complement, so complement and PMNs will go to work with their inflammatory processes in the most vulnerable part of the kidney, damaging the delicate membranes and wrecking normal function. As a result the patient, having recovered from the throat infection, goes down with acute kidney failure. Other infections that have a similar effect include hepatitis B and malaria, the damage occurring in the kidney, the skin, the lung, or the joints, depending on the disease.

It is important to realize that most of what has happened here is perfectly normal. Antibodies *should* bind to antigens, and PMNs and complement *should* respond to the resulting complex. All that has gone wrong is that it is happening in the kidney. Possibly there was simply too much antigen around at one stage of the infection, or perhaps the normal complex-removal pathway – mainly in the liver – was overloaded or not working properly. Sometimes the antigen itself may have a tendency to bind to particular blood vessels. But one cannot help concluding that there is a design fault here somewhere. The problem is not restricted to humans; in fact the mechanism of *immune complex disease* was originally worked out in rabbits, and there are strains of mice that get it spontaneously.

## T lymphocytes and granulomas

Here we shall take tuberculosis as our example. The problem has already been hinted at in earlier chapters. *Mycobacterium tuberculosis*, the tubercle bacillus, is very tough by bacterial standards, with a waxy cell wall that resists many chemicals which would kill other bacteria. It has also developed to a fine art the ability to live inside macrophages – the graveyard of so many other pathogens. But in the presence of a normal population of helper T lymphocytes, the growth of tubercle bacilli can be kept in check by attracting sufficient numbers of macrophages to the site and keeping them in a state of activation by releasing appropriate cytokines – interferon gamma (IFNγ) being the most important of these. In the process an ever-increasing clump of macrophages and lymphocytes accumulates to form a *granuloma*, which eventually becomes surrounded by fibrous tissue laid down by the host, often with the deposition of calcium. The bacteria, though still alive, are effectively walled in, thanks to a protective reaction which is at the same time a *chronic state of inflammation*. These little nodules are often visible on the X-ray of people who have recovered from a primary infection which they may not even have realized they had.

So far, so good. However, in patients whose T lymphocytes are not at full strength – perhaps because of some other disease such as AIDS, or malnutrition, or over-enthusiastic treatment with steroid drugs – the balance may tip in favour of the bacilli. They can break out and set up new foci of infection, either elsewhere in the lung or in distant organs such as bone or kidney. The immune system is now in a real quandary, because if every new focus is turned into a granuloma, substantial areas of normal tissue will be replaced. Destruction of the adrenal glands in this way used to be the main cause of adrenal failure, though nowadays this is more often autoimmune. Large, poorly formed granulomas can break down and form cavities, especially in the lung (this is where the blood on the handkerchief comes from). So too much immunity is almost as bad as too little. The same problem is seen with leprosy, with some fungal infections, and with the eggs of the schistosome worm when they lodge in the liver. Here, too little cellular immune reaction leads to liver damage – because the eggs are designed to destroy tissue as part of the process of getting out into water and into the intermediate snail host – while too much leads to granulomas that block blood flow through the liver. Sometimes the immune system just cannot win. The answer to tuberculosis is good nutrition and good general health, plus good drugs when needed; the answer to schistosomiasis is not to paddle in water containing snails.

I mentioned cytotoxic T lymphocytes as a generally safe way of removing virus-infected cells. But in hepatitis B infection, destruction of liver cells by cytotoxic T lymphocytes is thought to be the main cause of the liver damage. The virus does not itself kill the infected cells, but an over-vigorous immune response can actually kill the patient, whereas when for any reason the immune response is inadequate, the patient can go on carrying and transmitting virus permanently, becoming a *carrier*. So a successful outcome depends on the cytotoxic T cells getting it exactly right. It is thought that the generalized bleeding that is such a frightening feature of Ebola and other haemorrhagic virus infections is mainly due to immune destruction of virus-infected blood vessels, rather than to the virus itself. In fact one case was successfully treated by *suppressing* the immune response – a daring experiment in the true Pasteur tradition.

## Cytokines – again

Most dangerous of all T lymphocyte responses are those to *superantigens*, notably those from staphs and streps. These strange molecules don't obey the general rule of stimulating one T lymphocyte in every 100,000 or so, but instead stimulate as many as 1 in every 5 to release a virtual torrent of cytokines (see 'cytokine storm', above). A lot of research is going into ways to inhibit the effects of superantigens, but also to use them therapeutically – for example in treating tumours. The staphylococcal exotoxin TSST-1, trigger of the *toxic shock syndrome* is the best known superantigen but there are many others. It has recently been found that viruses too can trigger excessive cytokine release, and this may be the cause of the sudden unexpected worsening that can occur in such diseases as flu and SARS. Superantigens are suspected of being involved in many conditions, from food poisoning to asthma, eczema, and diabetes and possibly AIDS.

## Autoimmunity

Paul Ehrlich posed his famous question (*Why does the immune system not attack the body's 'self' antigens?*) on the basis that, as far as he was aware, such a thing never happened. He even coined the term 'Horror autotoxicus' to describe this unthinkable prospect. However, over the next half century it gradually became evident that *sometimes it did*. First a form of anaemia, then a disease of the thyroid, and then one disease after another, were found to be accompanied by *autoantibodies* – antibodies that quite clearly recognized self antigens. Even in some immune complex diseases such as lupus, the antigens turned out to be self molecules. What was going on?

At the time when I became an immunologist, this question was on everyone's lips. In fact it was the challenge that lured me away from more orthodox medicine. It became almost a standing joke at ward rounds that every mysterious symptom was 'autoimmune'. We all had the feeling that some deep secret lay hidden, perhaps in the thymus, which had also burst into prominence just about then, and that some lucky scientist was going to solve it and acquire fame and riches (well, fame anyway; scientists seldom become rich, unless they set up companies and sell out before they collapse).

As discussed towards the end of Chapter 3, there was no single answer – just a series of compromises. The nearest thing to a deep secret was the demonstration by Peter Medawar in 1959 that lymphocytes which met an antigen very early in their existence were deleted – and obviously such antigens are likely to be 'self'. It was the fact that Macfarlane Burnet's clonal selection theory explained this so neatly that helped the theory itself to be accepted. According to Burnet, non-reactivity to 'self' was due to *clonal deletion*, starting in fetal life. A lymphocyte that displayed a receptor for 'self' would simply not be allowed to 'grow up' – which in modern terms means allowed out of the thymus or bone marrow. One could compare the bone marrow and thymus to particularly brutal schools in which youngsters with antisocial tendencies were quietly strangled.

Burnet's theory implied that lymphocytes would have to respond differently to antigen, depending on whether they were 'young' or 'adult'. This seemed far-fetched to a lot of people, but turned out to be quite true. A newly produced lymphocyte is extremely sensitive to elimination if it meets 'its' antigen. Autoantibodies could still be explained, because the B lymphocyte genes that code for antibody molecules might have a high rate of *mutation*. Mutations are random changes in DNA, and a mutation in an antibody molecule could make it better at recognizing some pathogen, but it also could make it recognize 'self' – in other words, become an autoantibody (T cell receptors do not mutate, so the problem doesn't arise). Again, Burnet was right. Antibody genes do mutate. Burnet, like Ehrlich, seems to have had the rare knack of making the correct prediction on the flimsiest of evidence.

You may be wondering what all this rather academic discussion has to do with infection. If, as many scientists used to think (and some still do), the production of self-recognizing T or B lymphocytes is just a glitch in the system, the answer would be: not much. But more and more people, and I include myself, believe that in most cases autoimmunity is actually *caused* by infection. The classic example was the same Group A streptococcus described above in connection with kidney damage. This bacterium has on its surface a protein very similar to one found on human heart muscle. Following repeated strep throats, antibodies are made that bind to both the bacterium *and heart muscle*. Now the heart is treated as a pathogen and attacked. In the days when streptococcal infections were frequent and untreated, *post-streptococcal myocarditis* was the commonest cause of heart valve disease.

Autoimmune myocarditis was for long thought to be an isolated phenomenon. But now that the full structure of most human and microbial molecules is known, a large number of unexpected similarities (official name: 'cross-reactions') have turned up. In the acute neurological disease known as the Guillain–Barré syndrome, autoantibodies occur against molecules on nerve cells which are also found on the bacterium *Campylobacter jejuni* and two herpesviruses, Epstein–Barr virus and cytomegalovirus. And sure enough, the Guillain–Barré syndrome practically always follows infection with one or other of these pathogens. In the liver disease primary biliary cirrhosis antibodies are found against enzymes from the *mitochondria*, which you may remember from Chapter 2 are thought to be the descendants of bacteria that established themselves in eukaryotic cells over a billion years ago. If for some reason the immune system reacts against certain bacteria, there is the risk of damaging mitochondria as well.

Probably these conditions are only the tip of the iceberg. Coeliac disease, diabetes, multiple sclerosis, adrenal autoimmunity, and some forms of arthritis, could all be caused in this way. The problem is by no means solved, however, because it still remains to be explained why only some people respond to these relatively common infections by making autoantibodies. And even when they do, there is often no proof that it is the autoantibodies that cause the disease. In Type I diabetes, for instance, despite the presence of several types of autoantibody, it is T cells that actually destroy the insulin-producing cells in the pancreas – perhaps stimulated by a virus *superantigen* (see above). Like allergies, autoimmunity tends to run in families, so there is probably a large genetic predisposition at work too. I can imagine that one day people identified as carrying particular susceptibility genes will be warned, or even vaccinated, against those micro-organisms most likely to trigger their autoimmunity.

Before leaving the subject of autoimmunity, I should mention a topic that occasionally gets confused with it, namely *autotoxicity*. This was the theory, emanating from the great Metchnikoff in his declining years, that absorption of toxins from bacteria in the colon was responsible for all the ills of old age. As a result thousands of colons were unnecessarily removed during the period around the First World War. Bernard Shaw, always on the lookout for medical absurdities, made great fun of the whole concept in *The Doctor's Dilemma* in the person of the surgeon Cutler Walpole, who makes a fortune removing a totally imaginary organ, the nuciform sac.

## The MHC, choosing a kidney, and choosing a mate

A special form of pathology, which Nature cannot be blamed for not having foreseen, occurs when foreign cells or tissues are deliberately introduced to the body. Obvious examples are blood transfusions and transplants of kidney, heart, and bone marrow – all intended to save life. Unfortunately, a kidney transplant must look, to the immune system, like the arrival of an outrageously large pathogen, to be got rid of as rapidly as possible. Admittedly, the new organ is *human*, but it is not *self*. The T lymphocytes will spot this at once, because of the *MHC molecules*, whose role in molecular haulage I described in Chapter 4. The MHC molecules on the new cells are not just slightly altered (as they would be if the cells contained, say, a virus); they are *completely different*. The purpose of *tissue typing*, which really means MHC typing, is to make this donor–recipient difference as small as possible. But there will always be a difference, except between identical twins, because virtually everybody's set of MHC molecules is unique.

Exactly why this should be has intrigued immunologists for decades. One theory, put forward in the 1970s by Lewis Thomas and Macfarlane Burnet, was that it was to ensure that children did not catch cancer from their grandparents! I think that both these great men are entitled to their one lapse. Today's favoured explanation would be that different MHC molecules handle and transport different pathogens differently. Yours might be just slightly better at handling a particular antigen from flu, mine might be better at plague or the SARS virus. So even a new pathogen that wipes out vast numbers of individuals will come up against someone somewhere who can deal with it. And since MHC genes are inherited from both parents, six from each, you will have a bigger selection if your parents have completely different sets of MHC genes. Increased resistance to infection is probably one element in the *hybrid vigour* observed when breeding mice and racehorses (and sometimes lacking in royal lineages).

There is one other theory, based on evidence that MHC differences play a part in the selection of mating partner – in mice anyway (but also, some claim, in humans). Given the choice, mice will mate with an MHC-different rather than MHC-identical partner. Hybrid vigour again – but how do they know? A clue may be that MHC molecules are excreted in the urine; they certainly appear to be what tracker dogs use in following a single quarry among thousands of others. A fascinating thought . . . do we really choose our partners by *smell*? Perhaps not, after all, since – leaving aside perfumes from a bottle – it is surely skin and gastrointestinal odours that we tend to notice when meeting in normal circumstances, rather than the smell of urine.

 **Visible pathology**

A friend of mine from medical school days, with whom I kept in touch through 40 years of playing together in amateur orchestras, once explained to me his reasons for specializing in dermatology, as follows: his patients seldom died of their disease, but they also seldom recovered rapidly, they never called him at night, and their disease was visible to the naked eye, which usually made diagnosis fairly easy. All four reasons seemed logical, but for the purposes of this book, the last is the interesting one. One look at a measles or chickenpox rash is enough. Of course a skin rash does not always mean infection: many rashes are due to allergy, drugs, or other causes, and even more are *idiopathic* – that useful synonym for 'nobody knows'.

Rashes can be caused by all classes of pathogen (Table 7.2), as well as by skin-burrowing insects or *ectoparasites* ('outside parasites'). Their pathology can be either direct or immune-mediated. To take a few examples: the 'red-on-red' rash of scarlet fever is a direct effect of a streptococcal toxin, while the fluid-filled vesicles of chickenpox and herpes are the result of skin cells being killed by the virus, and the common wart is due to stimulation of skin cell growth by the papilloma virus. On the other hand the rash of measles is due to a T lymphocyte response to virus in the skin, and, as already mentioned, the skin can be affected by immune complex disease, as in the rashes of typhoid and hepatitis B infection. In typhus, dengue, and other 'haemorrhagic' fevers, probably both direct and immune-mediated mechanisms contribute to the rash. A rash in meningococcal meningitis is a danger sign, indicating that bacteria are spreading through the bloodstream. This and other haemorrhagic rashes are due to blood that has leaked into the skin, so that pressure on the lesions does not cause them to blanch as it would if they were merely inflammatory – that is, due to increased blood flow.

### Skin testing

Because they are so visible, inflammatory reactions in the skin can sometimes be used to assess immune status to particular antigens. The *delayed* (Mantoux) reaction for tuberculosis is one example (see Chapter 2) and there are also *immediate* reactions that detect allergies. These mostly employ animal and plant extracts, house

**Table 7.2 Some skin rashes of infectious origin**

| Pathogen/disease | Type of rash/comments |
|---|---|
| Herpes simplex virus types 1, 2 | Vesicles (HSV type 2, mainly genital) |
| Chickenpox | Vesicles; may recur as shingles |
| Measles | Rash due to immune response |
| Rubella | Rash due to immune response |
| Hepatitis B | Rash due to immune response |
| Dengue | Haemorrhagic (non-blanching on pressure) |
| Typhoid | Rash due to immune response |
| Typhus | Haemorrhagic |
| *Meningococcus* | Haemorrhagic |
| *Streptococcus pyogenes* | Toxic (scarlet fever) |
| Syphilis | In secondary stage |
| Leprosy | Pathology depends on type of immunity |
| Anthrax | Black ulcer at site of infection |
| Dermatophyte fungi | Ringworm; athlete's foot |
| *Leishmania* (cutaneous) | Ulceration; some immunity to reinfection |
| Schistosomiasis | Dermatitis follows infection |
| Hookworm | Dermatitis follows infection |
| Onchocerciasis | Skin nodules contain worms |
| Scabies | Mite burrows and lays eggs in skin |

dust etc., but allergy can occur to fungal spores and worm antigens too.

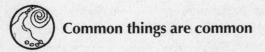 **Common things are common**

To curb our youthful zeal for exotic and improbable diagnoses, our hospital consultants had a saying: 'common things are common;

rarities seldom occur'. Table 7.3 lists some of the more likely causes of common types of infection.

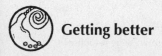 **Getting better**

Recovery from an infectious disease is a question of (1) recognizing and disposing of the pathogen and (2) repairing the damage – to both of which should be added the caveat *if possible*. The previous two chapters have discussed point (1), but point (2) is worth a few comments here, since the extent to which complete recovery is achieved varies considerably from disease to disease. A typical upper respiratory virus infection should recover completely, since the surface cells of the nose, throat, and airways are easily replaced. Skin should also repair itself almost invisibly, but healing a large boil or abscess may require a certain amount of *fibrosis* and leave a visible scar. The same applies to the liver, where the fibrosis is called *cirrhosis* and can, if extensive, impair liver function, although the liver cells themselves can regenerate. However, destruction of neurons in the brain is irreversible, which is why the paralysis of polio is for life.

In the lung, for example after extensive tuberculosis, fibrosis is the best that can be hoped for, but there will inevitably be some loss of lung function. For large cavities it used to be the practice to help the healing process by letting air into the space between the lung and the ribs and deliberately collapsing the lung – the technique of artificial *pneumothorax*. In streptococcal pneumonia, on the other hand, there is no destruction of lung tissue, only fluid and cellular congestion, and once that has cleared up, recovery should be complete.

**Table 7.3 Common infections and their likely causes**

| Colds and sore throats | Bronchitis and pneumonia | Ear infection | Eye infection | Meningitis and encephalitis | Gastroenteritis | Urinary infection |
| --- | --- | --- | --- | --- | --- | --- |
| Rhinovirus | Influenza; parainfluenza | Mumps virus | Adenovirus | Herpes simplex virus | Rotavirus, Norwalk virus | Escherichia coli |
| Coronavirus | Respiratory syncytial virus (RSV) | RSV | Measles virus | Chickenpox virus | Salmonella | Proteus |
| Adenovirus | Measles virus | Streptococcus pneumoniae | S. pneumoniae | Measles virus | Shigella; E. coli | Staphylococcus |
| Echovirus | Adenovirus; rhinovirus | | Trachoma* | HIV | Cholera* | Sexually transmitted |
| Coxsackie virus | S. pneumoniae | | Toxoplasma* | Polio virus* | Campylobacter | |
| Epstein–Barr virus | Bordetella pertussis (whooping cough) | | Onchocerca* | Rabies virus | Helicobacter | HSV types 1, 2 |
| Influenza virus | Haemophilus influenzae | | | West Nile virus | Entamoeba histolytica* | HIV |
| Streptococcus pyogenes | Staphylococcus aureus | | | Tuberculosis | Giardia | Hepatitis B |
| Haemophilus | Tuberculosis | | | Haemophilus | Cryptosporidium** | Genital warts |
| Diphtheria* | Legionella | | | Meningococcus | Strongyloides** | Gonococcus |
| | Pseudomonas** | | | Malaria* | (Food poisoning) | Syphilis* |
| | | | | Toxoplasma** | S. aureus | Candida |
| | | | | Trypanosomiasis** | Bacillus cereus | Trichomonas |
| | | | | | | Chlamydia |

Finally, a brief reminder that *feeling* better does not necessarily mean that the infection has been eliminated. Long-term pathogen persistence without symptoms is a feature of herpesviruses, tuberculosis, syphilis, and some forms of malaria. Typhoid and hepatitis B can lead to a *carrier* state – healthy but still infectious – while in brucellosis and relapsing fever, periods of apparently normal health alternate with fever and obvious illness. And of course all these patterns of recovery can be thrown out if the immune system itself is not working properly, as the next chapter illustrates.

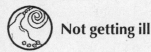 Not getting ill

The germ theory linking microbes to disease was summed up in Robert Koch's famous 'postulates' of 1891 as follows: (1) the organism should be found in all cases of the disease; (2) the organism should be grown in culture; (3) it should reproduce the disease when introduced to a healthy animal; (4) it should be recoverable from this second host. The first disease he worked on, anthrax, illustrated these principles perfectly. But one of the earliest objections to this theory was that not everyone exposed to a known pathogen got the same symptoms – or indeed any symptoms. One of Koch's sceptical colleagues, a Dr Von Pettenkofer, drank a vial of cholera bacilli and remained healthy, proving to his own satisfaction that the bacilli alone were not the whole cause of cholera. He was very lucky, and I can only assume that either the bacilli were mostly dead or dying or his gastric acidity was very high that day (it takes about 10 000 000 000 organisms to cause cholera with a normal gastric acidity, but only 10 000 if the acid is neutralized). However, a similar phenomenon occurs with almost all infections. I remember being the only boy at my boarding school not to get measles during an epidemic – not counting those who had had it previously (this was in the days before the vaccine). I still haven't had it. Why not?

Lack of sufficient exposure is an unlikely explanation, as infection is via airborne droplets and I certainly carried on breathing throughout the epidemic! I could have had a rare *subclinical* infection with no rash, passed off as a cold and leaving me immune. Or I might, by great fortune, have had just the right MHC and T lymphocyte receptor molecules to mount ultra-rapid antibody and cytotoxic T lymphocyte responses to measles. I doubt if my cells lack the receptor for the measles virus (CD46) – at least I hope not, because that molecule is also involved in regulating the complement system. Supporters of holistic medicine might say that I had an unusually 'positive' attitude, but from what I can recall of my pre-teenage self this sounds most improbable. In any case I had a bad attack of another virus infection, chickenpox, the following year and I have always had my share of colds and flu. So, like Dr Petternkofer, I was probably just lucky. Had the epidemic been of EBV, flu, tuberculosis, or even plague, not getting ill would be less remarkable since there is a considerable chance of a symptomless infection, while with poliovirus or the meningococcus, disease with serious symptoms is restricted to a minority of those infected, for reasons that are not clear. One possibility would be that they have an undetected, possibly transient, immune defect (see next chapter). So although there is much that is not understood about the development of pathology during infection, nothing has happened since Koch's day to question his fundamental insight that each disease had its own microbe. In those postulates he was careful *not* to say that the microbe in question must always induce the disease in everyone, regardless of any other factors. The seed was essential but it still needed the right soil. Koch, a meticulous and rather obsessive personality, emphasized the 'seed' while his opponents put more emphasis on the 'soil'. Science often benefits from personality differences like this, as long as there is some degree of truth on both sides – as in this case there was.

 ## Infectious – or not?

Knowing what we do now, it is quite hard to imagine medicine before Koch. Even when it was accepted that microbes (that is, bacteria) existed, that they caused decay, and that they could be found in diseased bodies, most doctors continued to believe that they did not actually cause disease, and certainly not in a one-to-one fashion. The pattern of a disease, even an obviously contagious one, was felt to be entirely determined by the patient, not the contagion – the latter being generally visualized as a vague miasma that brought out whatever disease the patient was prone to. Even the great Virchow never fully accepted Koch's ideas. But before we smile at such ignorance, we should remember that there are a number of important diseases today about which we are still uncertain whether they are infectious or not. In sarcoidosis and Crohn's disease there are granulomas reminiscent of tuberculosis. Are they due to some as-yet unidentified mycobacterium? Many arthritic conditions have been vaguely linked to viruses, mycoplasma, and bacteria, again without definite proof. I have mentioned the possibility that autoimmune diseases such as diabetes might be triggered by infection. These and a long list of other diseases have been found to be slightly commoner in people with certain MHC types, and given the 'haulage' role of MHC molecules in T lymphocyte responses (described in Chapters 4 and 5), this has aroused suspicion that a pathogen is involved somewhere. And after all, not so long ago, the idea that gastric ulcers and Creutzfeldt–Jakob disease might have an infectious cause was unheard of. So the story of infection and disease has by no means reached its end, though thanks to Koch and his followers I would imagine we are about three-quarters of the way there.

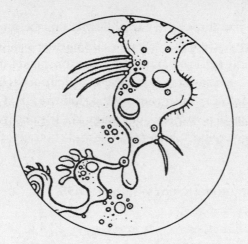

# 8  Immunodeficiency

Like a toothless clawless tiger,
Like an organ-grinder's bear.
Like a knight without his armor,
Like Samson without his hair.
  My defenses are down –
  I might as well surrender
  for the battle can't be won . . .
Irving Berlin, *Annie Get Your Gun*, 1946

If there were people who had never thought much about
immunodeficiency, or indeed about immunity at all, the AIDS
epidemic must have opened their eyes. For immunologists, it was a
nightmare come true. Here as we watched, fascinated and horrified,
was the proof of all the things we had been teaching our rather
bored students for years – that you needed T lymphocytes to control

tuberculosis, that there were parasites that only became pathogenic when immunity failed, that one animal's harmless parasite could be another's deadly pathogen, that one infection could influence another, that vaccines were not always straightforward to make. It was all true! In the quarter century that followed, HIV has become more notorious than any previous plague. T lymphocyte levels are monitored as closely as blood pressure and cholesterol.

 **Immunodeficiency before AIDS**

Even before 1981, however, there was quite a lot to say about immunodeficiency. Odd cases had already made history. In 1952 a US Army doctor, Colonel Ogden Bruton, using the brand-new technique of measuring proteins in serum, had shown that a boy who was suffering repeated attacks of pneumonia lacked the fraction which normally contained antibodies. And in 1965 a New York paediatrician, Angelo Di George, had found that babies who had developed fatal cowpox after the normally harmless vaccine had completely absent thymuses. With the widespread use of drugs to suppress chronic inflammatory diseases, cancer, and the rejection of kidney grafts, new infections started to appear – including most of those later to become everyday names because of AIDS. As immunological screening tests became standardized and available in every hospital, it was realized that quite a number of people had some immunological defect or other (about 3 per 100 000 in the UK, or up to 20 times that number if abnormal tests with no obvious clinical effect were included). In tropical countries, especially where malnutrition was rife, whole populations were discovered to be immunologically below par. In specialist departments, sophisticated treatments were devised to keep babies alive who would certainly have died in earlier times. There were the usual indignant protests about 'disturbing the balance of Nature' – as if that was not what doctors had been trying to do ever since Hippocrates.

Just as problems with your car can be due to errors built in at the factory or to your own mistakes – driving into a tree or forgetting to fill up with oil – immunodeficiency can be due to a *genetic* predisposition ('primary') or to *external* factors ('secondary').

 **Immunodeficiency in the genes**

Primary immune defects are mostly single recessive mutations in some gene that affects the development of an immune component. An example would be the absence of one of the complement proteins or one of the enzymes in the phagocyte (*recessive* means that the defect will not show up if there is also a normal copy of the same gene is also present; a mutation is a change in the DNA). Such a mutation would not be *inherited* unless it occurred in the *germ-line* – that is, an ovum or sperm cell destined to form an individual of the next generation (note: no connection whatever with the *germs* of this book's title). A mutation in any other cell is called *somatic*; it only lasts for the lifetime of the individual and has no evolutionary effect.

For genes in the germ-line, two inheritance patterns are possible: *X-linked* and *autosomal*. An X-linked mutation is one lying on the X chromosome (the one that females have two of and males only one). This gives the interesting result that females are generally not affected by the mutation, because they will almost certainly have a normal gene on their other X chromosome, but they are *carriers* of the gene and can pass it to half their children (on average, half will get the mutated chromosome and half the normal one). Males carrying the mutation, on the other hand, will show the disease effect, not having a normal X chromosome to compensate for it. However, *their* children, whether boys or girls, will get a normal X chromosome from their mother, and will be unaffected, except in the rare cases where an affected male marries a carrier female. So the normal inheritance pattern is: *mother to son* – exactly the same as for red-green colour blindness, or the clotting disease *haemophilia*, which Queen Victoria, a carrier, donated to 13 male members of the royal families of Europe through her numerous offspring. A daughter will be affected only if her father is affected and her mother is a carrier – a fairly rare event.

I stressed this rather confusing bit of genetics because in fact several of the primary immune defects *are* X-linked, which means that the bit of the X chromosome which is different from the Y chromosome (parts of it are the same) must carry several genes important for proper development of the immune system. By the same token, females will lack any genes that are unique to the Y chromosome. This may explain the small but definite difference in certain immune responses between the sexes – although the sex hormones play a part in this too. Autosomal mutations (that is, not on the X or Y chromosome) will affect both sexes, but only if they are *dominant* or if both parents carry them, and even then not all children will be affected.

Primary immunodeficiencies are likely to show up quite early in life, with repeated infections, unusual infections, or perhaps a failure to respond to vaccination. Let us look at some of them, system by system.

## External defences

There are undoubtedly person-to-person differences in the antibacterial secretions of the skin, lungs, and other body surfaces, but it has been difficult to pin them down. They can be trivial, or really serious, as in those unfortunate victims of repeated skin infections whose only hope is almost continuous antibiotic treatment. Better understood is *cystic fibrosis*, where there is a fault affecting the mechanism for washing particles out of the air passages in the lung. A single gene is responsible, and mutations are quite common; however, since they are recessive, a defective gene from both parents is needed to cause the disease. Cystic fibrosis is one of the top candidates for genetic testing and possible gene replacement therapy.

Antiviral defences evidently vary too, since some people are constantly getting colds and others never do, even though they probably all consider themselves normal. It would be very interesting, but very expensive, to investigate the reason for these minor differences. Some of them, of course, may be due to lifestyle, diet, etc., in which case they would count as *secondary*.

## Innate immunity

Here we are on surer ground. In the *complement* system, practically every component can be absent or reduced in level. A lot can be learned about the real importance of each component by following affected individuals. Surprisingly, the five components responsible for punching holes in bacteria ('lysis') seem only to be important in infections by *Neisseria* (gonorrhoea and meningitis); this tells us that for all other bacteria, phagocytosis is a more important disposal mechanism than lysis. Defects of other components lead to problems with *immune complex* disease, and yet another causes an unpleasant condition called *hereditary angioedema*, with recurrent swelling of the larynx and difficulty in breathing. In this case the complement cascade is *over*active, the defect being in one of the natural inhibitors by which it is regulated. The gene is autosomal but *dominant* – which is why the disease is hereditary.

*Phagocytes* are also susceptible to a number of defects. They may fail to 'home in' on inflammatory sites – the aptly named *lazy leucocyte* syndrome. They may lack the receptors that normally attach them to blood vessel walls as a preliminary to leaving the circulation. Or they may lack one or other of the killing molecules stored in their internal granules. One enzyme has dramatic effects, being subject to several mutations that block the killing pathway based on hydrogen peroxide formation. The result is that bacteria such as staphylococci and fungi such as *Aspergillus* grow unchecked, leading to abscesses. T lymphocytes are called in and granulomas form, which is how the disease came to be named *chronic granulomatous disease* (CGD). Sometimes the phagocytes are normal but there are not enough of them. In the disease *cyclic neutropaenia*, the numbers of PMNs in the blood fluctuate periodically, with recurrent skin and throat infections. However, the majority of neutropaenias are secondary (see below).

Primary *cytokine* defects are beginning to be detected, particularly among the interferons. These are not always as serious as might be

expected, because so many different cytokines have approximately
the same activities. In other words there is an excess *redundancy* in
the system – rather in the way that a message with some words
missing can still more or less make sense. Nevertheless, studies of
people with different susceptibilities to diseases such as
tuberculosis and malaria have shown a link with slightly different
versions of the same cytokine gene, particularly IFNγ and TNFα.
It might be tempting to label the more susceptible individuals
'immunodeficient', but it also might turn out that the same gene
actually confers resistance to some other disease – on the principle
that you can't always have the best of both sides. This would tend to
keep the two different versions of the gene in the population, an
example of balanced polymorphism (like sickle-cell disease). As
genetic analysis becomes simpler, faster, and cheaper, enormous
amounts of data on genes and disease susceptibility are going to
accumulate for the statisticians and epidemiologists to get to work
on.

## Adaptive immunity

Lymphocytes have a very complicated development, being
generated from *stem cells* in the bone marrow via (if they are to
become T lymphocytes) the *thymus*, undergoing various genetic
rearrangements to produce their *receptors*, roving the body to meet
their *antigens*, and, finally, proliferating into clones, with secretion
of antibody or cytokines, which turns them into useful elements in
defence. Practically every step in this long pathway can be defective.
We will start at the beginning.

A number of general defects can hit lymphocytes as well as other
cells. There may be a total stem cell failure in the bone marrow, with

no production of any blood cells, which would rapidly be fatal. Defects in DNA repair and cell movement will impair both B and T lymphocyte function. Defects in the enzymes that break down *purines* allow the build-up of molecules toxic to lymphocytes – another candidate for gene replacement. Absence of the receptor for a key cytokine (IL-2) prevents lymphocyte development (this is one of the X-linked conditions). The last two defects cause a similar overall picture and are referred to as *severe combined immune deficiency*, or SCID – one of the diseases for which gene therapy is under trial.

Defects occurring later along the development pathway affect T and B lymphocytes separately. Absence of the thymus (Di George syndrome) completely prevents T lymphocytes developing. The *parathyroid* glands, which arise close to the thymus in the embryo, are also absent. The parathyroids regulate calcium levels, and affected babies usually present with *tetany*, due to low blood calcium (not to be confused with the bacterial disease tetanus). Because of the missing T lymphocytes, they are vulnerable to intracellular infections, and several have died from the normally well-controlled cowpox and BCG vaccines. If they catch measles, instead of getting a skin rash, they die of disseminated disease. This proves two things: recovery from measles depends on T lymphocytes but *so does the rash*. One obvious possible treatment, which has had some success, is a graft of normal thymus.

The B lymphocyte equivalent is Bruton's disease, in which there are no B lymphocytes and therefore no antibodies. Antibodies reside in the serum fraction known as gammaglobulins, so an alternative name for this disease is *agammaglobulinaemia* ('no gammaglobulins in blood'). This is another X-linked disease, and results in repeated extracellular infections, particularly pneumonia. A commoner and less severe form gives rise to *hypogammaglobulinaemia* ('not enough gammaglobulins in blood'). Even milder antibody defects consist merely of the temporary lack of one *class* of antibodies, IgA being the most affected. Strangely enough, this often passes quite unnoticed. In other cases there are raised levels of IgM or IgE, suggesting a malfunction of the mechanism by which B lymphocytes switch production from one class to another. All in all there are probably hundreds of minor primary defects, many of which remain to be identified.

### Treating primary immunodeficiency

Fortunately there is a simple treatment for antibody deficiencies: injection of gammaglobulins from normal donors once a month, which keeps the patients healthy. This, incidentally, is reassuring proof that normal people have protective levels of antibody against common infections. Otherwise the day-to-day requirement for an immunodeficient individual is that infections be treated as they occur – generally a question of antibiotics. But sooner or later the issue of *replacement therapy* will arise. Is it possible to replace the missing cell or the abnormal gene? Sometimes it is. Severe combined immunodeficiency (SCID) has been successfully treated by transfusions of normal bone marrow, which should in theory be able to restore normal lymphocyte production, though there may be complications due to MHC mismatch unless the donor is an identical twin. A more recent idea is to replace the abnormal gene, which is technically possible but also has its dangers. Bone marrow cells will find their own way to where they are needed, but an inserted gene may not end up in its normal site and may have unforeseen effects on other genes. Nevertheless this approach, too, has been successful in cystic fibrosis and in some cases of SCID.

 **Immunodeficiency from the environment**

You are probably getting tired of being reminded that HIV is about the worst cause of immunodeficiency imaginable – equivalent in motorway terms, it has been said, to a massive fatal crash occurring in agonizingly slow motion. The *opportunistic* infections that eventually carry off the patient are listed in Table 2.6. So I will say no more about AIDS for the moment, and instead concentrate on the many other causes of secondary (acquired) defects. Unlike the primary defects, these often affect more than one system, so we will take them cause by cause, pointing out where the defect lies, if this is known.

### Malnutrition and dietary supplements

For an immune response to occur, cells must divide and molecules by synthesized. This requires considerable metabolic energy, so immunity suffers when food intake falls below a certain level. Both total calories and protein are important. Antibody production is generally the first to decline, followed by T lymphocytes, complement, and phagocyte function. Pneumonia, ear infections, and diarrhoea from a variety of pathogens become rampant, leading to appalling infant mortality – a million a year from measles pneumonia alone. Occasionally a disease is found to be *less* severe in the malnourished. I remember, in the 1960s at a WHO workshop, hearing an elderly survivor of the Siege of Leningrad (as it then was) in the Second World War, tell us that the incidence of many bacterial infections actually fell during the siege. His slides were in Russian and his talk made little impression at the time, but his results are all that I recall from that particular meeting.

One element with a special influence on immunity is *iron*. Iron is required by the immune system for many of its microbe-killing pathways. On the other hand, bacteria, fungi, and protozoa also require iron for their own growth. As they are parasites, it must come from the host. So there is competition for the available iron, with a tug of war between host and microbial iron-binding molecules. Both iron deficiency (from inadequate diet or blood loss) and iron overload (as in the disease *haemochromatosis*) can impair immune function. An exception to this rule is malaria, where a degree of iron deficiency can reduce infection by slowing the growth of the parasite in red cells, while in sickle-cell anaemia the abnormal haemoglobin S also confers partial resistance.

Zinc, selenium, and some vitamins (A, B, C, and E) are also thought to be necessary ingredients for normal immune function, and a visit to any chemist will suggest that the pharmaceutical industry would like us to believe there are many others. Our cat pellets, the label assures us, contain 'a higher level of vitamin E for a healthy immune system'. Perhaps so, but when dispensing them I always wonder what scientific experiment supports this claim. Of course it would be rash to say there are not genuinely beneficial immunostimulants yet to be discovered, but the evidence will need to be more than just anecdotal. It always amazes me that people who take a pill and feel better automatically put it down to an effect on their immune system. In some cases it may be, and it is good to see detailed immunological studies being published, in reputable journals, on the plants, mushrooms etc. of traditional – especially Oriental – medicine. But let us for a moment imagine that a new 'wonder' immunostimulant does appear on the shelves. We will call it Mongolian Morning Mulberry – MMM for short. According to the blurb, *MMM stimulates phagocytes, T lymphocytes, and antibody, raising immune defences to heights you never dreamed of before. Mmm! You will never have felt so get-up-and-go* . . . etc., etc.

Would MMM really be such a blessing? Not necessarily. Permanently stimulated phagocytes would release inflammatory cytokines to the point where you would feel you were going down with flu all the time. Increased levels of antibody would increase the danger of immune complex disease and autoimmunity. Overactive T lymphocytes would create granulomas at every infected site. There could be side effects, not tested for, outside the immune system. A year ago, a drug designed to stimulate a special population of T lymphocytes has made six volunteers to its first clinical trial dangerously ill. And one should remember that the 'normal' immune system is already being stimulated by the viruses, bacteria etc. that bombard us all the time. In other words, the immune system, in most people most of the time, is set at about the right balance between immunodeficiency on the one hand and immunopathology on the other. Deliberate immunostimulation ought really to be kept for those individuals shown to have some detectable immune defect, however minor. So the trend, I hope, will be towards cheaper and more sensitive outpatient tests for immune functions, both innate and adaptive.

## Infection

Plenty of pathogens besides HIV cause immunosuppression, presumably as part of their own survival strategy, and, as would be expected, they tend to be long-term ('chronic') infections. I have already mentioned the herpesviruses and malaria. In the case of viruses, quite often they infect cells of the immune system itself – either T lymphocytes (HIV, measles, EBV, adenoviruses) or macrophages (HIV, CMV, rubella) – or they disrupt the cytokine signalling system. Since cytokines are not antigen-specific, interfering with their function can protect other pathogens from destruction too. For example immunosuppression following a normal attack of measles can cause a flare-up of previously dormant TB.

Immunosuppression by chronic malaria has been shown to have two far-reaching effects: it reduces the response to the quite unrelated pneumococcal and meningococcal vaccines, and it impairs the immune control of EBV, contributing to the development of *Burkitt's lymphoma*, a tumour of B lymphocytes common in areas where malaria is endemic. In fact the precise correlation on the map of Africa between malaria and the tumour led Denis Burkitt in 1961 to suggest that the causative agent (it was not yet known to be a virus) was spread by the same mosquito as malaria – a very reasonable hypothesis, but wrong as it turned out. Burkitt, a tireless traveller and observer, also established the very important link between colon cancer and low dietary roughage, so I think he is entitled to his one minor mistake. Burkitt's lymphoma also occurs in patients on immunosuppressive drugs (see below).

### Trauma

Burns, blood loss, septic shock, even major surgery, are often followed by a greatly increased susceptibility to infection. This seems odd, since these are just the times when infection is most likely. Probably what happens is that after the violent inflammatory response to the initial injury, compensatory mechanisms are switched on to damp it down, so that the patient is actually immunosuppressed for a few days. The inhibitory cytokines IL-10 and TGFβ seem to be mainly responsible, showing how the cytokine network is involved in *regulation* and not just stimulation of immunity.

A special situation is removal of the *spleen*, usually carried out because of accidental rupture or for certain blood diseases. Surprisingly, for such a large organ, life without a spleen is perfectly normal, except for difficulty in dealing with certain bloodstream infections with bacteria or protozoa – including one, *Babesia*, which normally infects only dogs and cattle. The spleen has two roles here: production of antibody and removal of antibody-coated material from the blood. At one time there was a theory that removing the appendix would impair immunity, but the evidence was never convincing, I am glad to say.

### Tumours and drugs

All blood cells come ultimately from the bone marrow, so their production can be crowded out by tumours of the bone marrow

such as leukaemia. Unfortunately, most of the drugs that kill
tumour cells also damage normal bone marrow, the worst hit cells
being those with the shortest lifespan – the PMNs. X-irradiation
has the same effect unless sufficient bone marrow is shielded.
Cortisone and similar drugs that are used to suppress inflammatory
diseases (arthritis, etc.), and the drugs used to prevent rejection of
grafts (e.g. kidney), will also suppress useful immunity unless great
care is taken with the dose. By a strange coincidence the fungal
product *cyclosporin*, extracted from a parasite of insects and under
investigation as a possible antibiotic for human use, turned out to
be strongly immunosuppressive. This ruled it out as an antibiotic
but led to its introduction in 1976 as one of the safest
immunosuppressive drugs known. It blocks the effect of the
important cytokine IL-2, though why an insect fungus should
inhibit human IL-2 is not obvious.

## Other diseases

Immunodeficiency is a frequent complication of kidney failure and
especially the condition called *nephrosis*, in which large amounts of
protein are lost in the urine. Antibodies and complement
components are proteins, so they are lost too. Diabetes is another
disease in which infections are common; here the problem is mainly
with the killing of bacteria by PMNs, which are weakened by the
two biochemical consequences of diabetes: too much sugar in the
blood and too little insulin.

## Stress

The relation between immunity and *mental state* has been the
subject of much debate. Infections are unquestionably commoner

at times of 'inescapable stress' such as bereavement and depression, when measurable decreases in T lymphocyte numbers and responses can be detected. Sitting exams is said to have the same effect, and evidence is beginning to accumulate that prolonged space travel may also lead to immunosuppression (the stressful isolation, radiation, and lack of gravity have all been blamed). Respiratory viruses seem to be the most affected. Raised levels of steroid hormones such as cortisone may partly explain this, but there is probably more than that to the mind – immunity association. Brain cells and lymphocytes respond to many of the same chemical stimuli, including both hormones and cytokines. Allergic skin reactions have been convincingly shown to be inhibited under hypnosis, mainly through an effect on small blood vessels, and the same mechanism may explain the occasional apparent cure of warts. It all seems to point, however hazily, at something interesting.

It has been traditional at international immunology congresses to devote one session to the whole field of *psychoneuroimmunology*, and I always used to go along out of interest. It was extraordinary to see the passions aroused – from furious rejection of the whole concept to an almost mystical belief in the immunological benefit of 'positive thinking' and even in the eventual prospect of total control of immune responses by the mind.

Time, I suppose, will tell who is nearest to the truth, but as with homoeopathy, it will be very hard to convince the sceptics. It is difficult enough to prove the beneficial effect of a new drug – let us say an antiviral claimed to reduce the frequency of colds. You would need a large group of people treated with the drug and another 'control' group given a dummy ('placebo') treatment, ideally without they or you knowing who had which treatment until the trial was over ('double-blind'). One cannot predict with certainty the arrival of a cold, so the trial would have to last long enough for the expected number of colds in both groups, *on average*, to be the same. Now imagine a similar trial where instead of a precise dose of a chemically pure drug, the therapeutic agent being tested is 'positive thinking'. The problems would be almost insuperable. Are two people's positive thoughts equally strong? Is it possible (or ethical) to persuade the control group to maintain 'negative' thoughts? How could patients possibly not know which group they were in? I am afraid that neither the enthusiasts nor the sceptics are likely to change their minds on this in the near future.

The lack of scientific proof does not mean, of course, that a treatment is not worth trying. All doctors are aware of the placebo effect – significant benefit from a sugar pill that the patient believes to be a potent drug. Many patients claim to have been helped by psychoanalysts, 'healers', mediums, witch doctors, and so on, although I don't think any scientific evidence has ever been produced in their favour. So I would be the last to pour cold water on positive thinking, provided it is not relied on to the exclusion of statistically validated standard treatments such as vaccines and antibiotics, as described in the next chapter. The real human benefits of the germ theory, as it struggled into existence with Pasteur and Koch and the rest just over a century ago, were not just in the diagnosis and understanding of disease but in providing a scientific basis for its *prevention* and *cure*.

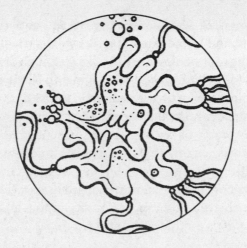

# 9 Controlling pathogens

Medicine has never before produced any single improvement
of such utility. You have erased from the calendar of human
affliction one of the greatest . . . Future nations will know by
history only that the loathsome small-pox has existed and by
you been extirpated.

Thomas Jefferson, letter to Edward Jenner

We are the only animals that have consciously interfered with the
balance between ourselves and our pathogens. Admittedly there are
reports of chimpanzees eating the right parts of the right plants to
get rid of their worm infections, but that is a far cry from draining
swamps, building hospitals, designing vaccines, and synthesizing
antibiotics. Nowadays, even when a totally new infectious disease
appears, the experience and the techniques are in place to identify
the pathogen and work out how best to control it – drugs, a vaccine,

or simple public health measures. This may of course take time, but our overall success can be measured by human life expectancy – in the developed world, more than twice what it was a century and a half ago, when infectious disease accounted for about half of all deaths (the figure now is about 5%). In this chapter we will look at how this has been achieved.

 **Public health**

Some diseases are so clearly contagious that it was always obvious that they were spread from person to person by something, though what that *something* was had to wait until the micro-organisms already glimpsed in the microscopes of Robert Hooke (1664) and Anton van Leeuwenhoek (1684) were definitively linked to disease by Robert Koch in 1876. It seems surprising to us that it took so long, but the notion that disease came straight from God had a grip that took a lot of loosening, and even when 'germs' were recognized as occurring in diseased tissue, it was assumed that they arose by spontaneous generation, despite lone voices of dissent such as Lazzaro Spallanzani (1763) and Theodore Schwann (1845). It took the combined genius of Pasteur and Koch in the 1860s and 1870s, and the general acceptance of the germ theory, to lay this ghost for ever.

Nevertheless the idea that diseased people should be isolated for the good of the community goes back at least to the Middle Ages, when lepers were forced to live apart in lazarettos and leprosaria. The famous siege of Caffa in 1347, when the Tartars catapulted plague corpses into the town, shows a good understanding of the spread of infection and the principles of germ warfare. The British were to use the same technique against the American

Indians in 1763 with gifts of smallpox-infected blankets. By then
military authorities knew that disease could be reduced by
burning the old clothes of new recruits, while the endless
scrubbing of everything that could be scrubbed on board ship
gave the Navy an enviable level of health. Florence Nightingale
famously made her Crimean War (1854–56) a 'war on dirt'. A step
forward was the demonstration in 1855 by the London doctor
John Snow, one of the unsung heroes of epidemiology, that
cholera was spread by drinking water. The provision of safe clean
water is still probably the most cost-efficient way of improving
health globally.

Other cheap and effective methods of limiting the transmission of
disease include hand-washing (especially in hospitals), mosquito
nets for malaria, condoms for sexually transmitted diseases,
screening of blood donors for hepatitis B/C and HIV, heating of
milk (pasteurization) for bovine TB, sterilization of surgical
instruments – plus, of course, proper sanitation and food-handling.
Breast feeding, by transmitting antibodies from mother to child,
significantly reduces the incidence of infantile diarrhoea and ear
infection. Fear of contact with infection can be carried too far, and
*germ phobia* is recognized as a particularly disabling form of
obsessive-compulsive behaviour, Howard Hughes and Glen Gould
being two famous examples. The proliferation of 'anti-bacterial'
creams, lotions, and sprays for use around the house shows that the
possibilities are not lost on the pharmaceutical industry.

More expensive but still worthwhile are the identification and
elimination of animal reservoirs of infection, insecticide spraying,
and campaigns to educate the public on how to avoid contact with
pathogens. For example, in a perfect world, schistosomiasis could

be prevented by forbidding children any contact with the nearby lake, or ordering the wearing of gumboots. However, like forcing city-dwellers to wear masks in the street during a flu epidemic, this calls for a level of public compliance that is unlikely except under the most fiercely authoritarian regime. This is one problem with the public health approach; the other is that it has to be kept up. As a disease declines, it is more and more difficult to maintain public enthusiasm for measures they may consider inconvenient and pointless. The same applies to some extent to vaccination, as we shall see.

## Categories and notification

Some pathogens are much more dangerous to handle than others, which has led to their classification for laboratory purposes into *categories*. Category 4, the most dangerous, contains those potentially fatal viruses where no treatment is available, for example Lassa, Ebola, Marburg, smallpox. These call for total isolation and maximum security. Category 3 includes viruses such as hepatitis, HIV, rabies, bacteria like *M. tuberculosis*, anthrax, and plague, and some fungi and protozoa; these are handled in separate laboratories. The remaining pathogens, treatable or easily prevented by vaccines, are worked on in safety cabinets; these are category 2. Category 1 are the non-pathogens.

As a precaution against spread in the population, most diseases in categories 2, 3, and 4, and all zoonoses (diseases caught from animals) are *notifiable*, meaning that a doctor is obliged to report every case to the local health authority, allowing contacts to be traced.

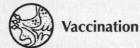 **Vaccination**

Credit for the first vaccine usually goes to Edward Jenner, a Gloucestershire doctor, who in 1796 inoculated 8-year-old James Phipps with material from a lesion of *cowpox* on a local milkmaid's hand. Jenner knew that milkmaids seldom developed smallpox and reasoned that cowpox might somehow protect against it. It worked and he became famous – luckily, because a certain Benjamin Jesty had done the same thing a few years earlier (but he was a farmer, not a doctor, and did not follow up his results on a large scale). At any rate, Jenner's method was far safer than the previous one, which was to use smallpox itself, taken late in the disease – the process of *variolation* – first practised in China about 500 years ago and brought to England from Turkey in 1718. This was risky, with a 3% death rate, compared to about one per million with the cowpox method. By the time Jenner died in 1823 his technique was established all over Europe, and in 1853 it was made compulsory in England. National leaders like Jefferson and Napoleon Bonaparte heaped praises on him although, particularly in America, religious groups mounted a vigorous opposition that has never quite died out. Ironically, the virus generally used, *vaccinia*, is not quite identical to cowpox or smallpox, and its exact origin is still unclear.

Clearly, the next step was to extend the method to other diseases, but in the absence of any scientific understanding of microbes or immunity, the way forward was not obvious. Unfortunately no other known human disease had an animal equivalent that could be used to protect, as cowpox could for smallpox. It was not until 1885, when Pasteur did his daring experiment on young Joseph Meister, who had been bitten by a rabid dog and was saved from rabies by inoculation with dried rabid rabbit spinal cord (!), that it was realized that a normal human virus could be *attenuated*, losing virulence but retaining the power to immunize. In modern immunological terms, we would say that it had retained enough *antigens* to induce the right T and B lymphocytes to respond, but had lost the ability to survive long enough in human cells to cause *pathology*. Cowpox, being related to smallpox but long-adapted to life in cows, behaved like attenuated smallpox. Rabies has nothing to do with cowpox (vaccinia), but Pasteur sensibly proposed that in honour of Jenner the name *vaccination* should be used to cover all such procedures. Naturally there are purists who insist that *immunization* is the only correct term.

### Attenuation; gambling with genes

To this day, the idea of using a normal animal pathogen to immunize against a related human one has never again had the success that cowpox had, though the possibility has been investigated for TB, using a mycobacterium from voles, and for the intestinal pathogen *rotavirus*. Attenuation, on the other hand, has turned out to be so successful that most of the viral vaccines in use today consist of attenuated viruses; measles, mumps, rubella, polio, yellow fever, and chickenpox are the chief examples.

Originally attenuation was a very hit-or-miss affair – 'genetic roulette' as it has been termed. Viruses were grown (or 'passaged') at unusual temperatures or in cells they were not accustomed to, and in attempting to adapt to these uncomfortable conditions by *mutating*, they would occasionally come up with a mutation that was less virulent but not less antigenic than the normal (or 'wild type') virus. Even if such lucky mutants only occurred once in millions of virus replications, these are so rapid that sooner or later one is likely to be spotted. To give an idea of the amount of work involved, the yellow fever vaccine took ten years to attenuate (1927–37) and 270 passages.

The problem was always that there was no way of knowing *how many* mutations there were in these attenuated strains, which is important because a mutation that can go one way can also go the other way, and if a potential vaccine virus has only very few differences from the wild type, there is a good chance that it will one day revert to full virulence, and then the vaccinated individual is going to get the full-blown disease. This has in fact happened on several occasions with the attenuated polio vaccine, which is one of the reasons for preferring vaccines consisting of killed viruses (see below). Another is that an attenuated vaccine which gives little or no pathology in normal individuals can be highly pathogenic or even fatal in someone who is *immunodeficient* (this, you will recall, is how Dr Di George first identified the lack of T lymphocytes in the syndrome that bears his name). So there is a general rule that live vaccines are never given to immunodeficient individuals, except after very careful calculation of the relative risks from the vaccine and the disease in question. In fact many babies with milder forms of Di George syndrome have been given attenuated vaccines without ill-effect.

Until recently, there was only one attenuated *bacterial* vaccine – against tuberculosis. This was produced by two French scientists, Albert Calmette and Camille Guérin, who between 1908 and 1918 patiently cultured bovine tubercle bacilli in the laboratory until they had lost their virulence for calves and, as it turned out, humans. The 'new' bacterium, christened *bacille Calmette–Guérin* or BCG, has remained non-virulent ever since, and is the most widely used vaccine in the world, being given (ideally) to all schoolchildren, or just after birth in countries where the risk of TB is high. The results are nowhere near as good as with the viral vaccines, but there is significant protection against TB – in some parts of the world more than others. An earlier attempt at a tuberculosis vaccine by Koch (1890), an uncharacteristically hasty experiment using a protein preparation he called *tuberculin*, was an embarrassing failure.

Thanks to the DNA revolution, there is no longer any need for these risky methods of attenuation. Nowadays the technique is to identify the genes you want to get rid of – for toxins or other 'virulence factors' – and simply remove them from the virus or bacterium. This has been applied to polio, cholera, typhoid, and many other pathogens, to create a whole new generation of 'tailor-made' attenuated vaccines. A more subtle approach is to damage the pathogen with X-rays or gamma rays so that it is still alive but unable to reproduce. This has given good results with a sheep vaccine against Schistosomiasis and has recently been tried with the bacterium *Listeria*.

### Dead vaccines and a deadly rivalry

Nevertheless, there are still some pathogens where neither old-style nor new-style attenuation has given satisfactory results, and here we have to rely on pathogens that have been killed, usually by chemicals. Examples include the viruses rabies, influenza, hepatitis A, and polio, and the bacteria *Bordetella pertussis* (whooping cough), cholera and typhoid (old-type), and plague.

You may have noticed that *polio* appears in both the attenuated and the killed list. This is the result of a race between two Americans, Albert Sabin and Jonas Salk, to produce the first polio vaccine. It was won in 1954 by Salk with his killed vaccine, which is still the vaccine of choice in Scandinavia (one of the accidents with the live vaccine mentioned above was in Sweden). But killed vaccines are known to be less powerful than attenuated ones, and Sabin's attenuated vaccine, produced in 1957, was also given a licence, and is preferred in most other countries. This is the only example where two completely different vaccines for the same disease are in use side by side. Each has its advantages and disadvantages. The Sabin vaccine probably gives longer-lasting protection but has occasionally caused outbreaks of full-blown polio. In one tragic episode, a batch of Salk vaccine was not properly killed and 11 people died. Sad to relate, the fierce competition between these two great men persisted until their deaths many years later, even then still hardly on speaking terms.

A third scientist, Hilary Koprowski, whose equally good attenuated vaccine was passed over in favour of Sabin's, had the further indignity of being more or less accused by a journalist, in a popular book, of having caused the AIDS epidemic by using infected monkey cells to grow polio virus. I am glad to say it has been proved that there is no truth whatever in this. Nevertheless the suspicion remains, particularly in some muslim communities, that polio vaccination represents a Western 'experiment' which should be boycotted. The tragic result has been the reappearance of polio in areas where it had been virtually eliminated. Polio is not the only vaccine to have given rise to controversy (see below).

### Little bits of pathogens

Since it is a vaccine's *antigens* that really matter in immunity, it is logical to use these rather than the whole organism where possible. Bacterial exotoxins illustrate this point well. With tetanus and diphtheria it is the toxins that cause the pathology, and antibody against the toxin is all that is needed to prevent this. Toxins can be *inactivated* by formaldehyde yet still retain their antigens; they are now called *toxoids*. Tetanus and diphtheria toxoids are given to all babies, normally with polio, the new pertussis toxoid, and antigens from *Haemophilus* (see below). Being 'dead' material which cannot reproduce as an attenuated virus can, these vaccines require further boosting every ten years or so, but they have undoubtedly saved millions of lives. All these 'non-living' vaccines are usually given with an alum (aluminium hydroxide) *adjuvant*, which was discovered 70 years ago to enhance and prolong their immunizing activity.

Another example where only part of the pathogen is needed are the bacteria with sugar-based *capsules* that block their uptake by phagocytes: the *Meningococcus*, *Pneumococcus*, and *Haemophilus influenzae* are examples. All that is needed to rectify matters here is a good antibody response against the capsule, so that the antibody molecule can do the attaching to the phagocytes. So the vaccines are composed of capsular material only. The only slight drawback is that very young babies do not make antibodies to sugar antigens, but this has been overcome in the case of *Haemophilus* by attaching a bacterial protein to make a *conjugate vaccine*.

## Genes without the roulette

The same idea can be applied to the protein *surface antigen* of the hepatitis B virus. In the first vaccine trials in 1982, surface antigen was laboriously purified from the blood of carriers, but it was later found possible to take the *gene* for this molecule and insert it into yeast cells, which promptly produced large amounts of surface antigen, uncontaminated with any infectious virus. This was the first *genetically engineered* vaccine, highly effective and much cheaper and safer than the blood-derived one. It paved the way for further applications of DNA technology. For example it is now possible to clone a gene for the desired antigen into some harmless virus or bacterium 'vector' and 'infect' the patient with it. The vector will travel to its normal site of infection and replicate for a time, and the antigen with it. Vaccinia and BCG are obvious possibilities as vectors, and there are even plans to put genes from half a dozen or more pathogens into one vector, to make a 'super-vaccine' which would simultaneously immunize against measles, mumps, polio, flu, TB, etc., etc. Genetically modified viruses are also being considered as biological control agents. For example a modified myxoma virus has been tried out in Spain, not to kill rabbits, as in the unsuccessful Australian trial, but to sterilize them – in effect a living anti-fertility vaccine. Given the objections to genetically modified plants, these new viruses can be expected to encounter vigorous opposition.

An even more audacious strategy is to use only the gene and inject it straight into the patient. If suitably done this can result in a steady production of the desired antigen from the body's own cells. I first heard about this at the 1992 International Congress (which took place during a ferocious heat-wave in Budapest), where it attracted equal amounts of curiosity and scepticism. Now fourteen years later, the 'DNA vaccine' is one of the front-runners among new-generation vaccines. Yet another idea is to put the microbial gene into plants to make an 'edible vaccine'; potatoes and bananas have been suggested as the cheapest and most widely acceptable vehicles.

Thanks to these exciting new developments, vaccine research has had something of a revival. In contrast to the apathy at that 1989 Berlin congress, meetings entirely devoted to vaccines are now quite common. I used to go every other year to Cape Sounion, a remote headland south of Athens, for the NATO vaccine conference where, in a charming modern hotel complete with tiny chalets half-smothered in vines and oleander, scientists from the worlds of immunology, microbiology, chemistry, and biotechnology would bring one another up to date on their latest work. Spouses and children would set off in buses for Athens or Delphi, sun themselves on the little beach, or climb to the ruined Greek temple to admire Byron's signature carved in the stone, while the rest of us crowded into the hot lecture theatre, held impromptu tutorials in the shade of olive trees, or quizzed eager young PhD students on their poster displays – always aware that one of them might be a future Albert Sabin or Jonas Salk.

Normally any meeting featuring immunology has an element of the cut-throat world of business, where you have to keep a watchful eye on who is up, who is down, who is worth cultivating, who is trying to steal your best student. But at the Sounion meetings the atmosphere was remarkably relaxed, with everybody looking much the same in shorts and tee-shirts – students, professors, and Nobel Prize-winners on first-name terms for a fortnight before going back to the more rigid hierarchies of their university departments or pharmaceutical companies or, in the case of the Americans, to do the rest of Europe. In the evening we would eat together at long democratic tables, or walk along the coast for fish and retsina at tavernas to continue the day's arguments. It would be nice to think that the spirit of Socrates was nodding approval somewhere.

## Problems, fears, and misconceptions

Even leaving aside accidents, supposed conspiracies, and the ancient prejudice against 'disturbing nature', vaccines still occasionally run into difficulties due to *side effects*, real or imaginary. The pertussis vaccine 'scare' in the 1970s caused a sharp drop in the numbers of children vaccinated in the UK (from 85% to 30%), following claims by doctors that the vaccine caused convulsions and even permanent brain damage. In 1998 a claim that the attenuated measles vaccine, normally given with mumps and rubella as MMR, caused some cases of juvenile autism, led to a similar drop in uptake. The risk with pertussis has never been totally disproved, but the risk of brain damage due to the vaccine, rather than to some other cause, is estimated at three per million children vaccinated, whereas the drop in vaccine uptake resulted in a substantial increase in cases of whooping cough – 20 000–30 000 in some years – with a fatality rate of about 1 in 600 cases. So dropping the vaccine may have led to some 50 deaths. The old vaccine has now been replaced by a safer toxoid (see above).

In contrast, the link between the measles vaccine and autism has utterly failed to stand the test of worldwide scrutiny and the 1998 paper has been retracted by the authors. But the damage to public trust had been done and some parents have exercised their right to have 'single-shot' vaccines omitting measles, often at considerable cost. I often wonder where they got the information in which they based this decision, which led to an increase of some 250 cases of measles per year in the UK. As the overall incidence of diseases like measles, whooping cough, and diphtheria falls, it is more important than ever to keep up vaccination; otherwise there will be a large non-immune population ready to go down with the diseases if they should reappear – that is, a collapse of 'herd immunity'. Following the break-up of the Soviet Union, where vaccination had been conscientiously monitored, the annual incidence of diphtheria rose from 800 to 50 000, with 1500 deaths. It always surprised me that the American public, normally so opposed to government interference, accepts compulsory vaccination as a prerequisite for school entry, whereas in Britain, with its centralized health service, it remains optional. Even the smallpox vaccine was no longer compulsory after 1907.

The most recent vaccine scare is the idea that the debilitating symptoms of the 'Gulf War syndrome' might be due to the unusual batch of vaccines that combatants were given in anticipation of the use of biological weapons such as smallpox, anthrax, and plague. Smallpox and anthrax are live attenuated vaccines, and would certainly be pathogenic in immunodeficient individuals, but it is most unlikely that 1 in 15 combat-ready troops were immunodeficient! However, it is conceivable that normal responses to the vaccines were affected by the extremely stressful conditions. As with all suspected vaccine toxicity, the connection would be very hard to prove beyond all doubt in the absence of a non-vaccinated 'control' group exposed to the same conditions – hardly an ethical prospect. So we may never know.

The moral is that it is best not to accept uncritically every sensational theory you read in books or newspapers or on the internet or hear from the pulpit but keep it in mind as a possibility, strong or weak as the case may be, until more evidence turns up, either for or against the idea. If you are not an expert, talk to someone who is. Eventually, after repeated testing, it should reach the point of being accepted as probably true, or as probably untrue. Scientists will then adopt it pro tem as a reasonable probability until someone shows convincingly that it is wrong, or dismiss it until someone revives the idea with new data. Scientists are not afraid to change their minds and they don't always agree on every point, and now and then they are wrong. I can think of at least four dramatic 'discoveries' during my time in immunology that turned out to be completely false, and although it is tempting to talk about 'scientific fakes', there were simply cases of a scientist being carried away by an odd result and an exciting theory, and temporarily blinded to objections that were fairly obvious to the rest of us. There is not much point faking a result these days, because you will probably be caught out within a year or two at most if the claim is an important one, and ignored if it isn't.

All this is not to deny that genuine side-effects occur, including redness and pain at the injection site, mild fever, and brief fainting episodes. Live attenuated viral vaccines (e.g. MMR) may sometimes cause mild symptoms similar to the diseases they protect against, skin rashes being the commonest. The most serious, but extremely rare, is anaphylaxis, usually due to allergy to egg protein (many viruses are bulk-grown in eggs). Of course all medical treatments carry an element of risk, but this is particularly regrettable with vaccines, which, unlike surgery and drugs, are given to perfectly healthy people.

## When and how to vaccinate?

Vaccines are given at the time and by the route calculated to produce the strongest immunity. This is not the same for every disease. MMR is delayed for at least six months because babies are likely to have received some antibody against these common diseases from the mother before birth, and until this has all disappeared, it will inhibit the proper working of the vaccine. Where there is not much measles about, the vaccine can be left until about a year of age, when it will be at its most potent. Similarly, BCG is given immediately after birth in tropical countries, but not until the early teens in countries where TB is rare. The first dose of DPT is given a month or two after birth, but tetanus and diphtheria need a boost about 5 and 15 years later, because in the absence of any contact with either infection, antibody levels will have fallen below a protective level. Capsular vaccines do not induce good immunity until after two years of age, unless combined with a bacterial protein, as has been done in the case of *Haemophilus*. The pneumococcal vaccine is mainly reserved for the elderly. As mentioned above, living attenuated vaccines should never be given to immunodeficient individuals – though this must surely have happened occasionally in the past, when mild immunodeficiency was probably not diagnosed. One benefit of more careful screening for minor immune defects might be a reduction in vaccine 'accidents'.

Most of these vaccines are given by intramuscular injection, except for the Sabin (attenuated) polio vaccine, which is given by mouth. Not only is this a much pleasanter prospect for young children, but it also delivers the vaccine where it is needed because polio enters the body through the intestinal route. In the future all immunization against intestinal infections will probably also be given by mouth, once suitable antigen preparations are available.

## Why aren't there vaccines for HIV, and colds, and malaria, and worms, etc.?

In fact the list of diseases we don't have a vaccine for is longer than the list of ones for which we do. All types of cold, glandular fever, genital herpes, EBV, AIDS, the haemorrhagic viruses, staphylococcal infection, leprosy, syphilis, gonorrhoea, trachoma, *all* fungal, protozoal, and worm diseases . . . it goes on for ever. The reasons vary. To take a few examples: with cold viruses, there are just too many strains in the community, each of which would need a separate vaccine. With HIV the ceaseless antigenic variation makes it impossible to select the right antigen. A syphilis vaccine seems unlikely because the normal infection induces little or no immunity. When immunopathology is a feature of the disease, there is the worry that a vaccine could make it worse.

Protozoal and worm infections are the most obstinately resistant of all to vaccination, despite decades of work under the sponsorship of the World Health Organization, who year after year bullied rich countries to fund this commercially unprofitable field (you will probably not be surprised to hear that the Scandinavian countries have the best record in this area). The problem is that almost none of the eukaryotic pathogens induce protective immunity in the way measles or even TB do, so it is not easy to know even what *sort* of immunity to aim for. Vaccines against a few fungi have given protection in animals, but not yet in humans. A malaria vaccine has repeatedly seemed to be within sight, but the trials have shown only slight protection; the ever-changing stages of the life cycle and antigenic variation of the blood stage are the main stumbling blocks. A Colombian scientist achieved brief notoriety with a vaccine that seemed to work in Venezuelan army conscripts but was a failure in Africa. In one African village it was found that every single inhabitant had a different antigenic variant; no vaccine that can be imagined at present could protect them all. The same applies to the trypanosomes of sleeping sickness where antigens vary from week to week during the infection. With the worms, the problem is chiefly that they are hard to dislodge or destroy, even when immunity is boosted – plus the possibility that increased immunity, if it did not completely eliminate the infection, would merely increase the pathology. Only in a few infections of dogs and farm animals has an effective anti-worm vaccine been shown to be possible.

## What about bird flu?

Reading the grim reports of slaughtered chickens and the predictions of hundreds of thousands of human deaths, many people are mystified. Why not simply vaccinate the birds and us? Here, for once, there is genuine disagreement even among the experts. It would be theoretically possible to vaccinate every farmyard chicken, duck, and turkey against H5N1, but the cost would be fantastic and the organizers would need huge government subsidies. Moreover unless the vaccine used is exactly the same as the infecting strain, it could have the effect of preventing symptoms without eliminating the virus, so that apparently healthy birds would continue to spread it – that is, become *carriers* – and the same argument would apply to human populations. Moreover it would be out of the question

to vaccinate all the wild geese and swans whose migrations carry
the virus around the world. The alternative for the birds is to isolate
and cull (that is, kill) all stocks as soon as disease appears, an
approach that has worked well in some of the richer Far Eastern
countries. For humans there is the added problem that we do not
yet know the exact structure of the hypothetical mutated virus that
will, or might, infect us, and there is no point starting vaccine
manufacture until we do. The main alternative is an antiviral
drug (see Chemotherapy, below) but here the logistic problems
are just as bad; only one pharmaceutical firm currently makes
the drug of choice and the hundreds of millions of doses that
would be needed would take at least two years to produce, at a
cost that most countries could not afford, while production
elsewhere has been held up by patent restrictions. Clearly it is up
to supranational organizations like the WHO and WTA to bang
heads together.

## Immunity in a bottle

In the opening months of trench warfare in the First World War
tetanus killed 15 per 1000 British troops, until supplies of *antitoxin*
– serum containing protective antibodies taken from horses
immunized with tetanus – were rushed to the battlefront,
whereupon the mortality fell by 90%. The first antitoxins had been
made only two years after the discovery of antibodies in 1888, at
first in sheep and goats by von Behring and Kitasato, and a few
years later in horses by Emile Roux. The 60-year-old Von Behring
was awarded the Iron Cross for his role in saving lives on the
German side. Pharmaceutical companies used to keep fields full of
horses for immunization against tetanus, diphtheria, pneumonia,
gas gangrene, and snake venom. Tom, a handsome white horse

belonging to London University, was the source of the first British antitoxin against diphtheria in 1894.

But the future was in vaccines. The tetanus toxoid vaccine for humans was introduced, just in time for the Second World War, in which there were almost no deaths from tetanus, and as other vaccines became available, as well as antibiotics, the use of these pre-formed antitoxins, or *passive immunization* as it was known, gradually died out. But they are still kept in refrigerators for emergency use in patients *already exposed* to tetanus, diphtheria, gas gangrene, rabies, and snake bite.

One application of passive immunotherapy which is not outdated is the monthly injections of normal human serum to patients with agammaglobulinaemia (see Chapter 8). Another is the idea of vaccinating a mother during pregnancy to protect her baby when born; this could be the answer to neonatal tetanus, still a major killer in some tropical countries. It is conceivable that passive immunization might have to be revived for the treatment of new diseases in the period before vaccines can be developed – normally a question of several years. Passively transferred serum from a nurse who had recovered from Lassa fever was used to protect a laboratory worker. When the majority of patients do not die from an infection (e.g. with SARS) it should be possible to obtain fairly large amounts of 'post-recovery' serum and use it in this way. It has even been suggested in China that horses could be brought back into service to make antibody to the H5N1 avian flu – turning the clock back a hundred years.

Horse antibodies have their problems, while supplies of human serum will never be unlimited, however, and as well as the virus in question they have to be screened for other viruses such as HIV and hepatitis, so great interest was aroused when in 1975 it was discovered how to make absolutely pure antibodies in the laboratory, using B lymphocytes that had been cloned and made 'immortal', so that they poured out the same antibody for ever. These *monoclonal antibodies* have been fantastically useful in research of all kinds, but as treatments for infections they have been rather disappointing, because antibody against a single bit of a single antigen on a pathogen is less effective than the mixture of antibodies that occurs naturally during infection, and at present monoclonals are only in use against one virus (RSV) causing chest infections in children. Most of the monoclonal antibodies in regular use are anti-inflammatory or anti-cancer.

## What have vaccines achieved?

For all their limitations, vaccines have undoubtedly made the single biggest contribution to the reduction of infectious disease. They have eliminated smallpox and could quite possibly eliminate polio, measles, mumps, and rubella within the next decade. They have reduced the death rate from tetanus, diphtheria, influenza, yellow fever, hepatitis, meningitis, pneumonia, and rabies. The *Haemophilus influenzae* vaccine, introduced only 15 years ago, has cut the incidence of this dangerous childhood disease by 95%. It is no longer necessary for parents to have six or eight children in order for two to survive. The average inhabitant of the developed world is much more likely nowadays to die of heart disease or cancer than of an infectious disease. Vaccines have had no impact yet on fungal, protozoal, or worm infections, which means that their overall effect has been far less dramatic in the tropics, where these are among the worst health problems.

They have so far failed to get to grips with AIDS, though this may change. New infections will still turn up from time to time, and we cannot predict whether vaccination will work against them. Table 9.1 summarizes the established vaccines in use today. As you will see, there are slight differences in the schedules for different countries.

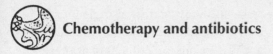 ## Chemotherapy and antibiotics

Everyone is familiar with the fact that chemicals can kill microbes. The introduction of the antiseptic *phenol* into the operating theatre by Joseph Lister (1867) instantly changed the pattern of post-operative infection, and surgery without sterilization of instruments would today be unthinkable. But phenol is a deadly poison if taken internally. Iodine, alcohol, and hydrogen peroxide are excellent antibacterials for reducing contamination of wounds, but still too toxic for internal use. So how can we attack, for example, tubercle bacilli in the lung or staphylococci in the blood, without damaging or destroying healthy tissue?

We have seen in earlier chapters how the immune system tackles this problem by using cells or molecules that specifically bind to pathogens, and how the amazingly prolific Paul Ehrlich worked out that this must be mediated by a system of specific *receptors*. At the same time he realized that it ought to be possible to make chemical poisons that only bound to pathogens; after all, there were already mixtures of dyes which would stain normal tissue one colour, let us say red, and bacteria another – blue. If the blue dye was toxic and the red one wasn't, you would have a safe antibacterial. And so began the history of *chemotherapy*.

## Table 9.1 Vaccines in common use today

| Pathogen/disease | Type of vaccine | Comments |
|---|---|---|
| **In general use** | | |
| Diphtheria | Toxoid (inactivated toxin) | |
| Tetanus | Toxoid | Usually given together |
| *B. pertussis* | Killed bacteria | |
| Measles | Attenuated virus | |
| Mumps | Attenuated virus | Usually given together |
| Rubella | Attenuated virus | |
| Poliovirus | Attenuated/killed virus | 3 types, given together |
| Tuberculosis | Attenuated bacterium (BCG) | |
| *Haemophilus* (HIB) | Bacterial capsule | Conjugated to protein |
| **Restricted use** | | |
| *Meningococcus* | Bacterial capsule (3 strains) | Travel; during outbreaks |
| *Pneumococcus* | Bacterial capsule (35 types) | Elderly; chronic heart/lung disease |
| Influenza | Killed virus | Elderly; during epidemics |
| Hepatitis A | Killed virus | Travel; contacts |
| Hepatitis B* | Recombinant surface antigen | Occupational risk |
| Cholera | Killed bacteria | Travel to tropics |
| Typhoid | Attenuated bacteria/capsule | Travel to tropics |
| Yellow fever | Attenuated virus | Travel to tropics |
| Chickenpox* | Attenuated virus | Leukaemics on chemotherapy |
| Rabies | Killed virus | Post-exposure; high risk |
| Anthrax | Attenuated bacteria/toxoid | Occupational risk (e.g. farmers; military) |
| Plague | Killed bacteria | Military |
| Smallpox | Vaccinia virus | Military |
| Rotavirus* | Attenuated virus | Recent (USA, 1998) |

*In general use in the USA.

Ehrlich chose to work on 'difficult' pathogens such as the trypanosomes of sleeping sickness and the spirochaetes of syphilis. He knew that certain metal compounds would kill them – arsenic, antimony, mercury – but these, of course, were well-known poisons for humans too. With his customary clarity, he set out the principle of *selective toxicity*: that it was going to be necessary to find and exploit *any* difference between the pathogen and its host, and concentrate the attack there – in other words to find a *chemical* with the same high degree of specificity already shown by the *antibody* molecule. It was the concept of the 'magic bullet' which, in German folklore, finds its way unerringly to the target (usually a werewolf). Ehrlich's first success, in 1910, the arsenic-containing molecule *salvarsan* for the treatment of syphilis, showed that this was a possibility. A few years later he produced an improved version, neo-salvarsan. The working titles of these drugs – 606 and 914 – give an idea of how many compounds he tested, and something of his obstinate humanity can be sensed in Edward G. Robinson's portrayal in the film *Dr. Ehrlich's Magic Bullet*, made in 1940 – a time when purely intellectual battles were still considered to have popular audience appeal. In 1935 another dye, Prontosil Red, was shown in the Bayer laboratories to kill streptococci, and the active portion was identified. This was *sulfanilamide*, the first synthetic molecule with wide antibacterial activity, and it opened the way to the present era, when chemotherapy of some kind is now the first choice of treatment for most infections.

The thorough and patient work of Ehrlich contrasts with the stroke of luck that led Alexander Fleming, in 1929, to discover *penicillin*, through the chance effect of some colonies of the fungus *Penicillium notatum* contaminating one of his bacterial culture plates. Evidently the fungus was producing something that killed bacteria. He did not follow this to its logical conclusion, and it was not until 1940 that, thanks to the work of Howard Florey and Ernst Chain in Oxford, penicillin became available to treat patients. Antimicrobial molecules like penicillin, produced naturally by micro-organisms as part of their own defence, are known as *antibiotics* – though they are still examples of chemotherapy. Several other fungi and bacteria produce useful antibiotics, notably the filamentous bacterium *Streptomyces*. Over 500 antibiotics are produced by species of *Streptomyces*, of which 50 have found a use in human or animal medicine, and culturing them has become a massive industrial process. It is estimated that in all there are about 5000 known antibiotics, and 300 new ones are discovered every year. Screening, production, safety-testing, and clinical trials of chemotherapeutic agents are time-consuming and costly (up to £500 million per drug in all), and less than 100 are in regular use. Table 9.2 lists a few of the best known and their origin.

Far the greatest success of chemotherapy has been in treating bacterial infection, so we will start there.

## Antibacterial drugs and antibiotics

The bacterium, with its prokaryotic cell design, has several points of difference from the eukaryotic human cell, and there are drugs that exploit each of these.

First of all there is the *cell wall*, a structure completely absent from mammalian cells. This is where the penicillins and their relatives the cephalosporins act, by blocking the enzymes used to assemble cell wall components. Unfortunately many bacteria, especially staphylococci, can destroy these enzymes and escape from the effect

**Table 9.2 Some important antibacterial drugs and their sources**

| Agent | Discovered | Source |
|---|---|---|
| Penicillin | 1929 | Fungus *Penicillium notatum* |
| Sulfanilamide | 1935 | Synthetic |
| Streptomycin | 1943 | Bacterium *Streptomyces (S.) griseus* |
| Chloramphenicol | 1947 | *S. venezuelae* (now synthetic) |
| Tetracycline | 1947 | *S. rimosus* |
| Cephalosporin | 1948 | Fungus *Cephalosporium* |
| Polymyxin | 1948 | *Bacillus polymyxia* |
| Erythromycin | 1952 | *S. erythrens* |
| Vancomycin | 1955 | *S. orientalis* |
| Methicillin | 1960 | Synthetic |
| Ampicillin | 1961 | Synthetic |
| Gentamycin | 1963 | Bacterium *Micromonospora* |
| Rifampicin | 1966 | Synthetic |
| Ciprofloxacin | 1983 | Synthetic |
| Teicoplanin | 1984 | *Actinomyces teichomyceticus* |
| Daptomycin | 1984 | *S. roseosporus* |
| Synercid | 1999 | *S. pristinaspiralis* |
| Linezolid | 1999 | Synthetic |

of penicillin (see below). Long before penicillin, Nature had evolved a way of attacking the cell walls of some bacteria, using the enzyme *lysozyme*, which is present in the granules of PMNs, and in blood, tears, and saliva (and also in egg-white). By a happy coincidence, it was Fleming who discovered this as well. It probably ensures that a large number of common bacteria are non-pathogenic.

Next is the *cell membrane*, more similar to the membrane of eukaryotic cells, but not identical; the polymyxin antibiotics exploit this difference. Bacterial *protein synthesis* is also slightly different from mammalian; this is where the widely used drugs tetracycline, streptomycin, and erythromycin act. The sulfonamides work by interfering with bacterial *nucleic acid* synthesis. Sulfonamides, being synthetic rather than natural molecules, are not strictly speaking antibiotics, but doctors are not too fussy about this rather pedantic distinction, particularly since many naturally occurring antibiotics can also be made synthetically. Calling them all antibiotics also avoids confusion with the *chemotherapy* used against cancer.

Finally, there is a separate group of synthetic drugs that are used mainly in tuberculosis and whose mode of action is still not fully understood. They have to be given over months or even years, whereas most courses of antibiotic are a matter of weeks.

There are two problems with antibiotics: *toxicity* and *resistance*.

## Toxicity

All drugs interfere in some way with normal functions, and the more they do so, the more they are liable to have potentially toxic *side-effects*. These side-effects are often unexpected and easily overlooked at first. For example it was a nasty surprise when streptomycin, which was so successful against tuberculosis, turned out to cause ear damage, dizziness, and even complete deafness. Chloramphenicol would be an excellent drug except for its inhibitory effect on the bone marrow. Tetracycline can cause diarrhoea by killing normal intestinal bacteria and allowing other bacteria, and especially yeasts, to replace them – and also stains the teeth of young children yellow.

A slightly different sort of side-effect is the tendency of antibiotics, especially penicillin and sulfonamides, to cause *immunopathology*. One has to remember that drugs are very definitely not 'self' molecules, and it is quite possible to make antibodies against them. This can lead to allergies (very common with penicillin), immune complex disease, autoimmunity, and dermatitis. It is because of the possibility of side effects that the introduction of a new drug takes so long and costs so much, and even so there is occasionally an unpleasant surprise.

### Resistance

When you consider that micro-organisms can escape from the immune system by various mutations, it is not surprising that they can also escape from the effects of antibiotics in a similar way. In the presence of the drug, any change that favours survival will be exploited. Within a few years gonococci had become resistant to sulfonamides, and many staphylococci to penicillin. How could this happen so rapidly, with a drug they had never encountered before? The answer is, by the same method by which the immune system can respond to a pathogen it has never previously seen: there is a regular rate of mutation, and resistant mutant staphylococci *were already there*, in tiny numbers – just as specific lymphocytes are in the immune system. When the right conditions came along, they seized their chance, multiplying while their antibiotic-susceptible neighbours died, and soon replaced them to become the dominant population. This is *natural selection* in action, and it has proved an enormous problem for doctors – though very profitable for the drug industry. It was while contemplating bacterial resistance that Burnet and Joshua Lederberg conceived the clonal selection theory of antibody formation.

The actual mechanisms used by bacteria to achieve resistance vary, and we will consider just two examples that show how well-designed these microscopic single-celled creatures are for survival in new and hostile conditions. Penicillin, as already mentioned, kills staphylococci and streptococci by preventing them constructing their cell walls. The 'target' molecule is one of the bacterial wall-building enzymes, which penicillin binds to, putting a block on its function. Occasional mutations in the bacteria produce enzymes that destroy penicillin as well as other antibiotics that act in the same way. What was the function of these mutations in the millions of years before Fleming? Remember that penicillin is a natural product of a fungus; presumably bacteria long ago had to evolve the means of surviving in the presence of fungi. Away from fungi (or antibiotics) the resistant population had no reason to take over, but the ability was there, ready for when the need arose.

Resistance to tetracycline is even more interesting because when it develops, in bacteria exposed to the drug, the bacteria simultaneously become resistant to chloramphenicol, streptomycin, and sulfonamides! These drugs do not all act in the same way, so one single gene could not account for this. What has happened is that several resistance genes occur together on the same detachable piece of DNA, known as a *plasmid*. Plasmids can be exchanged between bacteria, so resistance can spread rapidly within the bacterial population – almost like virus infections do in higher animals.

Because of the prolonged course of tuberculosis and the lengthy treatment required (at least six months), resistance is an increasing worry, particularly in those least able to comply – the homeless,

drug addicts, AIDS victims. Three or more drugs in combination
offer the best hope of avoiding complete resistance, but multiple-
drug-resistant (MDR) tuberculosis, first observed in Russia and
now in India, is increasingly a worldwide problem.

## Superbugs

The question is often asked whether pathogenic bacteria will
eventually be resistant to *all* antibiotics, which would mean the end
of the antibiotic era. Nobody can say this could not happen, and
even now the methicillin-resistant *Staphylococcus aureus* (MRSA)
is causing serious alarm. For a time intravenous vancomycin
seemed to be the answer, but resistance can develop to that too,
leaving the new drugs synercid and linezolid as the last resort.
Meanwhile, the best that can be done to prolong the effectiveness
of antibiotics is to use them carefully; this is mainly a question of
not using them when they are not needed (e.g. for virus infections)
but, once they are used, completing the prescribed course to ensure
that all the bacteria are killed. An inadequate dose is simply a way
to generate resistant strains. Another culprit is thought to be the
food industry. Feeding antibiotics to animals and plants can
improve their health and size, but the resistant strains of bacteria
that emerge will find their way into the food chain. The one
encouraging feature is that, in the absence of antibiotics, the
resistant strains usually grow slightly *less* well than the 'normal'
susceptible ones. So the 'superbug', properly handled, can still
be tamed.

### A new era?

The possibility of total resistance to conventional antibiotics has
directed attention to previously neglected alternatives. For example,

the tiny *peptide* molecules found in phagocytes and elsewhere (including the saliva of that ancient reptile, the Komodo dragon) and the *bacteriophage* viruses have been known for some time to destroy bacteria and have their enthusiastic supporters as potential therapeutic agents. Only time will tell if this enthusiasm is justified.

## Antiviral drugs

This brings us to the question of chemotherapy against viruses, a much more difficult problem. Viruses do not have to make their own cell walls or membranes, and their proteins arc madc mainly using equipment provided by the host cell, so the available targets for 'selective toxicity' are much reduced. But once again Nature has shown the way by evolving the *interferons*, which can inhibit viral replication without damaging cells. Interferon is now available commercially, and has proved valuable in treating persistent hepatitis and herpesvirus infections. It also has the quite separate effect of increasing the number of MHC molecules on infected cells, which makes them more likely to be killed by T lymphocytes. So the interferon system acts like a complete antiviral 'package'.

No drug has been found that acts exactly like interferon, but there are a few drugs that exploit weak points in the viral life cycle. One, *amantidine*, blocks the entry of influenza virus into cells and appreciably shortens the illness. The other main anti-flu drug *tamiflu* blocks the formation of surface neuraminidase (e.g. the N in H5N1). The most vulnerable points inside the cell are those enzymes that only viruses possess, such as the DNA polymerase of herpesviruses, which is blocked by *acyclovir*, and the reverse transcriptase of HIV, blocked by *zidovudine* (also known as azidothymidine: AZT). Effective control of HIV requires a combination of three drugs, a cumbersome and expensive treatment far beyond the reach of the worst affected populations in the developing world.

A novel idea is to design 'antisense' RNA or DNA that binds to viral genes and prevents them functioning; if it works, this might be the safest and most specific of all treatments. Like antibacterials, antiviral drugs show both *toxicity* (mainly to the bone marrow) and *resistance*. Even the naturally occurring interferons, if given in high doses, can have unpleasant side-effects, patients often complaining that they feel permanently 'flu-like'. For this reason, interferon is not used for minor virus infections, although it was shown in experiments at the Common Cold Research unit outside Salisbury to be able to prevent a cold – if given before the infection!

## Antifungal drugs

When we come to fungi, protozoa, and worms, we are dealing with eukaryotic pathogens, with a cell structure not so different from our own. In fungi there is one Achilles' heel, because the cell membrane contains *ergosterol* instead of cholesterol, the mammalian equivalent. So most antifungal drugs act here. Nucleic acid and protein synthesis are also possible targets, but with more danger of damage to host cells. Since fungal infections have come to prominence as serious pathogens in AIDS patients, the need for safe antifungals has become acute.

## Antiprotozoal drugs

Protozoa are such highly evolved and unique creatures that there are no drugs that kill them all. Some, like *Leishmania* and the trypanosomes, are extremely hard to kill without serious side-effects. Drugs containing arsenic and antimony are still in use, almost 100 years after Ehrlich's invention of salvarsan, which, though more effective against syphilis, was originally intended for trypanosomiasis.

The story of malaria is particularly frustrating. Over 300 years ago it was discovered that the bark of the cinchona tree was effective against 'fever' (which in tropical accounts usually means malaria). The active component was found to be *quinine*, still one of the best drugs for acute life-threatening malaria, despite its side-effects on the heart, eyes, ears, blood pressure, and blood sugar. Then during the Second World War the safer and more practical *chloroquine* was introduced, and it looked as if malaria was about to be vanquished. But within 20 years resistant parasites had emerged and by 1990 chloroquine-resistance had spread worldwide. Of the new drugs that have taken its place, the most promising is *artemisin*, derived from a traditional Chinese herbal remedy. It is quite curious that the only two plant-derived antibiotics in regular medical use are both active against malaria. Many other plants are claimed to have antimalarial, antibacterial, or antiviral activity, but at the moment their use is restricted to herbal practitioners (see below).

## Anti-helminthic drugs

With their large multicellular construction, worms might be expected to be the hardest pathogens of all to kill. However, a loophole has been discovered in, of all places, their nervous system; the drugs *ivermectin* and *levamisole* interfere with nerve–muscle conduction in worms but not mammals. A real magic bullet; Ehrlich would have been thrilled! So, ironically, drug treatment for many worm infections is safer and more effective than for protozoa.

This does not mean that worm infections are about to disappear, because in tropical countries the worm burdens are colossal, the drugs are expensive, and health budgets are tiny.

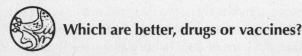 ## Which are better, drugs or vaccines?

In practice this choice very seldom arises, because their strengths are different. Most of the effective vaccines are against viruses, while most of the effective drugs are against bacteria. Vaccines have the great advantage that they only need to be given once or a few times; the immune system, with its built-in memory, takes over subsequently – but they take time to act. In contrast, antibiotics act straight away, but generally need to be given daily (or more often) for weeks or months. This, of course, makes them a more attractive financial prospect; in fact many pharmaceutical companies have abandoned vaccine manufacture as uncommercial. Indeed as I write this, one AIDS vaccine trial has been stopped in mid-course, purely on financial grounds. Drugs are more likely to be toxic than vaccines – but on the other hand there are (some) drugs against eukaryotes, but no vaccines. So really we are very fortunate to have both options. Only in a few cases, such as tuberculosis and flu, are both in regular use.

We should not forget the public health measures, however. For example, in looking at the huge reduction in tuberculosis in the UK between 1850 and 1950, it is tempting to ask whether this was mainly due to BCG or to streptomycin. The answer is: neither. Three-quarters of the reduction occurred before either of these was introduced, and was due to general improvements in nutrition and living conditions.

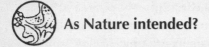 ## As Nature intended?

Nature seems to attract blame and credit in equal proportion. 'Doing what comes naturally' can be a convenient excuse for almost any disreputable behaviour, whereas living 'as Nature intended' usually means following whatever lifestyle its supporters happen to think worthy of admiration – vegetarian, ascetic, ruthlessly competitive, nudist, etc. Judging by the science shelf in bookshops, antibiotics are high on the blacklist of things that Nature is considered not to have intended. Usually they are contrasted with herbal remedies with their unblemished record of antibacterial, antiviral, immunostimulating, and generally life-enhancing properties, and their few or no side-effects. I have little direct experience of herbal antibiotics, but if they work that is excellent, and I certainly think we in the West ought to look seriously at any remedy that is widely believed to be effective, as fortunately we did with the Chinese antimalarial herb artemisia. Another Asian plant, duckweed, is reported to be effective in chronic hepatitis B, and remarkable curative powers are claimed for certain *lichens*, those curious symbiotic aggregations of fungi and green algae. The whole field of plant medicine (phytopharmacy) does seem to be finally attracting industrial interest.

However, I am never quite sure why it should be 'unnatural' to treat a bacterial infection with the fungal product penicillin, but 'natural' to do so with large doses of echinacea, wild indigo, or marshmallow. The strongest argument in favour of unpurified material is that it sometimes contains more than one component of value in treatment – though a similar effect should be obtainable, with patience, by using several pure drugs in combination. The disadvantage is that a plant extract containing hundreds of unidentified molecules could well include toxic ones we would be better off without. Remember that some of the most powerful poisons known are of plant origin. Darwinian principles would suggest that plants have evolved primarily to favour their own survival rather than to benefit humanity, which arrived, from their point of view, very late on the scene. So plant-derived antibiotics would be expected to work best against the viral, bacterial, fungal, and insect parasites of plants; this makes it all the more surprising that, as mentioned earlier, two plant products are among the most powerful antimalarials; I am still not sure what this is trying to tell us. Perhaps there is a clue in the surprising finding that several protozoa, including the malaria parasite, appear to have picked up genes from the chloroplasts of plants – emphasizing the fact that exchange of genes among different forms of life is far commoner than used to be thought.

 **Living without germs?**

No less a scientist than Pasteur stated that microbes were essential for normal life. He was right in the sense that animals deprived of their normal flora – particularly the bacteria in the intestine – or born and raised in the total absence of any form of micro-organism, show reductions in weight, metabolic rate, cardiac output, etc. They also have no antibodies in their blood, which shows that the normal level of some 20 grams of immunoglobulin (about 60 million million million molecules) per litre is due to stimulation by micro-organisms. However, such 'germ-free' animals *can* be kept alive and healthy (at great expense) provided they do not become exposed to pathogens; the same technology of total isolation is used as for the severely immunodeficient 'bubble babies'. But it is quite impossible to imagine the germ-free state coming about naturally to test the truth of Pasteur's statement.

On the other hand it is perfectly possible to imagine a world without higher animals, which after all did exist for billions of years – and could again, if the worst predictions of nuclear apocalypse, massive meteorite impact, nano-robot take-over, etc. ever came true. There are bacteria that can survive under extraordinary conditions of temperature (−12°C, 120°C), water and oxygen concentration (including none), salt concentration (up to 32%), radiation (up to 2000 times the lethal dose for humans), etc. The evolution of plants and animals would then presumably have to start all over again, which is an interesting thought. The question of whether it would be roughly similar or quite different seems to me one of the few reasons for going to the expense of looking for life on other planets. We saw in Chapter 2 how bacteria, in their role as chloroplasts and mitochondria, were the powerhouse for both plant and animal evolution – but suppose only the mitochondria managed it the second time round: could a world of animals without plants exist? There is material here for endless computer simulations. But assuming for the moment that this doomsday scenario doesn't materialize, let us end by looking at the more immediate prospect.

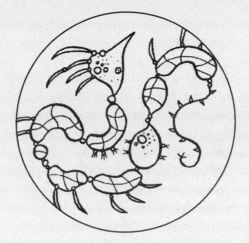

# 10 **A look ahead**

Human history . . . a race between education and catastrophe.
H. G. Wells

One last analogy: the host–pathogen relationship can be seen as a vast historical drama acted out simultaneously at a variety of different speeds and levels. In the remote distance, parasites and their hosts adjust to each other over millions of years, gradually reaching a mutually tolerable balance. In centre stage, on a scale of months, a pandemic rages across continents, pursued by drugs and vaccines. And at the front, pathogens battle from day to day to avoid elimination by the immune system for long enough to spread to another host. The script of the drama is by no means finished – indeed we are in the very middle of a period when new episodes are being added faster than ever before. By looking back at what has changed within living memory, perhaps it may be easier to imagine what might be coming next.

First the good news. Almost certainly there will be effective new vaccines and antibiotics. Measles, mumps, rubella, polio, and perhaps diphtheria and even leprosy, may be headed for extinction. With the mapping of the whole genome of all the major pathogens, a whole new range of targets for drugs should be identified. Given enough money and motivation, food and water supplies might reach adequate levels in the tropical world – though unfortunately research in this absolutely critical area does not have quite the glamour of drugs, genes, and vaccines. I am sure some herbal remedies will gradually come to be accepted in orthodox medical circles, while others will be shown to be useless. Either way, this would be progress. Perhaps the champions of positive thinking will convince the rest of us. The understanding of the immune system will no doubt improve by leaps and bounds, and my particular hope is that more attention will be paid to minor degrees of immunodeficiency, which might explain some of the individual differences in disease incidence and severity. Studies of the human genome will be most useful here. There is also the possibility of further slight improvements in our immune defences through evolution, as discussed in Chapter 5. But the bad news is a much longer list.

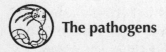 **The pathogens**

Since 1975, at least eight previously unknown pathogens have been identified: the bacteria causing Lyme disease, Legionnaire's disease, and gastric ulcer, two new hepatitis viruses, and three new herpesviruses. We can surely expect many more to come to light in the next quarter century. The problem of resistance to drugs has already been discussed; it is conceivable (though far from certain) that staphylococcal infection, tuberculosis, and malaria will one day be totally resistant to all antibiotics.

Equally worryingly, at least 20 viruses have crossed from animals to humans, with frequently fatal results. HIV is the only one of these *zoonoses* to have spread on a global scale, but there are also Lassa, Hanta, Ebola, Marburg, West Nile, Nipah, Hendra, Lyssa, monkeypox, the SARS coronavirus, avian flu, and several others capable of causing serious outbreaks – and there is no guarantee that one of them will not acquire a mutation that enables it to spread more widely. Although it is probably not a virus, we should include BSE/CJD. The chance of animal-to-human transfer is obviously increased where animal tissues are transplanted into humans, as is already happening with pig pancreas and brain cells (and large organ transplants have been proposed). So far no unwelcome viruses have been picked up from these procedures, but given the experience of HIV the risk seems rather terrifying. Once it happens, there may be no going back.

Then there are the *opportunists* which take advantage of the immunodeficient individuals, whose numbers are steadily rising because of AIDS, immunosuppressive drugs for transplantation, cancer, and immunopathological diseases, and better diagnosis and survival of children with primary immunodeficiencies. CMV, avian TB, *Pseudomonas*, *Pneumocystis*, *Candida*, *Cryptosporidium*, *Toxoplasma*, *Cryptococcus*, *Giardia*, and *Strongyloides* will in future have to be treated as dangerous pathogens. In the very long term, one could even imagine whole human populations with such reduced immune competence that these opportunists might have to reduce their own virulence in turn in order to survive along with their hosts. We want to live with our germs, but it would also pay them to live with us.

More alarming still are the totally new pathogens. Every time the flu virus plays its dangerous game of gene-shuffling, a potential pandemic is born. In 2003 a new respiratory disease, SARS, generated worldwide panic, again from a starting-point in China. It is caused by a variant of one of the common cold viruses, a coronavirus, probably of animal origin. As I write (2006), what may become an even more dangerous virus is threatening the Far East; this is the bird flu virus H5N1, which has been known since 1997 to be capable of infecting humans but may recently have acquired the ability to spread from human to human – a necessary step in giving rise to a pandemic.

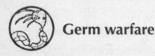 Germ warfare

Finally, there is the most frightening prospect of all: the deliberate use, or modification, of a pathogen for purposes of biological warfare. Several governments are known to have spent enormous sums on this, either (ostensibly) as a protective and monitoring measure (e.g. the US, the UK) or quite openly for aggressive purposes (e.g., at various times, Japan, Russia, South Africa, Iraq, North Korea). At least 25 pathogens have been considered as potential weapons, headed by anthrax, plague, smallpox, botulism, and the viral haemorrhagic fevers (see Table 10.1). In the case of smallpox, complete destruction of the few remaining stocks, which sounds at first like an excellent idea, would rule out the possibility of

**Table 10.1 Some candidate pathogens for biological warfare**

| Pathogen/disease | Type of organism | Comments |
|---|---|---|
| Anthrax | Bacterium | Easily spread; early treatment effective |
| Plague | " | " " |
| Tularaemia | " | " " |
| *Brucella* | " | Chronic but non-fatal |
| Botulism | " | Toxin more effective than organism |
| Q fever | Rickettsia | Usually non-fatal |
| Smallpox | Virus | Easily spread, but vaccine available |
| Ebola, Marburg | " | Easily spread; no treatment available |

ever learning anything more about the pathogen. The terrible 1918 flu virus was thought to have been lost for good, but the rescue of samples from frozen corpses is helping in the understanding of exactly what made it so virulent, which could make all the difference if and when we come face to face with another human-spread bird flu.

Anyway, with the current state of knowledge it would probably be possible to tailor-make a micro-organism to cause almost any desired kind of pathology, resistant to all drugs and vaccines. It might be as simple as creating a plasmid carrying a complete set of antibiotic and immune resistance genes, and allowing it to spread naturally; in fact precisely such a 'superplague' is said to have been manufactured in the Soviet Union. Or two viruses such as Ebola and Marburg could be genetically fused to make an even more lethal one. It might even be possible to construct pathogens that affect only certain ethnic groups. In fact the main stumbling block has proved to be the design of effective delivery methods. But anything a Hollywood scriptwriter can think up could probably be achieved in time, given sufficiently evil intent. And as with Internet viruses, it is extremely hard to see how such activities could be completely controlled without a 'thought police' of truly Orwellian proportions. On the other hand it would be virtually impossible to deliver such a pathogen to every single isolated community in the world, and unless the perpetrators were determined to die too, I do not see a real danger of total extinction by this route.

 **The host**

Human behaviour could undo some of the gains already made. The indiscriminate prescription of antibiotics ensures the spread of resistant strains of bacteria, while the threat of litigation deters doctors from withholding these drugs even when they consider them unnecessary. Their use in food plants and animals is a further stimulus to the emergence of resistance. Whether any international organization will be strong enough to stand up to vested interests in the food industry and the legal profession remains to be seen. Complacency, or active opposition, could lead to vaccine campaigns losing momentum unless – as they are in the US – enforced by law. The same goes for the maintenance of clean water, air, and food, which require constant monitoring and expense. When a new outbreak of infection occurs, it is tempting for embarrassed authorities to play down its importance or even deny its existence, delaying the start of proper methods of isolation and diagnosis, as happened with BSE in the UK and SARS in China. The huge increase in travel, especially by air, which means that an individual can board a tightly packed plane in South America, stop off in West Africa, and disembark in London, is a very efficient way of spreading pathogens to a population that is not prepared for them –

like a speeded-up replay of Cortez and the Aztecs. The 1999 outbreak of West Nile virus in New York and the spread of SARS to distant Toronto were chilling reminders of how fast a new pathogen can cross the world.

 **The planet**

One of the perils of *global warming* is likely to be the establishment of tropical diseases in countries from which they have long vanished. Mosquito-borne malaria and dengue are already creeping northward and southward from the tropics. Given the right temperature and the right strain of mosquitoes, there is no reason why malaria should not return to Northern Europe, in which case our immigrant populations, with their partial-resistance genes, might find themselves at an advantage. This is one ray of hope for the long term; human populations are genetically so diverse that whatever new infectious organism they are faced with, some of them somewhere will have the appropriate answer in their phagocytes, lymphocytes, and antibodies – as the Australian rabbits did to the myxomatosis virus. Could this genetic diversity be one reason why *Homo sapiens*, alone among hominids, succeeded in colonizing every corner of the globe – regularly confronted, as he must have been, by different animals and their pathogens? If enough DNA from Neanderthals is ever available, the analysis of their MHC diversity would be fascinating, because infectious diseases are often quoted as one possible reason for their extinction.

As for other planets, if we ever reach them and if life really did originate there, we shall be in for some real surprises. At the moment the main problem with space travel appears to be slightly decreased resistance in astronauts to our own pathogens on return. So while the future is highly unpredictable, I am reasonably confident that if the human race is wiped out it will not be by a 'normal' pathogen (but see Germ warfare, above).

 **Knowledge is power**

We can go further than this, I think. However much the battle with pathogens may look like going against us, we have one inestimably valuable weapon on our side: *intelligence*. Bacteria and viruses evolve fast, but human knowledge evolves faster still. We can identify problems, ask questions, do experiments, learn from the results, understand their meaning, and, if we are lucky, devise a solution – on a time-scale not of millions of years but of human lifetimes. Within two centuries of the first glimmerings of chemistry, Ehrlich had designed a drug that specifically killed the spirochaete of syphilis. A century after Jenner, Pasteur had shown that vaccines could be made to order, and Koch and Virchow had established the power of the microscope in diagnosis. Fifty years later, thanks to Gowans, Burnet, and the rest, a coherent picture of the immune system began to emerge.

Now, another fifty years on, microbiologists, immunologists, biochemists, molecular biologists, pharmacologists, geneticists, and mathematicians routinely collaborate to explore, computer-model, and manipulate every gene, every protein, every molecular angle and crevice of pathogen antigens and immune receptors, as virus, bacterium, protozoan, lymphocyte, and phagocyte yield up their innermost secrets. Each result, positive or negative, is a step forward and almost instantly accessible worldwide. This year's discovery is next year's undergraduate lecture. The age of hit-and-miss in the treatment and prevention of infectious disease is effectively over.

This does not mean that microbiology and immunology have become automated – that the scientist merely mans a machine. Far from it. Science is not like car manufacture. Of course scientists have to learn their trade and earn a living, often by teaching or hospital work or in an industrial research programme. But outside these duties they are free individuals in a world of ideas – closer to the artist than the factory worker. For me Koch, Pasteur, and Ehrlich are the Bach, Mozart, and Beethoven of infectious disease.

So, far from being 'time to close the book on infectious diseases', as that Surgeon General rashly declared, this is the best possible time for young scientists to enter the field. As I hope this book has shown, immense challenges still face them. But never before has there been available to help them so much technology and so much knowledge, and in the words of Francis Bacon – who did so much to establish the scientific method 400 years ago – 'knowledge is power'. Of course power can be a good or a bad thing, depending on who wields it. In the hands of deadly rivals, it can set progress back. And while it would be over-optimistic to say that scientific rivalry is, or ever will be, a thing of the past – it is, after all, one of the driving forces of progress – there are signs that it may be receding to more civilized proportions. It took two years to identify the virus of AIDS, in an atmosphere of mutual secrecy and suspicion; the virus of SARS was identified in 15 days, thanks to the firm insistence by the WHO that national laboratories should share their skills and resources. I have a feeling that this may turn out to be, in the words so beloved of politicians, 'a defining moment of the twenty-first century'. Today bird flu is being watched from minute to minute in the full glare of newspapers and television. Whatever the virus does, we shall have to find out how to live with it.

# Glossary and abbreviations

| | |
|---|---|
| **Adaptive** | (of immunity) Lymphocyte-based, showing high specificity and memory |
| **Aerobic** | Growing in the presence of oxygen |
| **Aerosol** | Airborne water droplet which may contain viruses, bacteria, etc. |
| **AIDS** | Acquired immune deficiency syndrome |
| **Allergy** | Pathological antibody response resulting in acute inflammation |
| **Amino acids** | The building blocks of proteins |
| **Anaerobic** | Growing in the absence of oxygen |
| **Anaphylaxis** | Extreme form of allergy, often resulting in shock |
| **Antibiotic** | Naturally occurring antimicrobial agent |
| **Antibody** | Lymphocyte-derived protein molecule contributing to immunity |
| **Antigen** | Portion of foreign object (e.g. pathogen) recognized by a lymphocyte |
| **Antitoxin** | Antibody preparation for neutralizing toxin |
| **APC** | Antigen-presenting cell |
| **Attenuated** | (of vaccine) Living but with absent or reduced pathogenicity |
| **Atypical** | (of bacteria) Lacking some component of normal bacteria |
| **Autoimmunity** | Immune response (cellular or humoral) against 'self' components |

| | |
|---|---|
| **Autosomal** | (of mutation) On a chromosome other than X or Y |
| **AZT** | Azidothymidine (also known as zidovudine) |
| **B cell** | Bone marrow-derived lymphocyte |
| **Bacillus** | Rod-shaped bacterium |
| **Bacteriophage** | Virus specialized for infecting bacteria |
| **BCG** | Bacille Calmette – Guérin (the attenuated TB vaccine) |
| **Biofilm** | Layer of bacteria growing as a unit |
| **BSE** | Bovine spongiform encephalopathy |
| **Capsule** | Anti-phagocytic outer coat, e.g. of bacterium, usually composed of sugars |
| **Carrier** | Symptomless individual infectious to others |
| **CD** | Cluster of differentiation; numbering system for cell surface molecules |
| **CDC** | Centers for Disease Control (USA) |
| **Cell** | The basic structural element of animals and plants |
| **Cellular** | (of immune response) Mediated by T lymphocytes but not antibody |
| **CGD** | Chronic granulomatous disease |
| **Chemotherapy** | (of infection) Treatment by natural or synthetic antimicrobials |
| **Chloroplast** | Organelle in plant cell containing respiratory enzymes |
| **Chromosome** | Structure along which a cell's genes are organized |
| **Cirrhosis** | Destruction of liver tissue by fibrosis |

| | |
|---|---|
| **CJD** | Creutzfeldt–Jakob disease |
| **Class** | (of antibody) Subdivision with particular biological function (see Ig) |
| **Clonal selection** | Mechanism by which lymphocytes responding to a particular antigen are expanded into a larger number (originally a *theory*) |
| **CMV** | Cytomegalovirus |
| **Coccus** | Spherical bacterium |
| **Combining site** | (of antibody) Region that binds to antigen and defines specificity |
| **Complement** | Series of serum proteins involved in immune defence |
| **Complex** | (immune-) Combination of antigen and antibody |
| **Cyst** | (e.g. of protozoa, worm) Hollow structure facilitating survival |
| **Cytokine** | Molecule mediating cellular interactions in the immune system |
| **Cytopathic** | Causing damage to cells |
| **Cytoplasm** | Contents of cell, other than the nucleus |
| **Cytotoxic** | Able to kill cells; also a subdivision of T lymphocytes, usually carrying CD8 molecules |
| **DNA** | Deoxyribonucleic acid; genetic material, composed of nucleotides |
| **Dominant** | (of mutation) Producing effect in single dose |
| **DPT** | The triple diphtheria–pertussis–tetanus vaccine |

| | |
|---|---|
| **Dysentery** | Diarrhoea containing blood |
| **EBV** | Epstein–Barr virus |
| **Endemic** | (of infection) Constantly present in a population |
| **Endotoxin** | Toxin released by dead organism, usually bacterium |
| **Enzyme** | A protein that catalyses a particular chemical reaction |
| **Eosinophil** | A white blood cell containing granules toxic to, e.g., worms |
| **Epidemic** | (of infection) Occurring at an unusually high frequency |
| **ER** | Endoplasmic reticulum; a membrane system in eukaryotic cells |
| **Exotoxin** | Toxin secreted by living organism, usually bacterium |
| **Eukaryote** | Single or multi-cellular nucleated organism, e.g. protozoan, mammal |
| **Fibrosis** | Replacement of normal tissue structure by fibres of, e.g., collagen |
| **Fimbria** | (pl. fimbriae) Bacterial attachment organ similar to pili |
| **Flagellum** | (pl. flagella) Thread-like organ of, e.g., bacterial movement |
| **Gene** | Unit of heredity, composed of DNA |
| **Genome** | The total of all genes in the cell or animal |
| **Germ-line** | (of mutation) In sperm or ova and therefore inherited |
| **Germ theory** | Theory proposed by Koch that microbes caused specific diseases |

| | |
|---|---|
| **Granuloma** | Chronic inflammatory focus mainly composed of macrophages |
| **Helminth** | A name covering the parasitic classes of worms |
| **Helper cell** | Subdivision of T lymphocytes that activate B lymphocytes, macrophages, etc. by secreting cytokines; usually carries CD4 molecules |
| **Herd immunity** | Freedom from infection of the unprotected minority in a mainly immune population |
| **HIB** | Haemophilus influenzae type B |
| **HIV** | Human immunodeficiency virus (two types, HIV-1 and HIV-2) |
| **Hormone** | Molecule regulating cell functions, e.g. insulin, thyroxin |
| **HSV** | Herpes simplex virus (two types, HSV-1 and HSV-2) |
| **Humoral** | (of immune response) Mediated by antibody |
| **Hybrid vigour** | Improved qualities produced by crossing two different strains |
| **IFN** | Interferon |
| **Ig** | Immunoglobulin (e.g. IgM, IgG) |
| **IL** | Interleukin (e.g. IL-1, IL-2) |
| **Immune** | (to a pathogen) Resistant to infection (to an antigen) Able to mount an enhanced response |
| **Immune complex** | see Complex |
| **Immunity** | State of being immune |
| **Immunize** | To induce immunity, e.g. by vaccination |

| | |
|---|---|
| **Immunoglobulin** | Synonymous with antibody (see Ig) |
| **Immunopathology** | Tissue damage caused by the immune system |
| **Inflammation** | Local tissue response to injury or infection, with increased blood flow and pain |
| **Innate** | (of immunity) Unchanging, non-lymphocyte-based |
| **Interferon** | Family of antiviral cytokines |
| **Interleukin** | Numbered member of the cytokine family (see IL) |
| *In vitro* | In laboratory culture (literally: 'in glass') |
| *In vivo* | In the living animal |
| **Latent** | (e.g. of virus) Persistent but symptomless |
| **Lipid** | Fat-based, water-insoluble molecule |
| **LPS** | Lipopolysaccharide, the major bacterial endotoxin |
| **Lymphatic** | Vessel transmitting fluid and lymphocytes from tissues to lymph nodes |
| **Lymphocyte** | White cell of blood, the cell of adaptive immunity |
| **Lysis** | Damage-induced leakage of cell contents |
| **Lysosome** | Intracellular vesicle containing killing and digestive material |
| **Lysozyme** | An enzyme in blood, tears, and saliva that kills some bacteria |

| | |
|---|---|
| **Macrophage** | Large phagocytic cell, mainly found in tissues |
| **Mast cell** | Tissue cell containing inflammatory mediators |
| **MDR** | (e.g. of tuberculosis) Multiple-drug-resistant |
| **Memory** | (in immunology) Ability to respond more vigorously to a second identical stimulus |
| **Meninges** | Lining layer between skull and brain |
| **Messenger RNA** | RNA carrying information to make protein |
| **Metabolic** | Related to biochemical processes in the cell |
| **MHC** | Major histocompatibility complex, a set of highly diverse genes; MHC molecules are responsible for transport of intracellular proteins for recognition by T lymphocytes (and thus also for graft rejection) |
| **Miasma** | Hypothetical medium transmitting infection (before germ theory) |
| **Mitochondrion** | Intracellular organelle containing respiratory enzymes |
| **MMR** | The triple measles–mumps–rubella vaccine |
| **Molecule** | Chemical unit of (in biology) protein, carbohydrate, or fat |
| **Monoclonal** | (of antibody) Produced by a single clone of identical B lymphocytes |
| **mRNA** | see Messenger RNA |

| | |
|---|---|
| **MRSA** | Methicillin- (or multiple-) resistant *Staphylococcus aureus* |
| **MTB** | Occasional abbreviation for *Mycobacterium tuberculosis* |
| **Mutation** | Inheritable change in DNA |
| **Mycosis** | Fungal infection |
| **Natural selection** | Evolution based on mutation and survival of fittest variants |
| **Network** | In immunology, a set of interacting cells or molecules (e.g. cytokines) |
| **Neutropaenia** | Low or absent level of neutrophils in the blood |
| **Neutrophil** | see PMN |
| **NK cell** | Natural killer cell |
| **Normal flora** | The microbial contents of the normal body (intestine, skin, etc.) |
| **Nucleic acids** | see DNA and RNA |
| **Nucleolus** | Structure within nucleus, rich in RNA |
| **Nucleotide** | A single unit of a nucleic acid (purine or pyrimidine) |
| **Nucleus** | Membrane-bound region of eukaryotic cell containing chromosomes |
| **Opportunist** | Organism pathogenic only in immunodeficient host |
| **Opsonin** | Molecule capable of enhancing phagocytosis, e.g. antibody, complement |
| **PAMP** | Pathogen-associated molecular pattern |
| **Pandemic** | A worldwide epidemic |

| | |
|---|---|
| **Parasite** | A living organism depending on another for some or all of its requirements. |
| **Passage** | (pronounced as in French) A cycle of growth *in vitro* or *in vivo* during, e.g., the attenuation of a vaccine |
| **Passive** | (of immunity) Transferred from another source, e.g. by serum |
| **Pathogen** | Parasite that causes disease |
| **Peptide** | Molecule composed of two or more amino acids |
| **Phagocytosis** | Ingestion of particles by, e.g., protozoan or phagocytic cell |
| **Pilus** | (pl. pili) Thread-like bacterial attachment organ |
| **Plasma** | Blood minus cells |
| **Plasmid** | Non-chromosomal DNA, e.g. in bacterium |
| **PMN** | Polymorphonuclear neutrophil, the major phagocytic cell of blood |
| **Polymorph** | see PMN |
| **Polymorphism** | Coexistence in a population of two or more versions of the same gene |
| **Polysaccharide** | Complex sugar molecule |
| **Primary** | (of immune response) Following first contact with antigen (of immunodeficiency) Genetically determined |
| **Prion** | Infectious particle containing protein only (see BSE, CJD) |

| | |
|---|---|
| **Prokaryote** | Single-celled organism without nucleus, e.g. bacterium |
| **Prostaglandins** | Family of small lipid molecules involved in inflammation |
| **Protein** | Molecule composed of amino acids and coded in DNA |
| **Purine** | One type of nucleotide (pyrimidine is the other type) |
| **Receptor** | Molecule on cell surface to which virus, cytokine, etc. binds |
| **Recessive** | (of mutation) Producing an effect only in double dose |
| **Recognition** | (by immune cell or molecule) Specific binding |
| **Recombinant** | (of DNA) Combined from two or more sources |
| **Reservoir** | (of infection) Alternative (e.g. animal) source of infection |
| **Retrovirus** | RNA virus able to insert DNA into host cell genome |
| **Reverse transcriptase** | An enzyme used by retroviruses to transcribe their RNA into DNA |
| **Ribosome** | Site of protein synthesis from messenger RNA template |
| **RNA** | Ribonucleic acid; intermediary between DNA and protein synthesis, composed of nucleotides |
| **RSV** | Respiratory syncytial virus |
| **SARS** | Severe acute respiratory syndrome |
| **SCID** | Severe combined immune deficiency |

| | |
|---|---|
| **Secondary** | (of immune response) Following second or later contact with antigen (of immunodeficiency) Environmentally caused |
| **Self** | (of antigen) Derived from host |
| **Septicaemia** | Invasion of the bloodstream, usually by bacteria |
| **Serum** | Blood minus cells and clotting factors |
| **Sex-linked** | (of disease) Occurring in one sex only; see X-linked |
| **Shock** | Vascular collapse, with low blood pressure and often organ failure |
| **SIV** | Simian immunodeficiency virus |
| **Somatic** | (of mutation) In cell other than germ-line; not inherited |
| **Specific** | In immunology, denoting restriction to one or a few antigens |
| **Spleen** | Large abdominal organ with haematological and immune functions |
| **Spore** | Resistant resting form of bacteria or fungi |
| **Staph** | Common abbreviation for staphylococcus |
| **Stem cell** | Cell able to give rise to many or all other cell types |
| **Strain** | Genetically identical subdivision of a species (e.g. mouse, staphylococcus) |
| **Strep** | Common abbreviation for streptococcus |
| **Symbiosis** | Association between living organisms beneficial to both |

| | |
|---|---|
| **T cell** | Thymus-derived lymphocyte |
| **Taxonomy** | Science by which living organisms are classified |
| **TGF** | Transforming growth factor, a mainly inhibitory cytokine |
| **Thymus** | Lymphoid organ in neck, the source of T lymphocytes |
| **TNF** | Tumour necrosis factor, an inflammatory cytokine |
| **Tolerance** | (in immunology) Unresponsiveness to a normally antigenic stimulus |
| **Toxin** | Microbial product, usually protein, able to damage host cells |
| **Toxoid** | Inactivated toxin able to induce immunity |
| **TSST** | Toxic shock syndrome toxin |
| **Vaccine** | A preparation able to induce immunity, usually a killed or attenuated micro-organism or portion thereof |
| **Vacuole, Vesicle** | Membrane-bound, fluid-containing intracellular structure |
| **Vector** | (of pathogens) Transmitting insect or animal<br>(of genes) Transmitting element, e.g. plasmid, bacteriophage |
| **Vibrio** | A group of curved bacteria, of which *V. cholerae* causes human disease (cholera) |
| **Virulence** | Ability of a pathogen to survive in and/ or damage host |
| **VZV** | Varicella–zoster virus, the virus of chickenpox and shingles |

| **WHO** | World Health Organization, based in Geneva |
| **Wild-type** | Normal or predominant (e.g. not mutant) type of organism |
| **X-linked** | (of disease) Due to mutation on X chromosome |
| **Zoonosis** | Animal disease which can affect humans |

# Biographies

**Some important scientists mentioned in the text.**

**Behring, Emil Von** (1854–1917). German bacteriologist and immunologist. Nobel Prize 1901 for work on diphtheria and tetanus antitoxins.

**Bruton, Colonel Ogden** (1908– ). American paediatrician. Agammaglobulinaemia 1951.

**Burkitt, Denis** (1911–93). British surgeon. Extensive practice in Africa. Burkitt's lymphoma 1957.

**Burnet, Sir Frank Macfarlane** (1899–1985). Australian virologist and immunologist. Clonal selection theory 1959, Nobel Prize 1960.

**Calmette, Albert** (1863–1933). French bacteriologist, With **Guérin** produced BCG vaccine for tuberculosis (1906 bovine, 1924 human).

**Chain, Sir Ernest** (1906–79). German-British chemist. At Oxford, with **Florey,** purified penicillin 1941. Nobel Prize 1945.

**Creutzfeld, Hans** (1885–1964). German neuropathologist. With Jakob first described Dementia named after them 1920.

**Crick, Francis** (1916– ). English molecular biologist. DNA structure with Watson, 1953. Nobel Prize 1962.

**Dawkins, Richard** (1941– ). English zoologist and religious sceptic, Oxford. Proponent of 'selfish gene' theory.

**Di George, Angelo** (1921– ). American paediatrician. Thymus and cellular immunity 1965.

**Doherty, Peter** (1940– ). Australian immunologist. Role of MHC in cell collaboration, with Zinkernagel. Nobel Prize 1996.

**Ehrlich, Paul** (1854–1915). German medical scientist. Breslau, Berlin, Frankfurt. Histological staining, toxins and antitoxins, chemotherapy. Nobel Prize 1908, Salvarsan for syphilis 1910.

**Fleming, Sir Alexander** (1881–1955). Scottish bacteriologist. Worked in London. Typhoid vaccines, lysozyme, penicillin 1928. Nobel prize 1945.

**Florey, Sir Howard** (1898–1968). Australian pathologist. At Oxford, with **Chain,** purified penicillin 1941. Nobel Prize 1945.

**Gajdusek, Carleton** (1923– ). Slovak-American paediatrician. Studies on Kuru. Nobel prize 1976.

**Good, Robert** (1922– ). American paediatrician. Thymus and immunodeficiency.

**Gowans, Sir James** (1924– ). British experimental pathologist. Role of lymphocyte 1959.

**Guérin, Jean Marie** (1872–1961). French bacteriologist (see **Calmette**).

**Hooke, Robert** (1635–1703). English chemist/physicist. Microscopy 1662, also many physical discoveries.

**Jakob, Alfons** (1884–1931). German neurologist (see **Creutzfeldt**).

**Jenner, Edward** (1749–1823). English physician. Smallpox vaccine 1796.

**Kitasato, Shibasabura** (1852–1931). Japanese bacteriologist. Worked with Ehrlich and Von Behring in Berlin on antitoxins. First identified plague bacillus.

**Koch, Robert** (1843–1910). German bacteriologist. Wollstein, Berlin. Confirmed bacterial cause of anthrax, tuberculosis, cholera. Extensive travels in Africa. Nobel prize 1905.

**Koprowski, Hilary** (1916– ). Polish-American virologist. Oral polio vaccine 1950.

**Leeuwenhoek, Antoni Van** (1632–1723). Dutch microscopist 1671.

**Lister, Joseph Lord** (1827–1912). British surgeon. Introduced antiseptic surgery.

**Mantoux, Charles** (1877–1947). French physician. Intradermal tuberculin test for TB 1908.

**Medawar, Sir Peter** (later Lord) (1915–87). British zoologist and immunologist. London. Immunological tolerance. Nobel Prize 1960.

**Metchnikoff, Ilya** (1845–1916). Russian biologist. Phagocytosis 1882.

**Miller, Jacques** (1931– ). French-Australian immunologist. Role of thymus, 1961.

**Pasteur, Louis** (1822–95). French chemist, microbiologist. Strasbourg, Lille, Paris. Crystal structure, alcohol fermentation, silkworm diseases, anthrax, rabies vaccines. Disproved 'spontaneous generation' of bacteria. Pasteur Institute 1888.

**Pauling, Linus** (1901–94). American chemist. Instructive theory of antibody. Nobel Prizes 1954 (chemistry), 1962 (peace).

**Petternkofer, Max Von** (1818–1901). German chemist and hygienist. Quarrel with Koch over cholera germ theory.

**Prusiner, Stanley** (1942–   ). American neurologist. Prion theory. Nobel Prize 1997.

**Roitt, Ivan** (1927–   ). British immunologist. Autoantibodies in thyroiditis.

**Roux, Emile** (1853–1933). French bacteriologist. Diphtheria toxin 1894.

**Sabin, Albert** (1906–93). American microbiologist. Live oral polio vaccine 1959.

**Salk, Jonas** (1914–95). American virologist. Killed polio vaccine 1953.

**Schwann, Theodor** (1810–82). German physiologist and pioneer of cell theory.

**Snow, John** (1813–58). English epidemiologist. Cholera spread by water 1848. Anaesthetized Queen Victoria 1853.

**Spallanzani, Lazzaro** (1729–99). Italian biologist and early opponent of 'spontaneous generation' theory.

**Thomas, Lewis** (1913–93). American physician and essayist.

**Virchow, Rudolf** (1821–1902). German pathologist, politician, anthropologist. Cell theory 1858.

**Watson, James** (1928–   ). American geneticist. DNA structure with **Crick**, 1953. Nobel Prize 1962.

**Wright, Sir Edward Almroth** (1861–1947). English bacteriologist. Typhoid vaccine 1897, opsonins.

**Zinkernagel, Rolf** (1944–   ). Swiss immunologist. Basel, Canberra, Zurich. Role of MHC in cell collaboration (with Doherty). Nobel Prize 1996.

# Suggested further reading

**Infectious disease: general**

McNeill, William H. "Plagues and people"
  Basil Blackwell, Oxford 1977
  A historian's view. Scholarly, but a little out of date now.
Waller, John "The discovery of the germ"
  I Can Books, UK 2002   197 pp
  Very detailed and accurate. By a Wellcome historian.
Scientific American (eds) "Understanding germ warfare"
  Warner Books, New York 2002   132 pp
  Sixteen short update articles on infection, vaccines, drugs.
    The title is misleading; it is *not* only about
    bioterrorism.
Wilkins, Robert "The fireside book of deadly diseases"
  Robert Hale, London 1994
  Good stories in a racy style, with some lurid pictures.
Madigan, M. T., Martinko, J. M. & Parker, J. "Brock: biology of
microorganisms"
  Pearson Education, 10th edn 2003
  My favourite microbiology textbook (American).
    Very comprehensive, but for the serious student
    only.
Mims, C. A., Nash, A. & Stephen, J. "The pathogenesis of infectious
disease"
  Academic Press, 5th edn 2001
  Another excellent student-level textbook, concentrating on
    disease mechanisms rather than organisms.

Ayliffe, G. A. J. & English, M. P. "Hospital infection: from miasma to MRSA"
   Cambridge University Press, 2003    274 pp
   A thorough history of the subject.

## Viruses

Crawford, Dorothy H. "The invisible enemy"
   OUP 2000    275 pp
   A natural history of viruses. Vivid, with plenty of fascinating
      background stories.
Oldstone, Michael B. A. "Viruses, plague, and history"
   OUP 1998    227 pp
   Detailed and authoritative, though not very lively.
McCormick, Joseph B., Fischer-Hoch, Susan "The virus hunters"
   Bloomsbury 1996    379 pp
   Category 4 viruses in an exciting autobiographical setting by CDC
      staff.

## Bacteria

Dormandy, Thomas "The white death"
   The Hambledon Press 1999    433 pp
   A magisterial discussion of TB in all its aspects by a world expert.
      Good bibliography.
Postgate, John R. "Microbes and man"
   Cambridge University Press, 3rd edn 1992    295 pp
   Mainly about bacteria, medical and non-medical. A classic for
      many years.
Cantor, Norman F. "In the wake of the plague"
   Simon & Schuster, London 2001    245 pp
   The 1347 epidemic and its effects.

Porter, Stephen "The great plague"
  Sutton Publishing, Stroud 2003    170 pp
  A thorough historical account of the 1665 epidemic.


## Other pathogens

Zimmer, Carl "Parasite rex"
  The Free Press, NY 2000    298 pp
  By an American science writer. Detailed and sensational.
    Includes protozoal and worm diseases.
Rhodes, Richard "Deadly feasts"
  Touchstone Books 1998    278 pp
  CJD and prion diseases – a little out of date now.


## Immunology

Baxter, Alan G. "Germ warfare. Breakthroughs in immunology"
  Allen & Unwin, St Leonards, NSW, Australia 2000    220 pp
  A detailed history of immunology, with numerous biographies,
    from an Australian viewpoint. Again, the title is
    misleading.
Frank, Steven A. "Immunology and evolution of infectious disease"
  Princeton University Press 2002    348 pp
  A detailed, critical, and up-to-date account of the role of mutation
    in antibody and pathogen molecules. Heavy going for the
    non-scientist.
Rabin, Bruce S. "Stress, immune function, and health. The
connection"
  Wiley-Liss, New York 1999    341 pp
  A calm non-sensational appraisal to a controversial subject.

Goldsby, R. A., Kindt, T. J., Osborne, B. A. & Kuby, J. "Immunology"
WH Freeman 5th edn 2003
A comprehensive textbook, for students only. There are many
others, mostly excellent, but the non-expert will find the
language difficult.

## Vaccines

Ada, Gordon & Isaacs, David "Vaccination. The facts, the fears, the
future"
Allen & Unwin, St Leonards, NSW, Australia 2000   241 pp
A comprehensive and accurate account by Australian experts in
the field.
Bakalar, Nicholas "Where the germs are. A scientific safari"
John Wiley & Sons, Hoboken 2003   262 pp
A useful chapter on vaccines.

## Antibiotics

Mann, John "The elusive magic bullet"
OUP, Oxford 1999   209 pp
A scholarly and detailed history of antimicrobial drugs.
Rocco, Fiametta "The miraculous fever-tree"
HarperCollins 2003   348 pp
Everything you could possibly want to know about quinine and
malaria – a literary as well as a scientific delight.
Shnayerson, Michael & Plotkin, Mark "The killers within"
Time Warner Books UK 2003   328 pp
A thorough, detailed, up-to-date account of antibiotic resistance.
Chaitow, Leon "The antibiotic crisis"
Thorsons 1998   233 pp
A good review of microbial resistance.

McKenna, John "Alternatives to antibiotics"
    Gill & Macmillan, Dublin 1996    155 pp
    The case for herbal treatment, by a herbal practitioner.
Buhner, Stephen Harold "Herbal antibiotics"
    Newleaf 2000    135 pp
    Herbs as wonder drugs.


## Germ warfare

Mangold, Tom & Goldberg, Jeff "Plague wars"
    Pan/Macmillan, London 1999    402 pp
    A detailed and well-researched history of biological warfare
Barnaby, Wendy "The plague makers"
    Continuum, NY 2000    208 pp


## General interest

Porter, Roy "The greatest benefit to mankind"
    Fontana Press, London 1997    833 pp
    The classic monumental history of medicine – probably the best
        ever written.
Loudon, Irvine (ed.) "Western medicine. An illustrated history"
    OUP, Oxford 1997    347 pp
    Nineteen chapters by experts. Excellent.
Fortey, Richard "Life. An unauthorised biography"
    Flamingo, London 1998    399 pp
    A personal and highly readable account of 4 billion years of
        evolution by a leading palaeontologist.
Thomas, Lewis "The wonderful mistake: notes of a biology watcher"
    OUP, Oxford 1988    291 pp
    Meditations on biology, including infection, by an American
        poet/immunologist – full of odd facts and insights.

Sontag, Susan "Illness as metaphor" and "AIDS and its metaphors" (Farrar, Strauss & Giroux)/ Penguin 1991   180 pp
  TB, cancer, AIDS as seen by a non-scientist. Scholarly but rather wordy.

# Index

Note: page references in **bold** indicate figures or tables.

acne 28
actinomyces **22**, 39, 62, **229**
activation 131, 151, 171
agammaglobulinaemia 194–5, 233
AIDS 6, 48, 60–1, **68**, 130, 187–8
    immunosuppression and 149–50
allergies 62, 167, 168–9, 218
    skin testing for 179–80
Alzheimer's disease 67
amoebae 54, 59
anaphylactic shock 168
ancylostoma 65
anthrax 34, 183, 207, 244
antibacterial drugs 228–9
antibiotics 225–37
    resistance to 231–3
    toxicity of 230–1
antibody 81, 85, 106–9
    avoidance 152
    classes 107–8
    horses and 222–3
    monoclonal 224
    production of 123–7, **127**
    structure **107**
antigenic drift 145, 146
antigenic shift 144–6, **146**, **147**
antigenic variation 145, 146
antigens 107, 173, 213
antitoxins 81, 222–3
antiviral drugs 234–5

APCs 115
artemisin 236
arthritis 185
ascaris 63, 65
aspergillus 164, 192
athlete's foot 60
attenuation 209–11
Austen, Jane 30, 109
autism 216
autoantibodies 173, 174–6
autoimmunity 14, 130, 144, 167,
        173–6
autotoxicity 176

Bacon, Francis 249
bacteria 19–20, **21**, **22**
    nomenclature 27
    pathogenic 26
    probiotic 25
    reproduction 22
    survival 240
bacteriophages 52
balanced polymorphism 57, 193
BCG 210–11, 219
Benveniste, Jacques 169
Berlin, Irving 187
beer 62
bilharzia 63
biofilms 153
biological warfare 34

bird flu 48, 145, 221–2, 244
birds 103
black death 35–6
blastomycosis 37, 61
bone marrow 103
bordetella 30, 78, 211
borrelia 36
botulism 31–2, 244
brain 119
bread 62
breast-feeding 206
brucellosis 36, 161–2
Bruton, Ogden 188, 194
BSE 66
Bulgakov, Mikhail 32
Burkitt, Denis 199
Burkitt's lymphoma 46, 51, 199–200
Burnet, Macfarlane 101, 103, 174,
        177, 231

Caffa, siege of 205
Calmette, Albert 210
campylobacter 175
cancer 44, 51
candida 60
capsule **21**, 88, 139, 213
carbon 88
carriers 158, 221
catalase 139
cats 57, 122–3
CD4, CD8 128–30
cells 20–3
    bacterial **21**, 21–3
    membranes 21, 229–30
    NK 117, 152
    walls 21, 228–9
Chagas' disease 58

Chain, Ernst 228
Chapin, Charles V. vi
chemotherapy 225–37
    alternatives 233–4
    anti-bacterial 228–9
    anti-fungal 235
    anti-helminthic (anti-worm)
        236–7
    anti-protozoal 235–6
    anti-viral 234–5
    resistance to 231–3
    toxicity of 230–1
chickenpox 44, 46
China 48, 63, 208
chlamydia 38, 163
chloramphenicol 230
chloroplast 23
chloroquine 236
cholera 32, 183
chromosomes 21
chronic fatigue syndrome 47
chronic granulomatous disease
        (CGD) 192
chronic infections 140
cirrhosis 49, 175, 181
CJD 66
clones (lymphocytes) 100–1, 116
clonal deletion 174
clonal selection **101**, 101–2, 114–15,
        174, 173
clostridia 31–2
CMV 47
coccidioides 61
cold sores 44, 47
colds 52, 235
collaboration 91–2, 121–2, 130–1
combining sites 99, 106–7

communication 80, 92
communication molecules 124, 126,
    131
complement 90–1, **91**, 140
    deficiency 191–2
concealment 142–3
congenital infection **73**
coronavirus 48–9
cowpox 208
Creutzfeldt-Jacob disease 66
Crohn's disease 185
cryptosporidia 57
cyclic neutropaenia 192
cyclosporin 201
cystic fibrosis 76, 191
cysts 143
cytokines 112, 126–7, 131–5, 152–3,
    172, 193
cytomegalovirus (CMV) 47, 175
cytopathic virus 162–3
cytoplasm **24**
cytotoxicity 112, **113**, 113–14

decoy molecules 140–1, **142**, 152–3
defence analogy 12, 74–5
Defoe, Daniel 35
deletion 114–15
dengue 50, 247
Di George, Angelo 188
Di George syndrome 194
diphtheria 33, 45
disease, acquisition 15
disposal 80
DNA 20, 43
dogs 36, 50–1, 65–6
Doherty, Peter 110
dracunculus 64–5

*Dr Ehrlich's Magic Bullet* (film) 227
dysentery 33, 59

EB (Epstein-Barr) virus 46–7, 51,
    175
Ebola fever 50, 172
echinococcus 65–6, 143
Ehrlich, Paul 6, 37, 82, 89, 96–7,
    121, 173, 227
elephantiasis 64
endemics 47
endosymbiosis 23
endotoxins 163, 165–6
entamoebae 54, 59, 164
eosinophils 89
epidemics 47
escherichia (E)coli 33
eukaryotes 23–4, 54
exotoxins 163–4, **164**

faecal-oral spread 59, 63, **70**
*Fantastic Voyage* (film) 13
farmer's lung 62
fevers 36
fibrosis 181
filarial worms 64
fimbria 21
flagellum 21
fleas 35
Fleming, Alexander 6–27, 216
Florey, Howard 228
flu, *see* bird flu; influenza
Fortey, Richard 106
fungi 60–2

Gajdusek, Carleton 67
gastric ulcer 33

gastro-enteritis 49
gene therapy 53, 194
genes 133-6
    immunodeficiency in 189-93
germ-free animals 239-40
germ theory 34, 203
germ warfare 244-6, **245**
German measles 45, 46
giardia 59
glandular fever 46
global warming 247
God, disease from 35, 205
gonococcus 76
gonorrhoea 37
Good, Robert 103
Gowans, James 95
granulomas 170-2
Guerin, Camille 210
Guillain-Barre syndrome 175
guinea worm 64-5
gulf war syndrome 217

haemoflagellates 57
haemophilus 30-1, 213
Hansen, Armauer 35
helicobacter 33, 76
hepatitis 51, 172
    carriers 44, 49, 158, 172
    viruses 49
herbal antibiotics 236, 238-9
herd immunity 46, 217
hereditary angioedema 192
heredity 20
herpesviruses 44, 46-7, 140-1,
        152-3
H5N1 (bird flu) 48, 145, 221-2, 244
histoplasma 61

HIV 48, 149-50, 155, 234-5
    variation in 145
homoeopathy 168-9
Hooke, Robert 205
hookworms 65
hormones 131
horror autotoxicus 130, 173
hybrid vigour 178
hydatid disease 65-6, 168
hydrogen peroxide 139
hypogammaglobulinaemia 195

immune complex 169-70, 192
immunity 77, 108, 109, **118**
    adaptive 85, 98, 105, 114, 119,
        141-53, 166-78, 193-6
    cellular 102, 151
    evolution 105
    herd 46, 217
    humoral 102, 151
    innate 84, 86-93, 138-41, 191-3
    misdirected 151-2
    passive 223
    stimulation of 197-8
    suppression 149-50, 199
immunodeficiency 15, 38, 48, **73**,
        187-203
    environmental 196-203
    genetic 189-93
    incidence 188-9
    primary, treatment of 195-6
immunoglobulin (Ig)
    IgA 108, 195
    IgD 108
    IgE 108, 168, 195
    IgG 108
    IgM 108, 115, 195

immunology, history of 81–3
immunopathology 167, 231
immunosuppression **73**, 199
    AIDS and 149–50
    drugs 201
infections 140, 175, **182**, 199–200
    germ theory of 34
    recovery from 181–3
    spread of **73**
inflammation 79, 161–2, 171
influenza 47, 148
    variation 144–6, **146**
information transfer **24**
interferon 92–3, 117, 131, 140, **142**,
        170, 234
interleukins 131, 132, 161, 165
iron 197

jaundice 49
Jefferson, Thomas 204
Jenner, Edward vi, 16, 81, 208
Jesty, Benjamin 208

kidney failure 170, 201
kidney transplants 177
Kitasato, Shibasaburo 81
Koch, Robert 17, 28–9, 32, 34, 183,
        205, 211
Koprowski, Hilary 212
kuru 66

Lassa fever 50, 223
lazy leucocyte syndrome 192
Lederberg, Joshua 231
Leeuwenhoek, Anton van 205
legionella 31
leishmania 57, 58, 104

leprosy 35, 151
life, requirements for 20, 40
lipopolysaccharides (LPS) 87, 165
Lister, Joseph 225
listeria 38
lyme disease 36
lymph nodes 95
lymphocytes 85, 94–104
    and antibody production 124–7,
        130
    B 103–4, 105–6, 113, 115, 194
    defective, development of 193–4
    specificity of 96–8
    T 98, 103–4, 108, 109–13, 114–15
        in AIDS 150
        cytotoxic **113**, 128–30, 172
        deficiency 194
        and granulomas 170–2
        helper **127**, 128, 130, 149
lysis **91**, 191–2
lysosome **24**, 86
lysozyme 76, 78, 229

macrophages 61, 89, 127, **129**
magic bullet 227
malaria 7, 54–6, 58–9
    deaths **68**
    drugs for 236
    immunity to 156–7
    immunosuppression by 199
    life cycle 54–5, **56**
    as therapy 37
malnutrition 196–9
Mantoux test 29
Marburg disease 50
mast cells 168, 169
measles 13, 45, 46

Medawar, Peter 103, 174
memory 85
meningitis 31
meningococcus 31, 37
Metchnikoff, Ilya 81, 84, 176
MHC 24, 111–12, 113, 117, 125, 129
    and transplants 177
Miller, Jacques 103
mimicry 143–4
misdirected immunity 151–2
mitochondria 23, 175
MMR vaccine 216, 219
monkeypox 45
monoclonal antibodies 224
mosquitoes 49, 55–6, 58–9
moulds 60
MRSA 27, 233
MTB 28–9
mumps 45
Mussolini, Benito 58–9
mutation 22, 99–100, 145, 174,
    189–90
    and vaccines 209–11
mycobacteria 35, 170–1
mycoplasma 39, 163
mycoses 60
myocarditis 175

natural killer (NK) cells 117, 152
neisseria 31, 37, 152, 192
neurotoxins 32
Nightingale, Florence 206

onchocerca 64
opportunistic organisms 38, 60, 65,
    73, 157–8, 243–4
opsonins 81, 91

pandemics 47, 48
Papermaster, Ben 105
papilloma virus 51
paracoccidioides 61
paralysis 32
paramecium 54
parasites 8, 8–10, 38, 142–3
Parkinson's disease 67
Pasteur, Louis 17, 19, 34, 50–1, 81,
    208–9
pathogens 2, 8, 8–9, 12
    associated patterns (PAMPS)
        88
    categories 207
    escape 138–9, 154
    intracellular 109
    invasive 78
    new 244
    non-invasive 78–9
    spread 68–73
    survival strategies 138–9, 154
pathology 10–11
Pauling, Linus 102
penicillin 30, 62, 227
    resistance 232
Persian chessboard 116
phagocytes 81, 84, 86–8, 192
phagocytosis 86, 87, 89
pili 21, 37
pinta 37
plague 35–6, 244
plasma cells 106
plasmids 21, 40, 52–3, 232, 245
plasmodium 54–5
pneumococci 30, 148
pneumocystis 61
pneumonia 30–1, 39, 181

polio 45, 146
    vaccines 212
polyclonal activation 151
polymorphs (PMNs) 89, 95
poxviruses 141, 153
presentation 115–16
primary biliary cirrhosis 175
prions 66–7
prokaryotes 23
prostaglandins 162
protozoa 53–60, 235
Prusiner, Stanley 67
pseudomonas 38
psittacosis 39
psychoneuroimmunology 202–3
public health 205–7
PUO 161

quinine 236

rabies 50–1, 208–9
receptors **24**, 41–2, 88, 96–8, **97**,
        116, 128
    diversity of 98–100
    senses and 119–20
recognition 80, 113
recovery 181–3
relapsing fever 36, 49
replacement therapy 195
reproduction 11
retroviruses **43**
rickettsia 38, 163
ringworm 60, 61
river blindness 64
RNA 20, 43, 47, 87, 92
Roitt, Ivan 82
rotavirus 49, 209

roundworms 10, 64–5
Roux, Emile 222
RSV 224
rubella 45, 46

Sabin, Albert 212
saccharomyces 62
Salk, Jonas 212
salmonella 33
sarcoidosis 185
SARS 48–9, 244
scarlet fever 179
schistosomiasis 63–4, 143, 148, 171,
        206–7
Schwann, Theodor 205
scrapie 66
seed and soil metaphor 29, 37–8, 61,
        185
selective toxicity 227
selenium 197
septic shock 165
severe combined immunodeficiency
        (SCID) 194, 195–6
Shaw, George Bernard 81–2, 176
shigella 33, 70
shingles 46
sickle cell disease 56–7
side effects 14, 216, 230–1
SIV 150
skin 28, 75, 178–9
    rashes 179, **180**
sleeping sickness 57–8, 146–8
smallpox 45, 155, 205–6, 207, 244
smell 119, 178
Snow, John 206
sound 119–20
Spallanzani, Lazaro 205

specificity 97–8
spleen 200
sporozoa 54–5
staphylococci **22**, 27, 79, 104, 139
Stewart, William H. 17
streptococci **22**, 27–8, 104, 169, 175
streptomyces 228
streptomycin **229**, 230
stress 201–2
strongyloides 65
sulphonamides 230
superantigens 151, 173
superbugs 233–4
Swift, Jonathan 5
symbiosis 10
syphilis 37

taenia 65
tapeworms 65–6
tetanus 31–2, 156, 222
tetracycline **229**, 230, 232
TGF β 131, 132
Thomas, Lewis 94, 177
thymus 103, 114, 194
tissue typing 177
TNF 131, 132, 161, 165
tolerance 114
toxic shock syndrome 151, 165
toxins 27, 31–2, 88, 139, 163–4, **164**
toxocara 65
toxoids 32, 213
toxoplasma 57, 158
tracheotomy 32
trachoma 38–9, 64
transplants 177
trauma 200

treponema 37
trichinella 65, 143
trichomonas 59
trypanosomes 57–8, 104
    variation 146–7, **147**
tuberculosis 28–30, 35, 36, **68**, 102, 104, 170, 172
    vaccine 210
tularemia 36
tumours 200–1
typhoid 33, 158
typhus 38, **180**

ulcers 33
undulant fever 36

vaccination 208–25
vaccines 62, 108, **226**, 237
    attenuated 209–11
    DNA 215
    genetically engineered 214–15
    problems with 148, 216–18
    timing of 219–20
variation 144–6
varicella 45, 46
variolation 208
Vegetius, Flavius 74
Virchow, Rudolf 160, 166
viruses 8–9, 40–53
    and cancer 44, 51
    drugs 234–5
    killing **113**
    replication 42, **44**
    structure 41, **42**
vitamins 197
von Behring, Emil 81, 222
von Pettenkofer, Max 183

warts 52
Weil's disease 37
Wells, H.G. 241
whooping cough 7, 30
    vaccine 211, 216
wine 62
worms 62–6, 89, 104, 143, 148
    and allergies 168
    helminthicides 236–7
Wright, E. Almroth 81
wuchereria 64

X-linked immunodeficiencies
        189–90

yaws 37
yeasts 60, 62, 214
yellow fever 49–50, 148,
        209

zinc 197
Zinkernagel, Rolf 110
zoonoses 26, **72**, 207, 243

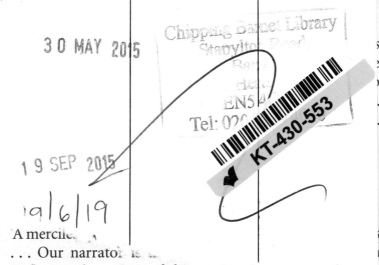
'A merciless ...
... Our narrator is a ...
Kafka novel ... One of the wittiest critiques of modern,
materialistic life that you'll read for a long while'

Fiona Wilson, *The Times*

'O'Neill has clearly set out in *The Dog* to broaden his
vision of the lost and lonely in *Netherland* to a much
grander scale: to the new elite of international, plane-
hopping white-collar brains servicing the planet's
affluent ... On page after page, O'Neill can still dazzle
as a compellingly intelligent writer. Everywhere you
look, there's a shimmering portrait of modernity
waiting to be glimpsed ... An ambitious, lucidly
thought-through novel'

Robert Collins, *Guardian*

'The sort of enraged, brutal, witty and at times brilliant
book that leaves you worrying about the mental state of
its writer ... Very funny ... Cumulatively, however, it
reads like a desolate cry for help.'

Lucy Atkins, *The Times*

'An impressive new novel . . . It would be wrong, though, to describe it as Kafkaesque: this compulsive account of a man rationalising his life with an intensity that at times resembles madness has an atmosphere all of its own'
Jonathan Beckman, *Literary Review*

'Joseph O'Neill is an extraordinary writer – his sentences are packed full of insight and humour and wit and brilliance.'
Elizabeth Day, *Saturday Review*, Radio 4

'The narrator's voice will hold your attention . . . The best comic novel I've read for ages'
*The Scotsman*

'The book's pleasures – which are dazzling . . . stem from the narrative voice'
*Literary Review*

'O'Neill is an extraordinarily gifted writer, the most interesting Irish novelist at work today. He is our only truly international writer . . . O'Neill's writing reflects the individual's concerns in our desolate modern world in prose that is illuminating, amusing, sometimes beautiful, but never showy. It's different and, once you get used to it, it's a joy to read . . . You can open the book anywhere and find sparkling sentences that perfectly describe what is momentarily in focus . . . The artificiality and absurdity of Dubai and of its expats and upper-class locals are mercilessly exposed in this novel, although it could be about many places in the world rather than this suspect Shangri-la. But it's really a wider commentary on mankind's moral progress, or lack of it . . . [O'Neill's] work is original and brilliant'
John Spain, *Irish Independent*

'It's satirical, often surreal . . . The savage, yet sometimes subtle, satire of O'Neill's novel is similar to Martin Amis's *Money* . . . *The Dog* is both laughably absurd and achingly real, reminding us that we are, even in the futuristic gleam of Dubai, primitive and brutal. O'Neill writes with great clarity and concision'

Christopher Jackson, *Irish Sunday Independent*

'With good-natured savagery, O'Neill draws us into a world where inter-human contact is mercenary and electronic, living standards are obscene at both ends of the scale, and morality is as archaic a concept as public transport. Bleak, black and brilliant'       Miranda Collinge, *Esquire*

'A finely crafted absurdist drama, written in thrillingly convoluted but never clunky prose'       *Metro*

'Genre-defying . . . Whilst neatly pricking the snobberies of expat life, O'Neill teeters between Douglas Coupland and Brett Easton Ellis'       *Monocle*

'*The Dog* is comic, and much more else besides. O'Neill, more than any other writer in English, inhabits a global world effortlessly . . . O'Neill's prose is never less than exacting and exalted'

Christina Hunt Mahony, *The Irish Times*

JOSEPH O'NEILL

# *The Dog*

FOURTH ESTATE • *London*

Fourth Estate
An imprint of HarperCollins*Publishers*
1 London Bridge Street
London SE1 9GF
www.4thestate.co.uk

This Fourth Estate paperback edition published 2015

1

First published in Great Britain by Fourth Estate in 2014

ISBN 978-0-00-727575-5

Set in Minion by Palimpsest Book Production Limited,
Falkirk, Stirlingshire

Printed and bound in Great Britain by Clays Ltd, St Ives plc

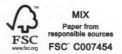

**MIX**
Paper from
responsible sources
FSC™ C007454

FSC™ is a non-profit international organisation established to promote the responsible management of the world's forests. Products carrying the FSC label are independently certified to assure consumers that they come from forests that are managed to meet the social, economic and ecological needs of present and future generations, and other controlled sources.

Find out more about HarperCollins and the environment at
**www.harpercollins.co.uk/green**

To M, P, O and G

Here's the smell of the blood still: all the perfumes of Arabia will not sweeten this little hand.

Shakespeare, *Macbeth*

I feel as a chessman must feel when the opponent says of it: That piece cannot be moved.

Kierkegaard, *Either/Or*

Perhaps because of my growing sense of the inefficiency of life lived on land and in air, of my growing sense that the accumulation of experience amounts, when all is said and done and pondered, simply to extra weight, so that one ends up dragging oneself around as if imprisoned in one of those Winnie the Pooh suits of explorers of the deep, I took up diving. As might be expected, this decision initially aggravated the problem of inefficiency. There was the bungling associated with a new endeavour, and there was the exhaustion brought on by over-watching the films of Jacques Cousteau. And yet, once I'd completed advanced scuba training and a Fish Identification Course and I began to dive properly and in fact at every opportunity, I learned that the undersea world may be nearly a pure substitute for the world from which one enters it. I cannot help pointing out that this substitution has the effect of limiting what might be termed the biographical import of life – the momentousness to which one's every drawing of breath seems damned. To be, almost without metaphor, a fish in water: what liberation.

I loved to dive at Musandam. Without fail my buddy was Ollie Christakos, who is from Cootamundra, Australia. One morning, out by one of the islands, we followed a wall at a depth of forty feet. At the tip of the island were strong currents, and once we had passed through these I looked up and saw an immense moth, it seemed for a moment, hurrying in the open water above. It was a remarkable thing, and I turned to alert Ollie. He was preoccupied. He was pointing beneath us, farther down the wall, into green and purple abyssal water. I looked: there was nothing there. With very uncharacteristic agitation, Ollie kept pointing, and again I looked and saw nothing. On the speedboat, I told him about the eagle ray. He stated that he'd spotted something a lot better than an eagle ray and that very frankly he was a little bit disappointed I wasn't able to verify it. Ollie said, 'I saw the Man from Atlantis.'

This was how I first heard of Ted Wilson – as the Man from Atlantis. The nickname derived from the Seventies TV drama of that name. It starred Patrick Duffy as the lone survivor from a ruined underwater civilization, who becomes involved in various adventures in which he puts to good use his inordinate aquatic powers. From my childhood I retained only this memory of *Man from Atlantis*: its amphibious hero propelled himself through the liquid element not with his arms, which remained at his sides, but by a forceful undulation of his trunk and legs. It was not suggested by anybody that Wilson was a superman. But it was said that Wilson spent more time below the surface of the water than above, that he always went out alone, and that his preference was for dives, including night-time dives, way too risky for a solo diver. It was said that he wore a wetsuit the colouring of which – olive green with faint swirls of pale green, dark green and yellow – made him all but invisible in and around the reefs, where, of course, hide-and-seek is the mortal way of things. Among the more fanatical local divers an underwater sighting of Wilson was grounds for sending an e-mail to interested parties setting out all relevant details of the event, and some jester briefly put up a webpage with a chart on which

2

corroborated sightings would be represented by a grinning emoticon and uncorroborated ones by an emoticon with an iffy expression. Whatever. People will do anything to keep busy. Who knows if the chart, which in my opinion constituted a hounding, had any factual basis: it is perhaps needless to bring up that the Man from Atlantis and his motives gave rise to a lot of speculation and mere opinion, and that accordingly it is difficult, especially in light of the other things that were said about him, to be confident about the actual rather than the fabulous extent of Wilson's undersea life; but there seems no question he spent unusual amounts of time underwater.

I must be careful, here, to separate myself distinctly from the milling of this man, Wilson, by rumour. It's one thing to offer intrusive conjecture about a person's recreational activities, another thing to place a person into a machine for grinding by crushing. This happened to Ted Wilson. He was discussed into dust. That's Dubai, I suppose – a country of buzz. Maybe the secrecy of the Ruler precludes any other state of affairs, and maybe not. There is no question that spreading everywhere in the emirate are opacities that, since we are on the subject, call to my mind submarine depths. And so the place makes gossips of us whether we like it or not, and makes us susceptible to gullibility and false shrewdness. I'm not sure there is a good way to counteract this; it may even be that there arrives a moment when the veteran of the never-ending struggle for solid facts perversely becomes greener than ever. Not long ago, I heard a story about a Tasmanian tiger for sale in Satwa and half-believed it.

Ted Wilson, it turned out, had an apartment in The Situation – the apartment building where I live. His place was on the twentieth floor, two above mine. Our interaction consisted of hellos in the elevator. Then, plunging or rising, we would study the Egyptian hieroglyphs inscribed on the stainless-steel sides of the car. These encounters reduced almost to nothing my curiosity about him. Wilson was a man in his forties of average height and weight, with a mostly bald head. He had the kind of face that seems to me purely Anglo-Saxon, that is, drained of all colour and features, and perhaps in reaction to this drainage he was, as I noticed, a man who fiddled at growing grey-blond goatees, beards, moustaches, sideburns. There was no sign of gills or webbed fingers.

The striking thing about him was his American accent. Few Americans move here, the usual explanation being that we must pay federal taxes on worldwide income and will benefit relatively little from the fiscal advantages the United Arab Emirates offers its denizens. This theory is, I think, only partly right. A further fraction of the answer must be that the typical American candidate for expatriation to the Gulf, who might without disparagement be described as the mediocre office worker, has little instinct for emigration. To put it another way, a person usually needs a special incentive to be here – or, perhaps more accurately, to not be elsewhere – and surely this is all the more true for the American who, rather than trying his luck in California or Texas or New York, chooses to come to this strange desert metropolis. Either way, fortune will play its expected role. I suppose I say all this from experience.

In early 2007, in a New York City cloakroom, I ran into a college friend, Edmond Batros. I hadn't thought about Eddie in years, and of course it was difficult to equate without shock this thirty-seven-year-old with his counterpart in memory. Whereas in college he'd been a chubby Lebanese kid who seemed dumbstruck by a pint of beer and whom everyone felt a little sorry for, grown-up Eddie gave every sign – pink shirt unbuttoned to the breastbone, suntan, glimmering female companion, twenty-buck tip to the coat-check girl – of being a brazenly contented man of the world. If he hadn't approached me and identified himself, I wouldn't have known him. We hugged, and there was a to-do about the wonderful improbability of it all. Eddie was only briefly in town and we agreed to meet the next day for dinner at Asia de Cuba. It was there, by the supposedly holographic waterfall, that we reminisced about the year we lived in a Dublin house occupied by college students who had in common only that we were not Irish: aside from me and Eddie, there was a Belgian and an Englishman and a Greek. Eddie and I were not by any stretch great pals but we had as an adventitious link the French language: I spoke it because of my francophone Swiss mother, Eddie because he'd grown up in that multilingual Lebanese way, speaking fluent if slightly alien versions of French, English and Arabic. In Ireland we'd mutter asides to each other in French and feel that this betokened something important. I had no idea his family was worth hundreds of millions of dollars.

Now he ordered one drink after another. Like a couple of old actuaries, we could not avoid surveying the various outcomes that long-lost friends or near-friends had met with. Eddie, with his Facebook account, was much more up to speed than I. From him I learned that one poor soul had had two autistic children, and that another had intentionally fallen into traffic from an overpass near Dublin airport. As he talked, I was confronted with a strangely painful idiosyncratic memory – how, during the rugby season, a vast, chaotic crowd periodically filled the street on which our house was situated and, seemingly by a miracle of arithmetic, went without residue into the stadium at the top of the road, a fateful mass subtraction that would make me think, with my youngster's lavish melancholy, of our species' brave collective merriness in the face of death. Out of the stadium came from time to time the famous Irish refrain,

*Alive, alive-o*
*Alive, alive-o.*

5

Obviously, I did not share this flashback with Eddie.

He removed a pair of sunglasses from his breast pocket and very ceremoniously put them on.

'You've got to be kidding me,' I said. The young Eddie had ridiculously worn these very shades at all times, even indoors. He was one of those guys for whom *Top Gun* was a big movie.

Eddie said, 'Oh yes, I'm still rocking the Aviators.' He said, 'Remember that standoff with the statistics professor?'

Yes, I remembered. This man had forbidden Eddie from wearing shades to his lectures. The interdiction had crushed Eddie. His shades were fitted with lenses for his myopia; having to wear regular spectacles would have destroyed him. I advised him, 'He can fuck himself. You do your thing. It's a free world.'

'He's a total bastard. He'll throw me out of the class.'

I said, 'Let him! You want to wear shades, wear shades. What's he saying – he gets to decide what you wear? Eddie, sometimes you've got to draw a line in the sand.'

Line in the sand? What was I talking about? What did I know about lines in the sand?

Young Eddie declared, '*Je vous ai compris!*' He persisted in wearing his sunglasses. The lecturer did nothing about it.

'That was a real lesson,' Eddie told me at Asia de Cuba. 'Fight them on the beaches. Fight them on the landing grounds.' Removing the Ray-Bans – he preserved them as a talisman now, and had a collection of hundreds of tinted bifocals for day-to-day use; on his travels he personally hand-carried his shades in a customized photographer's briefcase – Eddie told me that he'd taken over from his father the running of various Batros enterprises. In return I told him a little about my own situation. Either I was more revealing than I'd thought or Eddie Batros was now something of a psychologist, because soon afterwards he wrote to me with a job offer. He stated that he'd wanted for some time to appoint a Batros family trustee ('to keep an eye on our holdings, trusts, investment portfolios, etc.') but had not found a qualified person who both was ready to move to Dubai (where the Batros Group and indeed some Batros family members were nominally headquartered) and enjoyed, as such a person by definition had to, the family's 'limitless trust'. 'Hoping against hope,' as he put it, he wondered if I might be open to considering the position. His e-mail asserted,

> I know of no more honest man than you.

There was no reasonable basis for this statement, but I was moved by it – for a moment I wept a little, in fact. I wrote back expressing my interest. Eddie answered,

> OK. You will have to meet Sandro then decide. He will
> get in touch with you soon.

Sandro was the older of the two Batros brothers. I'd never met him.

Right away I came up with a plan. The plan was to fly New York–[Dubai]. This is to say, I had no interest in Dubai qua Dubai. My interest was in getting out of New York. If Eddie's job had been in Djibouti, the plan would have been to fly New York–[Djibouti].

Of course Djibouti pops into my head for a reason. The French Foreign Legion has long maintained a presence there, and among the earliest and most reprehensibly innocent manifestations of my wish to flee New York was a fascination with the *Légion étrangère*. The men without a past! They suddenly struck me as marvellous, these white-kepi-wearing internationals whose predecessors fought famously, as my online searches revealed, at Magenta and at Puebla and at Dien Bien Phu, at Kolwezi and Bir Hakeim, at Aisne and Narvik and

Fort Bamboo. *Vous, légionnaires, vous êtes soldats pour mourir, et je vous envoie où l'on meurt.* Unless the Wikipedia page misled, such were the exhortations that might drive into battle a fellow originating from any corner of the world yet beholden not at all to the compulsory systems of obligation of his native land. On the contrary, the legionnaire was bound only by the sincere comradeship into which he had voluntarily and humbly entered, a brotherly commitment captured with moving straightforwardness by his Code of Honour. I wanted to jump on a plane to Paris and sign up.

Though laughter would seem called for, I look back with astonishment and concern at this would-be soldier. How could this man, who had committed no crime and was guilty, to the best of my knowledge and belief, of not much more than the hurtfulness built into a human life – how could he find himself drawn to this absurd association of desperadoes and runaways? I remember how I yearned for a remote solitary fate causing shame and inconvenience to no one, for a life neither in the right nor in the wrong. Then along came Eddie Batros.

As the weeks passed and I heard nothing more from either Eddie or his brother and daily fought off the impulse to text Eddie for an update, it seemed that every five minutes brought mention of my new destination – Dubai. 'God, I could be in my swimming pool in Dubai by now,' groaned an English flight attendant during a runway holdup. The Albanian manager of my local hardware store said to somebody, 'They got a hotel at the bottom of the sea. They got millionaires, billionaires. Beckham lives there, Brad Pitt lives there, every day you got Lamborghinis crashing into other Lamborghinis, every day you got sunshine, the gas is basically free, they got no taxes, it's heaven on earth.' Dubai was suddenly everywhere, even in the office. A team from Capital Markets went over there for a two-day consultation that dragged on for ten days, and the whole thing turned into such a billing blowout that Karen from Administration was forced to look into it. The travelling partners, Dzeko and Olsenburger, reported that the quantum of fees and disbursements had to be seen in the relevant factual matrix, namely that the client had put the team up in a seven-star hotel in two-thousand-USD-a-night duplex suites offering a twelve-pillow pillow menu, a forty-two-inch plasma television set in a massive gold-leaf frame, a rain room, a butler service, and Hermès shower gel and shampoo and unguents. Also significant, for the purpose of establishing an appropriate billing benchmark, was the client's frankly carefree concierging of the hotel's Rolls-Royce chauffeur service and its further concierging, on more than one occasion, of the hotel helicopter service. Moreover, excessive billing reasonableness by the firm might be perceived as verging on underbilling, a practice evidently inconsistent, in the eyes of this client, with a law firm of world-class standing. Afterwards, getting hammered over cocktails, Dzeko more informally stated that these oil Arabs – he didn't want to generalize, there were other kinds of Arabs of course – these particular oil Arabs either had no understanding of how money worked, no idea about profit or value, or else knew all about it but just didn't give a shit and took a sick fucking pleasure in seeing these Westerners running around like pigs, snorting up cash on their hands and knees.

Dzeko was what we called a shovelhead, the kind of lawyer whose enormous industriousness is on the same intellectual plane as a ditch-digger's, so it was surprising to hear him come out with these speculations. But Dubai had called forth his inner theorist. Such was the provocative power of the brand, which was never more powerful, of course, than in 2007. In the middle of one of those agitated and sometimes frightening bouts of Googling with which, in those days, I would pass away my evenings, I finally entered 'dubai' in the search box rather than, say, 'fertility + ageing' or 'psychopathy' or 'narcissism' or 'huge + breasts' or 'tread + softly + dreams'.

I couldn't believe my eyes, in part because I was not actually meant to believe my eyes, or was meant to believe them in a special way, because many of the image results were not photographs of real Dubai but, rather, of renderings of a Dubai that was under construction or as yet conceptual. In any case I was left with the impression of a fantastic actual and/or soon-to-be city, an abracadabrapolis in which buildings flopped against each other and skyscrapers looked wobbly or were rumpled or might be twice as tall and slender as the Empire State Building, a city whose coastline featured bizarre man-made peninsulas as well as those already-famous artificial islets known as The World, so named because they were grouped to suggest, to a bird's eye, a physical map of the world; a city where huge stilts rose out of the earth and disappeared like Jack's beanstalk, three hundred metres up, into a synthetic cloud. Apparently the cloud contained, or would in due course contain, a platform with a park and other amenities.

The marketing strategists obviously were counting on me, the electronic traveller, to spread the word – Dubai! But if it's possible to have a proper-noun antonym of Marco Polo, my name would be that antonym. To me, this wonderland was the same as any other human place: it boiled down to a bunch of rooms. I had a theory or two about rooms. They were still fresh in my mind, those evenings when Jenn would pace in circles in our Gramercy Park one-bedroom in order to dramatize the one-bedroom's long-term impracticality and reinforce the analysis she was offering, namely that all would be well if she and I, first, mentally let go of our apartment, the historic and rent-stabilized location of our love; second, acknowledged that it made sense to buy a place that would more readily accommodate the kid or kids who, in contradiction to her earlier feelings on the matter, Jenn now definitely felt ready to try to have; and accordingly, third, that all would be well as soon as we got ourselves a place with *more rooms*. I must have said little. I certainly failed to mention the following insight: if you cannot identify a single room in the world entry into which will make you joyful – if you cannot point to a particular actual or imagined room, among the billions of rooms in the world, and state truthfully, Inside *that* room I will find joy – well, then you have found a useful measure of where you stand in the matter of joy. And in the matter of rooms, too.

One way to sum up the stupidity of this phase of my life, a phase I'm afraid is ongoing, would be to call it the phase of insights.

During my first internet encounter with Dubai I had a vision (a thing of a split second) of myself, somehow disembodied, hurrying from tall building to tall building and from floor to floor and from room to room, endlessly making haste through one space after another and never finding good cause to stay or even pause. I associated this ghostly hurrier with one of those computer worms, created by the Israeli and/or American security agencies, whose function is to pass without trace from one computer to another, searching and searching until it finds what it seeks – whereupon it does damage. As a corrective to this unpleasant notion, perhaps, I developed an intensely enjoy-able daydream of marooning myself on one of the outer islands of The World, say a fragment of 'Scandinavia' or 'Greenland', and living in a no-frills if comfortable almost-carbon-neutral cabin, alone except perhaps for a pet dog (one of those breeds that specialize in running into and out of water), a palm tree or two, and the odd visiting bird. I went through a period of islomania, the symptoms of which included discovering the word 'islomania', Googling 'bee + loud + glade' and 'islands + stream + Bee + Gees', and going to sleep every night listening to 'La Isla Bonita'.

Eventually I caved – I called Eddie for an update.

He told me everything was still on track but that the timeline was kind of wavy on account mainly of Sandro's scheduling issues but that bottom line everything was A-OK. 'Listen, I'm so sorry about this, I feel terrible, I'm going to take care of this right away, it's total bullshit.' He apologized at such length, incriminated himself so excessively, that I began to feel a puzzled guilt. Had I missed something? Had Eddie done something wrong? He had not; and, knowing Eddie as I now do, I can see this was probably a tactical mea culpa and he was just handling me the way one handles any problem. I'm not suggesting Eddie has a lowly nature; I just think he's not above preferring business objectives to personal ones. (He subsequently admitted this to me, indeed insisted on it. He said (on the phone), 'There's something we need to be clear on. I'm not going to nickel-and-dime you. You're going to get a sweet deal. Draft your own contract; do your worst. But you sign that dotted line, you're playing with the big boys. Same thing between me and my brother and my father: no favours. No mulligans. No quarter asked or given.' Eddie laughed a little, and I laughed a little, too, in part at the thought of my grown-up old friend raising the Jolly Roger of business. 'Got it,' I said. 'Absolutely.')

'No worries,' I said to him. 'These things always take time.' I was being sincere. I didn't hold the delay against Eddie. He wasn't to know that the passage of time was unusually painful for me, that my circumstances at work were unbearable now that Jenn and I had separated and had to spend our days dodging each other at the office and being downright tortured by the other's nearness.

(From what I gathered, in addition to the core pain of the ending of our partnership, Jenn was suffering horribly from 'humiliation' that was never keener than when she was at work, surrounded by the co-workers in whose eyes she felt herself unbearably lowered. I began to investigate this important question of humiliation, which I didn't fully understand (even though

I, too, found it almost intolerable to show my face at the office and there be subjected, as I detected or imagined, to unsympathetic evaluation by certain parties). It seemed to me that there had to be, in this day and age, a substantiated, widely accepted understanding of such an ancient mental state. I took it upon myself to visit websites dedicated to modern psychological advances and to drop in on discussion sites where, with an efficacy previously unavailable in the history of human endeavour, one might receive the benefit of the wisdom, experience and learning of a self-created global network or community of those most personally and ideally interested in humiliation, and in this way stand on the shoulders of a giant and, it followed, enjoy an unprecedented panorama of the subject. I cannot say that it turned out as I'd hoped. It would have been hard to uncover a more vicious and inflammatory collection of opiners and inveighers than this group of communitarians, who, perhaps distorted by a bitter private familiarity with humiliation and/ or by the barbarism in their natures, applied themselves to the verbal burning down of every attempt at reasoning and constructiveness. Frankly, it was grotesque and frightening to behold. Apparently the torch of knowledge, conserved through the ages by monks and scholars and brought to brilliance by the noblest spirits of modernity, now was in the hands of an irresistible horde of arsonists.)

In late March, I received a call from a woman speaking on behalf of Sandro Batros. She wanted to postpone the get-together until the morrow, Sunday.

'How do you mean, "the get-together"?' I said.

'I'm transferring you now,' she said.

I heard Sandro say how much he was looking forward to at last meeting his little brother's friend. He said, 'Listen, just a heads-up, I'm fat. Fat as in really big. Maybe Eddie told you. I just wanted to let you know. No surprises. Cards on the table.'

Next thing, the assistant was telling me the appointment

had been rescheduled to 10 a.m. at Sandro's suite at Claridge's hotel.

I said, 'Claridge's in London?' I heard no reply. I said, 'I'm in New York. I'm in the USA.'

'OK,' she said after a long pause, very absorbed by something.

I hung up, caught a plane to London, and took a taxi from Heathrow to Mayfair. I cannot extinguish from memory the terrifying racing red numbers of the meter. At 9.07 a.m., I arrived at Claridge's. I recall clearly that the taxi came to a halt behind a Bentley. I presented myself at the Claridge's front desk at 9.08. The receptionist told me that Mr Batros had checked out. She pointed back at the entrance. 'There he goes,' she said, and we watched the hotel Bentley pull away.

Sandro's assistant didn't return my calls. Neither did Eddie.

My return flight was not till the evening. What to do? It was a miserable, rainy day, and a walk was out of the question. Moreover this was London, a city I've never taken to, maybe because to visit the place even for a short time is to be turned upside down like a piggy bank and shaken until one is emptied of one's last little coin. I got the Tube back to Heathrow.

Looking up from my newspaper in the departure lounge, I saw two French-speaking little girls sneaking around histrionically as they tried to attach a paper fish to their father's jacket. The mother was in on the prank and the father was, too, although he was pretending not to notice. Something old-fashioned about the scene made me check the date on my newspaper. It was April 1st, 2007.

So long as I have adequate leg room, I like flying long haul. The trip back to New York was spent contentedly enough: watching Bourne movies, which for some reason I never tire of; drinking little bottles of red wine from Argentina; and mentally composing a series of phantasmal e-mails to Eddie Batros. Successively deploying modes of outrage, good humour, coldness, ruefulness and businesslike brevity, I let him know again and again about the London debacle and its inevitable consequence, namely, that I was withdrawing myself from consideration for the Dubai opening.

More than ever, I am in the habit of formulating e-mails that have no counterpart in fact. For example, currently I am ideating (among others) the following:

> *Eddie – I think we should have a talk about Alain. I completely understand that the boy needs help, but quite frankly I cannot be his babysitter. Could you please inform Sandro that he will have to make a different arrangement?*

And:

> *Sandro – Please confirm that, contrary to what I'm told by Gustav in Geneva, I am authorized to pay MM. Trigueros and Salzer-Levi for their work on the Divonne apartment. Mme. Spindler, the cleaner, is also indisputably owed money. Or is it our position that they are bound by contractual obligations and we are not?*

And:

> *Sandro – You cannot involve me in your yachting arrangements so long as you require me knowingly to make false representations to the crew. This is professionally and personally intolerable. Now I am instructed (so I understand) to inform Silvio that mooring costs at Bodrum are his responsibility, when such is not, has never been, nor could ever be, the case. My response to you therefore is: (1)*

15

*I will not say anything of the kind to Silvio; (2) this is the last straw; and (3) the first sentence hereof is repeated.*

And:

*Sandro — In answer to this morning's directive ('Make it happen'), I can only repeat that it is currently impossible to purchase Maltese citizenship for your cousins. Maltese law does not yet permit it, and I do not control the Parliament of Malta. I am ruled by the facts of the world.*

The reason I don't physically send, or even type, these e-mails is that it would be pointless. The Batros brothers are not to be influenced, never mind corrected. Even if they were, it would not be by e-mail and, even if by e-mail, then not by me. When I first took this job, I'd often write to them tactfully making points A and B or floating X or running Y up the flagpole or, finally, forcefully advising Z, and the consequence in all cases was nil. It's unsettling to be in a position where the performance of actions ceases to have the effect of making one an actor. This is a problem for all of us working on planet Batrosia, as we term it, and I'm sure I'm not the only Batrosian who, in reaction, composes phantom communiqués.

Arguably it is a little mad to covertly inhabit a bodiless universe of candour and reception. But surely real lunacy would be to pitch selfhood's tent in the world of exteriors. Let me turn the proposition around: only a lunatic would fail to distinguish between himself and his representative self. This banal distinction may be most obvious in the workplace, where invariably one must avail oneself of an even-tempered, abnormally industrious dummy stand-in who, precisely because it is a dummy, makes life easier for all the others, who are themselves present, which is to say, represented, by dummies of their own.

A strange feature of the whole Jenn thing was that when the news of our breakup got out – i.e., when Jenn got out her version of her news; I kept my facts to myself – some people at the office, and I don't think this is paranoia, emerged from their dummy entities. I'd be walking down a corridor in my basically upbeat office persona when it would become clear, from the hostile look I'd get from a passing colleague, that the normal dummy-to-dummy footing had been replaced by an unfriendly person-to-person relation – or woman-to-man, as I reluctantly came to believe. I had been educated to accept the factual, moral and legal invalidity of pretty much every constructed gender differentiation – and yet there existed, I think I discovered, a secret feminine jurisdiction authorizing the condemnation of men in respect of wrongs only men could commit! More than once my arrival in a room was followed by the sudden scattering of women and the stifling of their laughter, and wherever I went, it seemed to me, I was given to understand, from significant silences and mocking gestures of friendliness, that I'd been seen through – seen through all the way into my odious male nucleus. This subtle invasion of my being was my punishment. Meanwhile the men stayed in their shells – in hiding, was my impression. Though one time, in the restroom, there was a fellow who wordlessly slapped me on the back with a certain amount of sympathy.

It was ironic, this uncanny coming-to-life of my colleagues, because Jenn and I had been undone by the reverse develop-ment: at some point our bona fide human interaction had been thoroughly replaced by a course of dealing involving only our body doubles. The figure that gripped me, when I began to think about what was happening to us, was that we had been transformed into zombies controlled, it could only be, by evolu-tion's sorcery. Which is to say, the question of children having been (so we thought) answered – we couldn't reproduce without complicated medical intervention and so decided not to – our being together became a matter of outwardness, so that whether we dined wittily with friends or, in bed, felt for the other's body, we might as well have been jerking lifelessly down Broadway, flesh dropping from our faces, triggering panic; and by the time we, or rather Jenn, changed her/our mind about the baby, it was too late. In this sense, it came as a relief when it came to pass, late in the fall of 2006, that Jenn took sole possession of the rent-stabilized Gramercy one-bedroom and, after a brief crisis of relocation, I moved into a luxury rental with a view of Lincoln Tunnel traffic. This move, which involved some extraordinarily painful and exhausting and unbelievable scenes, at least brought what might be called spatial realism to our situation.

It was to this apartment of reality that I returned from the trip made in vain to London. I'd concluded that the most powerful statement I could make to the brothers Batros was to make no statement. Certainly it would have been self-contradictory to say to them that I had nothing more to say to them. Moreover, I was under no obligation of communication and indeed had just been so fucked over by them that it was hard to see what proper basis there might be for future communication on any subject. The salient point: I had no option but to put an end to my Dubai scheming – a suppression that cannot have been without side effects. It was around this time that, every evening after work, I tried to run from my building's lobby to my luxury rental on the eighteenth floor. My intention must have been to become fitter, feel more competent, clear my mind, etc.

I used the emergency stairway. To begin with, I could only run up to the third floor and would in effect creep up the rest of the way. Though I improved quickly, the going was always very hard after ten floors or so, and in order to push myself, I suppose, I fell into the habit of imagining that I was a firefighter and that a fire raged on the eighteenth floor and two young sisters were trapped up there in the smoke and the flames. The problem with this motivational fantasy was that it placed excessive demands on my real-world athletic capacities, so that by the time I finally reached my luxury rental I'd be in a state of very real distress because I was too late to save the two little girls, images of whose futile struggle for survival would pass through my mind in horrible flashes as I made my desperate, sweating ascent. A shower and a Bud Light would just about wash away this upset, but I doubt it was a coincidence that during this period I found myself brooding on the story of the Subway Samaritan – the New York construction worker who had, back in January, jumped in the path of an oncoming subway train to rescue a man who, in the course of a seizure, had fallen onto the tracks. Specifically, the Subway Samaritan had pushed the Fallen Traveller into the trench between the tracks and lain on top of him while the screeching train passed overhead.

I deeply envied this man, though not on account of the money and benefits in kind that immediately rained down on him. (The Subway Samaritan, who had acted for the benefit of a stranger, himself became the beneficiary of the largesse and assistance of parties personally unknown to him, including Donald Trump (ten thousand USD cheque); Chrysler (gift of a Jeep Patriot); the Gap (five thousand USD gift card); Playboy Enterprises, Inc. (free lifetime subscription to *Playboy* magazine (the Samaritan had worn a beanie with a Playboy Bunny logo during the rescue)); the New York Film Academy (five thousand USD in acting scholarships for the Samaritan's six- and eight-year-old daughters (the Fallen Traveller was a student at the Film Academy)); the Walt Disney World Resort (all-expenses-paid family trip to Disney World, plus Mickey Mouse ears for the girls, plus tickets to *The Lion King*); the New Jersey Nets (free season ticket); Beyoncé (complimentary backstage passes and tickets to a Beyoncé concert); Jason Kidd (signed Jason Kidd shirt); Progressive (gratis two years of Progressive auto insurance); and the Metropolitan Transportation Authority (one-year supply of MetroCards).) Nor was it the case that I envied the Samaritan his sudden celebrity and public glory: he could keep his Bronze Medallion from the city of New York and his appearances on *Letterman* and *Ellen*, and he was certainly welcome to his guest appearance at the State of the Union Address of George W. Bush, at which, bearing the title 'the Hero of Harlem' (like Lenny Skutnik, 'the Hero of the Potomac', before him), he was the object of congressional and presidential admiration and congratulation. No, my envy belonged to a less material though maybe no less indefensible plane: I coveted the Samaritan's newly earned and surely un-disputed privilege to walk into a room – an everyday room containing everyday persons – and be there received as your presumably decent human being presumably doing a pretty decent job of doing his best to do the right thing in what is, however you look at it, a difficult world.

But no – that privilege was disputed! It came to my notice that *even the Subway Samaritan* could not escape criticism from the online community, some members of which apparently didn't 'buy' the whole 'story', and suspected something 'fishy' was going on, and noted that at the time of the incident this man was escorting his daughters to 'their' (i.e., their mother's (i.e., not the Samaritan's)) home; had inexplicably and recklessly preferred the interests of a 'total' stranger to those of his daugh-ters; and (reading between the lines of even respectable threads) was a lowly African-American man and thus prima facie a parental failure and a person of hidden or soon-to-be-revealed criminality. I remember one electronic bystander invoking what he called the 'Stalin principle'. That is, he rhetorically asked if Stalin would be a good guy just because he'd once helped a little old lady to cross a road. More clever than this small-minded chorus, and more menacing to one's simple admiration of and gratitude for a brave and worthy deed, were those who questioned the whole 'heroism industry', who suggested that this kind of uncalled-for and disproportionately self-sacrificial intervention was ethically invalid because it could hardly be said that good people habitually did or should do likewise, and that moreover it was stupid retroactively to treat as virtuous an obviously reckless act that could very easily have had the consequence of depriving two children of their father. Another commenter even proposed that there was no point in looking for moral lessons in the behaviour of some unthinking instinctual (black) man whose actions, in their randomness and spontaneity and irrationality, were essentially akin to the motiveless pushing of persons onto the tracks that also occurred in the New York subway.

I was like, Who died and made these people pope?

One day, I ran the stairs in the morning. This was how I discovered that I wasn't the only runner in my building. There was another, named Don Sanchez. He was a physically and psychologically well-organized-, everything-in-order-, sanely-wry-professional-looking guy who wore sweat-wicking Under Armour shirts made from recycled plastic bottles. He had moved into our building not out of any fondness for his particular luxury rental but because, as he explained to me one day, he loved the high-quality run offered by the brand-new stairway, which had great handrails, bright-yellow-edged steps, and good lighting. Don told me, laughing, that he could no longer imagine living a life that did not include 'vertical athletics'. He had run the Empire State Building and dreamed of running Taipei 101 and Swissôtel The Stamford in Singapore. He ran with musical ladybirds in his ears. He was much faster and stronger than I, and quickly and easily made it to the top, twenty-sixth, floor. The little girls in my blazing luxury rental would always be saved if it were Don Sanchez coming to their rescue. I quit running in the evenings and instead woke at dawn to run with Don: falling quickly behind as he skipped up two steps at a time, I was able to trot steadily onward in the knowledge that all would end well for the endangered children. So reassuring was Don that I invited him down to my place for a drink. That was not a success. I had very few lamps in my luxury rental and only a few items of furniture, and what with the long shadows and the darkness it was as if I had contrived to place us in one of those grim, I want to say Swedish, movies my poor parents often co-watched, duplicating in the arrangement of their respective chairs the arrangement of silence, gloom and human separateness offered by the television. I confided various things to Don. He, in turn, disclosed that every year or three, he'd come across a staircase that would really grab him, and, other things being equal, he'd relocate to the building in question in order to run in it. He shared his physiological theories. He imparted his views on the different demands made by perpendicular and horizontal mobility, writing down for my benefit some relevant mathematical calculations. After a couple of somehow frightening evenings over the course of which each of us was, there can be little doubt, impressed more and more powerfully by the mental illness of the other, we restricted our friendship to the stairs.

By a meaningless accident, my current abode is also on the eighteenth floor, but of course it would be unheard of and frowned on and simply impermissible to race up and down the stairway at The Situation. The last thing The Situation needs is middle-aged guys running around and sweating hard in public and grunting and looking weird and signalling their pain and undermining our Ethos and putting under even more stress our already very stressed price-per-square-foot value.

There are plenty of high-rises here in the Marina district, but for valuation purposes the owners of apartments at The Situation – the Uncompromising Few, as TheSituation. com names us – need be concerned with only two comparators: The Aspiration, inhabited by the Dreamers of New Dreams, and The Statement, home of the Pioneers of Luxury™. We are all each other's Joneses. Because by design we exclusively occupy Privilege Bay – an elite creek or inlet of the planet's largest man-made lagoon – and, more important, because all three residential propositions have agreed on an Excellence Ethos (the tenets of which are published on our respective websites), our troika competes internally for the favour of an ultra-discerning micro-market of property investors – those who wish to reach The Far Side of Aspiration, in the terminology of TheAspiration.com. In principle, we three residential propositions proceed consultatively. In practice, it is like the three-way shoot-out in *The Good, the Bad and the Ugly*, and each will do whatever it takes to gain an advantage for itself, and each reacts like lightning to the slightest move made by another. When the cardio machines in the gym at The Aspiration were upgraded, those in The Situation and The Statement were at once replaced or renewed; same story when The Situation unilaterally began to offer complimentary sparkling water to visitors waiting in the lobby, and when The Statement without warning piped therapeutic aromas into its reception area. There is increasingly good if unexpected evidence that our rivalry has in effect been collaborative, in that it has functioned as a joining of forces against the great, strange waves that have attacked the Dubai property market. True, we have taken a massive hit, or haircut; but we float on. In our respective determination to not be outdone by the other two, we have, almost accidentally-on-purpose, cooperatively kept high our standards and morale and built up the frail composite brand conjured and encapsulated by the collective name we have given ourselves: the Privileged Three. I think of this brand as our little lifeboat. I think also of the bittersweet song I learned as a child from my mother:

> *Il était un petit navire*
> *Qui n'avait ja-ja-jamais navigué.*

That is, it may be that the same-boat strategy is no longer a good one. Soon, it may be every man for himself and dog-eat-dog and the horror of the *Medusa*.

Why? Because something weird is happening in the last vacant lot on Privilege Bay. This is the lot formerly dedicated to the Astrominium, which was destined to be the world's tallest residential building (at just over half a kilometre) and to offer the Ultimate Height of Luxury to the Ultimate Demographic. The Situation and The Statement and The Aspiration were developed with the Astrominium very much in mind. Those of us who acquired apartments in the Privileged Three did so on the footing (reflected in the purchase price) that we would in due course live next door to the Astrominium and that our residential propositions would draw value and kudos and identity from our huge neighbour even as they kowtowed to it.

Then – the *crise financière*. Soon after, the Astrominium site gave us the spectacle of the world's largest man-made hole in the ground, its colossal dimensions made vivid by the abandoned orange digger at the bottom of the chasm. I spent many hours looking at this digger from my apartment window, my mind turning always to the idea of a lost lobster. A few months ago, the digger disappeared; and a very peculiar thing occurred. If I happen to look out my window – if 'window' is the best noun for the immense glass wall that comprises the exterior perimeter of my apartment – I can see a new concrete platform on the sand, and on the platform there has risen a small concrete structure, about the size of a cottage, consisting of a concrete X that leans onto a cuboid concrete frame. Is it a sculpture? A monument? Is it the first part of an Astrominium-like edifice? More work apparently lies in store, because there's a bulldozer on site and a large pile of black dirt partially covered by tarpaulin. There's also a portable toilet. The indistinctness of what's going on is only deepened by the activity I've seen down there. Basically, from time to time a dozen management types in suits and dishdashas stand around and have a grinning conversation. Not one of them pays any attention to the structure. Then they leave. I keep waiting for construction crews to come in and take the project – which I have called Project X – forward to the next stage; it never happens. The structure remains inscrutable as Stonehenge. Nor is www.Astrominium. com any help: all we get is the assertion, by now more than two years old, that the 'building' of a 'building' will 'soon' be under way. This doesn't sound even linguistically right. It is unclear to me how the creation of a residential proposition suitable for Privilege Bay can be described as 'building' a 'building'.

I've got to find out what's going on. If the Astrominium plot isn't developed soon, and in accordance with the Excellence Ethos, the Privileged Three are sunk.

I do what I pretty much always do in Dubai when I need to know something. I ask Ali.

That's a Dubai joke – 'ask Ali'. When I first arrived here, I was given a couple of how-to books. The first was a how-to-work-with-Arabs guide titled *Don't They Know it's Friday?* The second was *Ask Ali*, on the cover of which the eponymous Ali, a cartoon individual in a dishdash, leans towards the reader, the back of his hand concealing his mouth, and mutters, 'Psst . . .' I permit myself a good laugh about the premise of *Ask Ali*, which is that, in order to learn about life in Dubai, you should follow a hissing informant to a hole-and-corner rendezvous where only things that are already matters of public knowledge will be disclosed to you on a hush-hush basis. Thus Ali will whisper in your ear about the local climate (hot), voltage (220), and body language:

> Whenever you see two [Middle Eastern] people speaking loudly or pointing at each other, relax and remember they are probably just chitchatting and having a good time.

25

I found my Ali, if I may be so possessive, soon after I moved into The Situation. I needed someone to fix me up with a personal VPN. A virtual private network, more than one expat had assured me, was the best and safest way to access Skype and other websites blocked by the UAE authorities. (Here the eyebrows of the expat would rise. Their import was not lost on me. I was really quite excited about re-connecting with the porn sites that, in my last USA years, had given me what felt like near-essential sustenance, presumably with Jenn's blessing, because she (who had once accused me of expecting her to be my 'concubine') was clearly counting on me (as I was on her) to be 97 or 98 per cent sexually self-sufficient, and must have understood that self-sufficiency of this kind would very possibly involve recourse to dirty movies. Even if she wasn't – even if Jenn was under the illusion that sexuality, like water left standing in a pot for years, somehow disappears over time – then surreptitiously making use of porn was clearly preferable to 'going outside the relationship' and creating a serious risk of emotional injury to Jenn and/or the third party. (There remained, of course, the problem of the welfare of the erotic performers. Any anxiety I might have felt on their behalf was eliminated almost completely by my preference for what seemed to be husband-and-wife porno acts (often mask-wearing or otherwise incognito) who gave the impression, accepted by me as bona fide, of offering up their intimate doings for money-making reasons, certainly, but on a voluntary and fun and expressly 'amateur' basis. In fact, if I felt guilty it was on account of my decision to not subscribe to these sites but instead to jerk off as a freeloader and so take the benefit of the product without doing the decent thing of compensating the entertainers for their valuable if hobbyistic efforts. I did not lose sleep over this wrong, it must be admitted, if it was a wrong, which isn't admitted. (Ideally, I should have found a way to content myself exclusively with cartoon porn, which is quite sophisticated in this day and age of digital technology, and in principle enables the viewer to erotically fuel him/ herself without any question arising of humans being harmed in the course of the filming. But what can I say? I'm a flesh- and-blood kind of person, and I'm really not turned on by the animation of certain scientifically impossible and/or violent scenarios, e.g., the rapture of human women by reptilian extra-planetary creatures, or the rape of cartoon women by cartoon rapists.)))

At any rate, someone was recommended to me for the purpose of installing an illegal internet connection in my apart- ment. To my surprise, this person, Ali, was an Emirati – a surprise because Emiratis (so I had been given to understand) were protected from the socio-economic factors that incentivize a person to undertake relatively menial work or, for that matter, to exert him- or herself in order to make a living, the upshot of which protection (according to expat lore) was a nation afflicted thoroughly by a peculiarly cheerful form of Bartlebyism. In substantiation of this stereotype, the only UAE national I could claim to know, Mahmud, who officially functions as the 'local service agent' of Batros Family Office (Dubai) Ltd and bears technical responsibility for the getting of licences, visas, labour cards, etc., was never to be found or, if to be found, failed to turn up for meetings or, if he did, turned up at his own convenience and in his own sweet time and to no effect. Mahmud was put on the payroll by Sandro Batros on account of his professed *wasta* – his clout with the Emirati authorities. To this day Mahmud, who is always good-natured and pleased about things, has yet to procure a single useful piece of paper. His workload consists, as far as I can tell, of accepting his Batros emoluments and hanging out with his pals at the Armani Caffè in Dubai Mall. I have spotted him there several times. He never fails to greet me jovially. Invariably he and his friends pointedly disregard a nearby group of standoffish Emirati young women who have not covered their pretty faces and whose head-to-toe black is offset by red or electric-blue trimming. In order to make a powerful impression on the women they're ignoring, the young men always talk gravely on the phone and urgently input their handhelds: each has placed two or three gadgets on the table. They work hard to generate for themselves a strong aura of possibility, as if the day were growing in excitement and they were in communication with some more interesting and important elsewhere and this interlude at the Armani Caffè was merely a parenthetical or trivial portion of some enormous indiscernible adventure. Whether in fact there exists such an exciting, adventurous elsewhere – this remains an open question. The question is especially open in Dubai, land of signs to nowhere: I have several times followed, in my car, signboards that direct you to roads that have yet to be built. Your journey fizzles out in sand. (The sand is natural. This is the desert. Disintegrated rock secretly underlies everything. It's almost nauseating to see the sand wherever the effort to cover it has not yet succeeded.) What's more, because of the velocity and immensity of the infrastructural operations, such roads as have been built are subject to sudden closure or transformation, and even old hands and taxi drivers are always getting lost and turned around. The U-turn is a huge manoeuvre here – and maybe not just because of the chaotic construction projects. Rumour has it that, in order to promote official control of the population, the traffic planning has been modelled on the oppressive urban development that apparently typified parts of Eastern Europe in the communist days, and it is no coincidence, say these rumourers, that cross-streets and turnoffs are strangely few and the driver who has missed his or her exit (very easily done) has nowhere to go but straight on, sometimes for a kilometre or more, until another interchange or roundabout finally permits a turning back, the total effect being a city in large part traversable only by peninsular, cul-de-sac-like routes of benefit mostly to the security forces, for whom life is much simpler if everyone is corralled into a near-maze from which there is no quick escape.

A clarification: I'm not seizing on this stuff as a gotcha. It isn't some great telling symbol of the shallowness and witlessness and nefariousness and wrongheadedness of the statelet. I do not align myself with the disparagers. I'll always remember a certain Western visitor who ominously murmured to himself, for my benefit, My name is Ozymandias, King of Kings – as if the poem were at his fingertips and the dude had not fortuitously run into it while browsing online for some bullshit reason; as if he habitually carried on with himself a quote-filled conversation steeped in the riches of Western civilization and by patrimonial cultural magic bore in his marrow the traces of Sophocles and Erasmus and the School of Salamanca. Oh, how these bozos make me laugh.

As for Mahmud: who can blame him? Sometimes I feel like high-fiving the guy. Here is someone who accepts without anguish his good fortune. Here is the hero for our times.

But Ali was the opposite of a Bartleby – a Jeeves. He turned up punctually; did the humble work he was asked to do; charged a reasonable fee; spoke good functional English. All of this was estimable. Outstanding was that he took it upon himself to fix the remote-control problem I was having with the ceiling fan and also, as I discovered after he'd left, to swap the bathtub and faucet characters so that faucet C no longer gave forth cold water, nor F hot.

Fittingly, it was while taking my first bath drawn with alphabetic correctness that I had my one solid-gold Dubai brainwave: I decided to hire Ali full-time, as my personal assistant. He has proven himself the perfect man for the job, which may be described as follows: to assist me with the challenge of day-to-day life in Dubai consisting of one goddamned glitch after another. (For example, the aforementioned bathtub had a built-in seat. I can only assume that this feature is highly sophisticated and aimed, like everything else in this country, at the mythic connoisseur, in this case the überbather who sits up in his tub and will not rudely immerse his/her head and torso in bathwater, i.e., bathe. I mentioned my dissatisfaction to Ali, and my wish was his command. He and a workman procured and installed a new, seatless, perfect tub.)

Even Ali is a glitch. Contrary to what his get-up led me to believe, he is not an Emirati. He is a 'bidoon' (Arabic for 'without', apparently), i.e., a stateless person, i.e., a person who is everywhere illegally present. I have not inquired into the whys and wherefores of Ali's situation, but, according to *The National*, there are tens of thousands of bidoons in the Gulf States. Most Dubai-based bidoons, I read, are the descendants of foreigners (from Iran, from other parts of Arabia) who settled here before the United Arab Emirates came into being (in 1971, I can declare off the top of my head) and who for whatever reason didn't register as citizens of the new state. Neither *jus sanguinis* nor *jus soli* avails bidoons. They are, as things stand, fucked.

Anyhow, none of this would be my problem if employing a bidoon were not technically cloudy. At Ali's own suggestion, he and I have left things on an informal basis, which I'm comfortable with. Income tax is in any case not payable in Dubai, so no question of tax evasion arises. Because he is not permitted to have a bank account, Ali receives compensation in cash dirhams from my office disbursement account, and quite frankly I treat as a sleeping dog the compliance nuances of this arrangement. *Los dos Batros* have been informed in writing of the payments and their purpose. Sandro has been introduced to Ali and is well aware of what he does. Since it is customary in the emirate to employ bidoons, I can with justi-fication proceed pro tem on the footing that all is hunky-dory or, since the case is not cloudless, that all is not not hunky-dory.

That's good enough for me. One can't be Utopian about these things.

I call Ali into my office. I have taken photos of Project X and I bring them up on my desktop and invite Ali to take a look. Over my shoulder, he says, 'What is this . . . building?'

'That's what I'd like to know. What do you think?'

This matter has no obvious bearing on my professional responsibilities, but I maintain that without Ali's miscellaneous assistance I wouldn't be able to begin to do my job.

Ali says, 'I do not recognize this.' He says, 'I will check this out.' What he means is, he will acquaint himself with the whispers and pass them on to me. I wouldn't actually know anything, but at least I would be in the know.

'No, thank you, Ali,' I say. 'That's OK. Don't worry about it.' Now I feel bad about having involved him. Ali is not, nor is he ever likely to be, a resident of Privilege Bay. He is never going to be one of the Uncompromising Few. He will always be one of the Compromising Many. My impression is that he lives somewhere in Deira, which is no great shakes but is very far from the end of the world. I will put it this way: I am socially acquainted with people who have lived for a while in Deira. Ali has volunteered very little to me about his personal circumstances and I am not about to stick my nose where it doesn't belong. (This is one of the great perks of living in Dubai: there are few places where one's nose does belong.) Nonetheless, I sometimes need to remind myself that I didn't write the citizenship rules and certainly didn't provide legal counsel to Ali's ancestors. I apprehend that Ali has applied for Emirati citizenship, but I haven't kept tabs on what must be, I don't doubt, a demoralizing process characterized by barely tolerable uncertainty, and I've never asked Ali about how it's going and don't intend to. What it boils down to is, I can't help it that Ali is a bidoon, and I can't help it that being a bidoon is what it is.

I say, 'Maybe we'll talk about this another time. Thank you.'

31

I am already intently perusing my e-mails, as if there isn't a minute to lose.

I doubt this performance sways Ali. He has seen for himself what my job entails, i.e., a couple of stressful hours of e-paperwork in the morning and an afternoon spent stressfully waiting around in case something should come up. The thought may have offered itself to him that I was crazy to quit what was, on the face of it, a secure and rewarding legal career at a good New York firm. (Ali knows a little about my old job, though he cannot be expected to appreciate what it means that I was of counsel, with a boutique but loyal private-client clientele.) I wasn't crazy, though. The reasonable man, put in my position, might very well have made, or seriously contemplated making, the decision made by me.

White as an egret, Ali exits and shuts the door. He will take a seat at his desk, which is just outside my office, in the reception area, and productively busy himself. (Often he will read a book in English, in a private effort of self-betterment. The luckless fellow is not permitted a higher education, and of course he cannot leave the country to seek his fortune elsewhere.) I swivel away from the desktop, put my feet on my desk, and hope my head is below the parapet.

It might seem hyperbolic to bring up the proverbial parapet, which calls to mind whistling bullets and, speaking for myself, the Alamo. I don't think it is.

At first sight, my job looks straightforward enough for a man of my qualifications and experience. As the Batros Family Officer, I am expressly charged (pursuant to the provisions of my contract of service, which I drafted) with the supervision of those specialized entities that perform the usual family office functions for the Batroses. These entities are (1) the Dubai branch of the multinational law firm entrusted with the

Batroses' personal legal affairs, many of which are governed by the laws of Dubai and the Dubai International Financial Centre (DIFC); (2) an elite wealth-management outfit in Luxembourg, which manages over two hundred million USD of Batros assets and devises the family's investment, tax and succession strategies; (3) the international concierge service, Fabulosity, whose task is nothing less than to make sure that the Batros living experience goes as smoothly as possible and that the family's huge wealth 'actually adds some fucking value to our fucking lives', as Sandro has put it; and (4) the Batros Foundation, which is principally operational in Africa but has its head office here, in International Humanitarian City. These supervisees are in a position to commit embezzlement or otherwise gravely fail the family. There is also the risk that a Batros will enrich himself at the expense of another Batros. My job is to make sure these bad things don't happen.

I have two main tools. First, I instruct a Swiss accountancy firm to spot-check and continuously verify the numbers generated by the activities of (1) to (4) above. The Swiss verifications are then verified by me, i.e., I roll a dull and unseeing eye over them. I am not and have never held myself out as professionally competent in the realm of financial scrutiny. I pointed this out to Eddie right at the beginning. He did that thing of waving away an imaginary flying pest and said, 'We've got experts to take care of all that. What we don't have is someone we can trust. That's where you come in – as our *homme de confiance*.' This brings me to my second tool: I am the General Expenditure Trustee of the so-called General Expenditure Accounts (GEAs). The GEAs are trust accounts held in the name of an Isle of Man trust company, Batros Trust Company Ltd. Monies funnel into the GEAs from all parts of the Batros Group, and the GEAs serve as a reservoir of money for the 'personal use' (per the relevant trust power) of Batros 'Family Members'. ('Family Member' means Eddie or Sandro or their father, Georges. Their

33

wives and children are not 'Family Members'.) If the trust powers are the dam, I'm the dam keeper: I am not empowered to authorize a GEA payment requested by a Family Member without the agreement of at least one other Family Member. In practice, this means that Georges and Eddie can withdraw as much as they want, because each has informed me that he agrees in advance to all GEA payments requested by the other; whereas Sandro, if and when he wishes to take out money, must go through the process of getting the permission of his father or his younger brother. In view of Sandro's history of profligacy and unsuccessful gambling, this process can be complex.

(Let me say this: I am of course aware of the technical risk of money laundering and/or tax evasion. The Isle of Man trust company is a red flag. Because I have no way to assess the risk, I have sought and received written assurances from each Family Member that to the best of his knowledge all sums credited to the GEAs have been lawfully gained and that all movements of money in and out of the GEAs have a lawful purpose and are free from any taint of illegality.)

There is a very high volume of requests for GEA money transfers, not least because the term 'personal use' is very broad and is to be construed, according to Batros custom, as encompassing personal use for a business transaction. The sensitivity and unavoidable complexity of Batros financial doings means that very often the form and/or function of a transfer is opaque or unexplained and involves collateral documents – deeds of trust, contracts, cheques, licences and other legal instruments – which are themselves opaque, written in foreign languages, etc., and to which I must also put my name. This last obligation is, unfortunately, of my own making. My self-written contract stipulates that I, the Family Officer,

> shall execute such [documents] *as pertain to* an authorized transfer [italics mine]

and I cannot argue in good faith that documents collateral or adjunctive to a GEA transfer don't fall within the ambit of 'pertain to'. A lot of the time I'm signing off on stuff that, to be perfectly honest, I barely, if at all, understand. I've made Eddie aware of this, too, and here again his response has been to laugh and tell me not to sweat it.

It's kind of Eddie to offer this reassurance, but mine is the inevitable fate of the overwhelmed fiduciary: inextinguishable boredom and fear of liability. To mitigate the latter problem, I am ordering customized stamps of disclaimer to use whenever I sign anything. The document in question will be stamped with a text delimiting the terms on which I lend my signature to it, the document. These stamps are still in the drafting stage. I am the draftsman, and I cannot say that I'm finding it easy: it is not my forte, as my father used to say. ('It would seem that reinsurance is no longer my forte,' he stated in 1982, when he was let go by Swiss Re and we left Zurich, where I was born and spent my first twelve years, and moved to Southbury, Connecticut, in the United States, that foreign country of my nationality. (I was so proud of my blue passport. *Mon petit mec américain*, Maman would call me, en route to the school in Zug.) 'International business machines are not my forte,' my father told me in 1992, when IBM fired him. More than once, after my mother had withdrawn to her bedroom, I heard him say softly, 'Boy, the female is really not my forte.' Fixing stuff around the house was not his forte, and neither was driving, nor understanding what was going on, nor doing crossword puzzles, nor playing games. A basketball in motion frightened him, as did Monopoly. I cannot forget one particular evening. I had forced him to play with me and some schoolfriends. The board was crowded with red hotels. My father's silver top hat was sent directly to jail, and for a while he was blamelessly and correctly exempt from the buying and selling and bankrupting and bargaining. He wore a huge smile throughout his captivity. If he was ever happier, I don't recall it.)

Perhaps my stamp should simply state:

NOT MY FORTE

Trying though these anxieties are, they come with professional territory I have voluntarily entered for reward. It doesn't end there, however. I have to deal, on an uncompensated basis, with extra-territorial bullshit. Every day, I get about two hundred unwarranted work-related messages. From every corner of Batrosia arrive complaints and inquiries and electronic carbon copies invariably written in non-English English or non-French French and/or bearing lengthy and complex attachments and/or referring to matters about which I have no clue. If somewhere a fuckup has occurred or may be about to occur and/or if there is an ass out there that needs cover, you can be sure that the relevant correspondence will be cc'd or forwarded to me. Word has somehow got out that there is a chump in Dubai into whose inbox every kind of trash may safely be dropped. Every day I delete about one hundred and fifty of these intruders. That leaves around fifty messages to defend myself against. How dearly I would love to re-forward them! But there's no one to send them on to: I am the final forwardee. Consequently I have become an expert in dead-end messages. For example, today I've written,

Hi, P – . Please particularize.

And,

This is beyond my ken, J – , but thank you. :)

And,

Many thanks, Q – . The inquiry as stated is premature.

36

And,

Hi. See previous e-mails, mutatis mutandis. ☺

I'll come right out with it: these incoming e-mails amount to nothing less than an around-the-clock attempt to encroach on my zone of accountability with the intention of transferring to that zone a risk or peril or duty that properly should be borne by the transferor. I've documented my predicament and brought it to the attention of the Batroses. They have not responded and, dare I say it, they don't care. It is not their function to care. On the contrary: they hired me precisely in order that I be the one who cares.

But what should I care about? That is the question. In order to clarify, circumscribe, and bring order to the scope of my liabilities and responsibilities, I'm drafting (in addition to the rubber-stamp disclaimers) what will be, I like to think, the ultimate e-mail disclaimer. One happy day, it will automatically appear in bold print at the foot of my messages and trounce the fuckers once and for all.

There remains another, I fear incurable, problem. My contract provides that the Family Officer

> shall comply with the reasonable instructions of the Family Members in relation to [. . .] other Family Office matters.

Innocuous, mechanically necessary stuff, I must have thought when I wrote this provision. But I had not reckoned on Sandro Batros. Sandro seems to be under the impression that I'm his majordomo. I cannot count the number of out-and-out inappropriate and frivolous demands on my time that he's made.

For example, he wants Bryan Ferry to play a private gig at

37

his fiftieth birthday party. OK, whatever. Sandro gets to do that, and it costs me nothing to tell him, 'I'll call Fabulosity.'

'No, no, no,' Sandro says. 'I want *you* to call Bryan Ferry. Not Fabulosity – you. This is very important. It isn't for me, it's for Mireille.' Mireille is his wife.

'Sandro, it's not my –' I cut myself off. I want to say that it isn't my job to call Bryan Ferry, but that would be wrong. It is my job, strictly speaking. The organizing of a social event is clearly capable of being described as a *Family Office matter*, and Sandro is a *Family Member* whose instructions in this instance (to personally book Bryan Ferry), though maybe unusual, are *reasonable*. Sandro is of course unconscious of the legal framework, but that does not negate the effect of the service agreement.

'OK,' I say. I will underhandedly contact Fabulosity and have them make the arrangements. Once everything is agreed, I will make a pro forma call to Bryan Ferry (i.e., to his agent) and tick the box created by my having uttered this 'OK' to Sandro. There are always more boxes to tick. It never ends. On paper, I am the hawk in the wind. Off paper, I am the mouse in the hole.

In theory, Eddie should be my ally.

> *Eddie – Is something the matter? I have e-mailed and called you many times these last six months and have not got a response. I know you're very busy, but no one's so busy that they can't even acknowledge e-mail. If you're feeling bad about having dropped me in it, vis-à-vis Sandro, don't. He's not your responsibility. And if it's the case that you can't stop him from making life difficult for me, so be it. But at least respond. Better still, look me up next time you're in Dubai and let me buy you a drink.*

I can't get too mad with Eddie. He and his brother have essentially stopped talking to each other, which from Eddie's viewpoint I totally get, plus Eddie lives far away, in Monte Carlo, plus there are issues, surely consuming and vexing, arising from his relations with his two ex-wives and their five (combined total) children. Plus he effectively runs the Batros Group. I might be hard to get hold of, too, if I were Eddie.

> *Dear Eddie – Sorry about that last, maybe somewhat officious e-mail. All I really meant to say is: Put yourself in my shoes, old friend.*

> *Eddie – Disregard my last e-mail, about the shoes.*

> *E – Never mind.*

The hard truth of the matter is that I don't have to ask Eddie to disregard my e-mails. He's already disregarding them. I have to respect this. You cannot coerce people into having relations they don't want to have. It's my job to give up on the idea that I can ask Eddie to take an interest in how I'm doing and what I'm up to.

I'll catch up with him before long. You cannot keep the world at bay. Exhibit A: Mrs Ted Wilson.

The reason I named her, right from our first encounter, 'Mrs Ted Wilson' was not because I find it whimsically gratifying to use a historically oppressive form of address but rather because this designation, while obviously a little old-fashioned, most accurately described the nexus between this person and me: from the outset, I dealt with her as the wife of Ted Wilson. And she set those dealings in motion. That's right – *she* came knocking. I answered the door as it were without prejudice (holding it open only by an inch or two, because visitors are always announced by a call from the doorman and it was the first time I'd heard a knocking on this particular door, and it was 9 p.m., and I was in fear, to be honest); and she held herself out as Ted Wilson's wife and *on this basis* sought admission to my apartment.

I had never met Mrs Ted Wilson or heard much about her. My information was merely that she'd remained in the United States after her husband had come to Dubai. In the Gulf, this is not an abnormal bargain. And if the arrangement had lasted for an unusually long time (it is not disputed that Wilson came to Dubai in 2004), who was I to question it?

Standing barefoot in my doorway in athletic shorts and T-shirt, I said to Mrs Ted Wilson, 'Can I help you?'

'Why – I don't know,' she said, looking at me as if I'd said something hurtful. 'I'd like to talk about Ted.' She told me she'd arrived in Dubai three days previously and that he'd failed to meet her at the airport and she had since found no sign of him, either at home or at work. 'He's just disappeared,' she said, not hiding her bewilderment.

I said, 'Yes, that must be worrying.' I said, 'I'm afraid I really have no idea where he might be.'

While true, this wasn't a comprehensive statement. Reports of people going AWOL were not extraordinary in 2009, which of course saw the beginning of the emirate's sudden depopulation and was the year the famous story went around of hundreds of expensive cars being ditched at the airport by fleeing debtor-foreigners – an understandable phenomenon, this being a legal regime in which financial failure, including the failure to make an automatic payment on a car lease, can amount to an imprisonable crime. (There are still such cars to be seen – brown ghosts, as I think of them, on account of the inch of sand in which they're uncannily coated. There's an abandoned Toyota Land Cruiser that's been sitting right here in Privilege Bay for at least a year.)

Again she looked at me with a pained expression. 'I thought you were friends. Don't you go scuba diving with him?'

I didn't answer, knowing full well that this was ambiguous. How she resolved the ambiguity was a matter for her. I surely wasn't under a duty to answer her questions or correct any misapprehensions she might have. If Ted Wilson had given his wife to understand that I was his diving partner – a flattering idea, incidentally, my being the buddy of the Man from Atlantis – that was between him and her. I had no wish and no obligation to be dragged into what was, as even a person of modest sensitivity could grasp, a private matter. And exactly what was this caller's status? She was the acquaintance of an acquaintance, which is to say, a member of a remote and almost unlimited class. It might be said: Wait a minute, she was your compatriot in a foreign land. Or, She was your neighbour. To the compatriotist I say, Give me a break. To the second speaker I say, A neighbour? Really? Number one, the Wilson apartment was two floors above mine; number two, Mrs Ted Wilson's permanent home was in Chicago, not Dubai; and number three, what's so special about neighbours? Since when is residential propinquity a basis for making demands? Let me put it this way: can I ring on the doorbells of those who happen to live in The Situation and expect special treatment? Can I burden random door-answerers with responsibility for my well-being?

She began to cry. This unsettled me, even as I was aware that crying is the oldest, most rotten trick in the book and one to which I have been only too vulnerable. But something else was spooking me. That very day, I'd read on my AOL home page of the death of the little girl who had inspired 'Lucy in the Sky with Diamonds'. This was news to me – that such an inspirational girl had existed. Her name was Lucy Vodden, née O'Donnell. The obituary reported that back in the Sixties, Julian Lennon, John's son, made a drawing of his

41

four-year-old classmate and brought it home to show his father and said, Lucy in the sky with diamonds. The cause of her death, at the age of forty-six, was lupus. This made me very angry. John Lennon being dead was bad enough – but Lucy, too? Little Lucy? No! I Googled 'Lucy Vodden' and came face-to-face with a very lovely, smiling woman in her forties with blonde shoulder-length hair whom for a moment I fell in love with and whom, only hours later, I briefly confused with another woman in her forties with blonde shoulder-length hair. I am convinced this hallucination played a part in what happened next: I allowed Mrs Ted Wilson to enter my apartment.

She sat in one of my armchairs and accepted a Kleenex. She struck me as a vision. How could she not? It was the first time I'd received a female visitor. That's right: in the year and a half I'd been there, not even a maid had crossed my threshold.

To be clear, the basis for the exclusion of female domestic help was not sex, and not even my finding it unbearable to have people entering my living quarters in my absence. (In New York, I had no such compunction. Returning home from work on Tuesdays, I looked forward to gleaming wood floors and ironed undershorts and a sparkling countertop, courtesy of Carla the cleaning lady. (What was her surname? Where is she now? How goes it with her no-longer-little daughter?)) The Situation offers its residents a 'White Glove Domestic Cleansing Service', but I don't avail myself of it. Why not? Here's why not.

When I first came to Dubai, I stayed for a week at the Westin hotel, which I remember mainly for its tagline – 'Between Being and Becoming'. From there I moved into a rented suite of rooms near the DIFC, on Sheikh Zayed Road. Beneath my window, six lanes of traffic bowled ceaselessly towards the distant skittles of Sharjah. This was a so-called serviced apartment. 'Serviced' meant that I'd come back from the office every evening to find all evidence of my occupation removed, as if I daily perpetrated a crime that daily needed to be covered up. Every one of my few belongings had been put out of sight; everything, down to the chocolate on the pillow, had been restored to the impeccable state in which I'd found the rooms when I first entered them. This was disconcerting, this non-accumulation of evidence of my existence. But what really rattled me was the mysterious population of cleaning personnel. The mystery lay not only in their alternative geography – theirs was a hidden zone of basements, laundry closets, staff elevators, storage areas – but in the more basic matter expressed in Butch Cassidy's question for the Sundance Kid: Who are those guys? That's not to say I viewed this tiny, timid population of women in maroon outfits as in some way hunting me down, as Butch and the Kid were, poor guys, all the way to Bolivia; but something wasn't right. To go back to Carla: I was aware that she originated in Ecuador, lived in Queens with a husband and a young daughter, got paid around seventeen USD per hour: of Carla I felt I could do the rough human math. (Carla, I'm so sorry.) The apartment-servicing crew, though, I couldn't work out. I couldn't place those strange brown faces – somewhere in Asia? Oceania? – and I certainly had no data about the bargains that presumably underwrote my room being clean and their hands being dirty. I was confronted with something newly dishonourable about myself: I didn't want to find out about these people. I did not want to distinguish between one brown face and another. I didn't want to know whether these persons were Nepalese, Guyanese, Indians, Bangladeshis, Sri Lankans, Kenyans, Malaysians, Filipinas or Pakistanis. What good did it do? How did it help anyone for me to know the difference? For their part, these women seemed not to want to be differentiated or even seen, because they always scurried away those few times our paths crossed. Therefore it was a situation governed by mutual avoidance. As the weeks went by, something appalling began to happen. I began to feel a fearful disgust at these scurriers as they intermittently appeared out of the walls and concealed spaces of the building. The feeling was elusively familiar. One morning, as an accidental encounter again dispersed a group of them into hiding, I recognized that my repugnance for these ladies was the repugnance one feels on coming upon vermin.

Out of shock at my monstrousness, I'm sure, I decided (in defiance of the house rules) to tip the service personnel. Easier said than done. My unknown cleaner or cleaners rejected the bills I left under my mattress (and placed them, folded, on my bedside table) and she/they ignored an envelope marked 'TIP! PLEASE TAKE! THANK YOU!' Evidently I would have to dispense the cash in person. The problem was, I couldn't make contact with a recipient. My long working hours – this was pre-Ali, when I was trying to single-handedly set up and operate the family office, an experience I never want to revisit – meant that I'd leave my suite too early and return too late to cross paths with the housekeepers, who moreover were trained to observe an extreme lowness of profile, the better to achieve their labour's almost magical effect. One Sunday morning, I finally spotted a distant uniformed figure hastening across the corridor. I practically sprinted after her. When I turned the corner, she was nowhere to be seen; yet, from somewhere behind the walls, a kind of poltergeist could be heard. I opened an unmarked door and found myself in a windowless room with a rough concrete floor and a whining service elevator. For some reason I felt a little frighened. I was on the point of turning back when a cart laden with sheets came in. A small lady was attached to it. There was an exclamation, followed by a statement that was linguistically impenetrable but very clear: my presence alarmed and dismayed her. I gave the lady a reassuring smile. 'Baksheesh, for you,' I said, and I pulled out a wad of dirhams and made to bestow them on her. She, who appeared to be equally in her thirties and fifties, made a negative hand gesture and, without meeting my eye, drove the cart into the elevator, whereupon she was as it were absorbed still more deeply by the building. I abandoned my quest to privately reward these workers. Apparently that would have been to put them in harm's way.

To avoid another such fiasco, I keep this place clean myself. It's no big deal; I like to mop my marble floor, the cleanliness of which I gauge by the blackening of the soles of my bare feet. When Mrs Ted Wilson came in, everything was spick and span.

She dabbed away her tears and her resemblance to poor Lucy Vodden.

She was intent on staying. Short of manhandling her, I saw no way to get her out. I must admit, I was curious about Ted Wilson; and inevitably I was curious about his wife, especially with her being a damsel, and in distress. But curiosity killed the cat. We all know of those gallant volunteers who rush towards a burning train wreck only to suffer lifelong trauma from the nervous shock caused by the scenes they witness, not to mention the lung disorders contracted from the fumes they inhale or the financial ruin resulting from lawsuits brought against them about what actions they took or failed to take. I resolved to keep as much distance between Mrs Ted Wilson and myself as was consistent with the basic civility that might reasonably be expected of me, the put-upon stranger.

She got up and wandered to the glass walls, and one might have thought she was going to step right out into the brilliant white tartan of the marina towers. After a contemplative moment, she gave her attention to the décor: large black leather sofa, two matching leather armchairs, big flatscreen, massive black leather massage chair, mezzanine bedroom, computer desk with computer, framed photograph of Swiss mountains. I'm sure she also took in the air purifier, and the ultrasonic humidifier, and the electronic salt and pepper mills, and the

3-D glasses, and the touchless automatic motion sensor trash can. 'This is basically exactly what Ted's place looks like,' she said. 'Do you guys shop together for furniture, too?'

Now she was inspecting my bookcase. She pulled out a volume of *Decline and Fall of the Roman Empire* and said, 'You even have the same books.' She said distractedly, 'You know Ted's a historian, right?'

I said, 'A historian?'

Mrs Ted Wilson took a seat. She related (unprompted) that when her husband initially went to Dubai it had been in order to teach for a year at the American University in Dubai. No one foresaw that he would almost immediately be offered the job with the advertising agency that was (as he saw it) his big chance to 'finally break the 70K barrier' and escape the 'humiliation' of an intellectual career that had left him teaching a course called 'The American Experience' in a place called Knowledge Village. (I pointed out that 'Knowledge Village' was merely the somewhat naïve-sounding (in English) designation given to Dubai's academic hub, but Mrs Ted Wilson didn't seem to hear me.) The Wilsons had spent most of the previous decade 'dragging' their two children (a boy and a girl) from one place to another, and now that both were in high school they agreed it was 'out of the question' to 'uproot' them again. Mrs Ted Wilson, meanwhile, had 'a project that I wanted to complete'. It was agreed that Ted would take the ad-agency job and the family would take things as they came, on the basis that 'life has a funny way of working out'. This plan now struck her as humorous, judging from the little noise she made.

By now her misconception about the quality of my association with Ted Wilson was beginning to trouble me. I said to her, 'Look, there's something you should know. I'm afraid I don't know your husband that well. I've just run into him here and there.' I further stated, 'I do, or did, scuba dive, but I've never dived with Ted.' As I made this disclosure, I was in the kitchen fiddling at opening a wine bottle, my back turned to her. This was my way of giving her space to take in my contradiction of her husband's story. After a moment, I approached her with a glass of white wine, which by virtue of having opened the wine bottle I was now obligated to offer her, God damn it.

I said, 'What was his field? As a historian, I mean.' I placed the wine glass within her reach.

Mrs Ted Wilson seemed dazed. 'German history,' she said.

Interesting. 'Which aspect?'

'Which aspect?' She seemed to be having difficulty. 'Sorry, you're asking me which aspect of German history Ted specialized in? You mean what was his dissertation about?'

'Sure, why not,' I said.

'Certain economic features of nineteenth-century Waldeck und Pyrmont.'

There wasn't much I could say to that.

I gave her my card. 'In case you need to get in touch,' I said. 'Thank you,' she said. She wrote her contact details on a piece of paper. 'Thanks,' I said, staying on my feet. As far as I was concerned, we were done.

But I'd forgotten about the glass of wine, and now she reached over and took a large mouthful of it and, for the first time, examined me. 'So what brought you here?' she asked.

I said, 'Oh, the usual.'

'You ran away,' she said. 'Everybody out here is on the run. You're all runners.'

It occurred to me that in all probability she'd had a few drinks earlier in the evening. 'I'm not sure that's entirely fair,' I said.

'Well, am I wrong?'

I said something about a unique professional opportunity.

'Oh, don't give me that shit.'

I was fully aware that this was a person in extremis. That didn't mean I had to give up the customary expectation of politeness. I said, 'Do you think you know me well enough to say that?'

'I know you well enough,' she said, motioning at my apartment significantly and, I must admit, infuriatingly. 'Ted told me about his diving buddy – you're some kind of New York attorney. And you still haven't answered my question.'

I understood her mania for enlightenment very well. Her life had become a riddle. I also suspect that she misidentified me as her husband, who was no longer available for questioning. It is fair to say that maybe I took Mrs Ted Wilson to be none other than Jenn, who was no longer available for answering. For a cracked, treacherous moment, I actually had the notion to tell this woman my story – to have my say at long last.

'I don't have to answer your questions,' I said – without hostility, to be clear.

There was that laugh again.

'Is something funny?' I said.

'You should see yourself. You're shaking. What is it? What are you hiding?'

'I'm not hiding anything. I don't have anything to hide.'

'I think you do,' she said, wagging the index finger of the hand that held the glass containing my wine. 'I think you have everything to hide.'

I said, 'You wag your finger at me? You come here uninvited, you throw yourself on my hospitality, and you wag your finger at me?'

She jumped up. 'How dare you. You pretended to be a friend of Ted. You deceived me. You lied. You lied to get me in here. Shame on you.'

I looked around for something to throw. To repeat, everything was spick-and-span. The only objects to hand were a copy of *Dwell* magazine and a plastic jar of Umbrian lentils. I picked up the jar, turned away from Mrs Ted Wilson, and hurled it against the wall. There was an unusual brown explosion as the jar burst.

'Get away from me,' she screamed.

'No, you get away from me,' I said. I was panting. I could hardly breathe. 'This is my apartment. If I want to throw stuff around in my apartment' – here I picked up the *Dwell* and flung it across the room – 'I get to throw stuff, understand? You don't like it, you're free to leave.'

She left, as was her right.

I swept up. Even so, for weeks afterwards I occasionally sensed a lentil underfoot.

It has to be said, my feet were in magnificent shape.


All credit for this goes to my old scuba buddy from Oz. One day, on the boat ride back to the shore, he, Ollie, said, 'You can't go around like that.' He was referring to my long, uneven, grey-and-yellow toenails and, especially, to my horribly fissured heels. Ollie said, 'I want you to drop by the spa, mate. We'll take care of you. My treat.'

Although a little jumpy at the prospect, I took Ollie up on his offer. Why not, after all? I wasn't to know (and would surely have been scared off if I had known) that he would personally handle the job, which is to say, handle me – wash my feet, trim my toenails, clip my cuticles, patiently carve slivers of skin off my heels with what looked like a miniature cheese-slicer, rub a pumice stone over the carved heels until they were pink and new-born. (Afterwards, his assistant manipulated my insteps and ankles, and, last but far from least, applied lotions to my feet, shins and calves.) Ollie was not even slightly queasy about any of this, not even about the flakes of dead skin accumulating like muesli on the towel on his lap. He spoke only in order to utter a kind of podiatric poetry about what action he was performing and which part of the foot was the planum, which the tarsus, and which the dorsum, consistently impressing upon me the enormous importance of feet, those great unsung

49

workhorses whose sensitivity and quasi-magical neural properties had been insufficiently examined and remained wrongly undervalued. What can I say? It was my happiest hour in Dubai.

Things have gone amazingly well for Ollie, I am very pleased to say. In a somewhat unreal turn, he has become an important and fashionable pedicurist who flies around the world to meet high-net-worth individuals who want important and fashionable pedicures: to this day he sends me gleeful, can-you-believe-this-shit texts from St Petersburg and London and New York. There is a downside, of course: Ollie got so busy he was forced to quit diving; and so I quit diving.

(I tried out another buddy but the guy was full of hot air and even underwater would clown around and bug me with pointless OK signs and make me feel unsafe. He boxed me in, somehow, even in the unpartitioned ocean. When Ollie and I dived, we stayed close; we accepted a severe duty of mutual care; but all the while we enjoyed the feeling of privacy that being underwater offers. This was fundamental to the undertaking, though of course there are those who understand privacy as a business of personal smells and locked bathroom doors.)

Ollie and I still have our jaunts, however. Sometimes, to blow off steam, we James-Bond-drive, as Ollie terms it, on the Gulf side of the Musandam peninsula. After we cross the Oman border and hit the new and almost empty highway, we notionally race to Khasab. It is no contest. I'm in my Range Rover Autobiography (2007 model, with a Terrain Response™ system designed for rough ground), and Ollie drives the bright-red Porsche Cayenne S that is his idea of a concession to family life. He zooms away almost immediately; from time to time, I catch sight of a pepper on a mountainside. Good luck to him. It is a joy merely to motor on this wonderfully engineered road, which curves between bare brown headlands and a blue bareness of open water, and whose rolled asphalt concrete is a kind of lushness. The road follows a dynamited zone of coastal mountain rock, and yet, as it has struck me again and again, my understanding never profiting from the repetition, this destroyed portion seems hardly different from the rest of the mountain, which itself seems to have been subjected to a vast natural blowing up. It is hard not to feel at one with the car advertisements as your vehicle adheres at speed to the surface of the earth, rushing through and over immense geophysical obstacles, then cresting at the pass, and then twisting down to a fjord so blue it seems technological. Who, a century ago, would even have dreamed of such transportation? We are practically in the realm of the incredible. Ollie sometimes urges me to rent something fast for the day – ideally another Porsche Cayenne S, to make a match of it – but I've never done that, chiefly because I don't want to be in an actual race, which would be frightening and dangerous and reckless. So as not to spoil his fun, I maintain that my choice of vehicle is strategic. I tell him, Remember the tortoise and the hare.

More usually, Ollie and I meet up when my feet feel dry. When that happens, I drive over to his salon at the Unique Luxury Resort and Hotel on the off chance that he or one of his helpers will be able to fit me in. It would feel wrong to make an appointment.

The morning after the run-in with Mrs Ted Wilson, my feet felt very dry.

There's more than one Unique. Ollie is based at the Unique on the Palm, and not the other, older Unique, which is in Jumeira. Driving along the Palm's main thoroughfare, the Trunk, always makes me think of Ceaușescu's Bucharest boulevards: visually coercive concrete apartment buildings that speak of broken Haussmannian dreams. A different gloom descends once I have passed through the tunnel and come to the west crescent, at the tip of which, near Logo Island, the Unique is situated. The west crescent consists mainly of the semi-abandoned construction sites of the Kingdom of Sheba and other failed waterside developments. One or two of the resorts give the appearance of functioning, but there is no getting around it: the drive is a downer. I cannot avoid recalling the automatic plenty of child-hood, when a pail and a patch of beach sand are enough to summon us into life's spell.

There is an important drawback to the Unique: I am known there by a false name. The (Assamese? Nepalese?) parking valets have no real interest in who I might be. Not so the pair of jolly, extraordinarily tall, and splendidly robed Nubian greeters whom all visitors must pass on their way into the hotel. (By 'Nubian' I am not making an informed reference to the ancient or modern people of the Nile, about whom I am ignorant. I am thinking of the Nubian in *Gladiator*, a very black good giant gladiator who is Russell Crowe's trusted friend in enslavement. Both greeters look like that Nubian.) I have never spoken to either of these gentlemen, and yet every time they see me they very loudly and gladly shout, 'Good day, Mr Pardew!' They have not gone mad. Mr G. Pardew is how, in a panic, I once identified myself to the front desk when presenting myself as a visitor of one of the female hotel guests.

I pulled into the hotel entranceway at the same time as a Maserati GranTurismo. I recognized the car. Its driver and his beautiful blonde female consort were paid to go from hotel to hotel in order to make an impression on tourists. I knew what would happen next: the Nubians would give their full attention to the performance of opening the doors of the Maserati GranTurismo. So it proved. I took the opportunity to sneak by unseen.

'Good day, Mr Pardew!' the Nubians called out.

I stormed past the front desk with a highly preoccupied air. 'Good morning, Mr Godfrey,' a receptionist said. I gave her an austere little bow of the head. This gesture was borrowed from and, I'd like to think, was a homage to the actual Godfrey Pardew, the octogenarian wills and trusts specialist who is my former mentor and remains the most senior partner at my old law firm and is the most correct, respectable, discreet and altogether old-school person I have ever met. In my assessment, he would rather disembowel himself than show his face at the Unique Luxury Resort and Hotel. I hasten to add that I would never try to pass myself off as Godfrey Pardew, Esq., of New York, New York, or any other actual G. Pardew. That would be wrong. G. Pardew is merely my Unique name.

I once tried to tell Ollie about this, but he raised a hand and said, 'I know nothing about Pardew. Nothing.' He knew, all right, but of course he didn't know, because what G. Pardew gets up to at the Unique is formally illegal. Of course, everybody knows that the Dubai authorities give sexual contractors a nod and a nose-tap and a say-no-more.

I walked past the Fountain of Ishtar and into the Hanging Gardens. The Unique has a Babylonian theme. What this imports, I do not know. My familiarity with Babylonian matters pretty much begins and ends with the words 'Ishtar', 'Hanging Gardens' and 'Nebuchadnezzar', this last item coming to me thanks to the (indoor swimming) Pool of Nebuchadnezzar, which one passes on the way down to the Unique Spa & Hammam. Here the Mesopotamian fantasia relents somewhat, although it may well be that high-net-worth Babylonians had light-flooded soaking pools and twelve-foot-long towels and whispering attendants dressed in white nursing uniforms.

I walked in – and there, in conversation with a technician, was Ollie! Hooray! 'Well, well, well,' Ollie said. 'Need a foot up?' This question is his catchphrase, and I will never tire of hearing it. It invariably prefaces half an hour or more during which I'll sit back and receive ministrations, and Ollie will tell me about his globetrotting adventures and fill me in on local excitements. He is extremely well informed, being the confidant of scores of Dubaian ladies. I am a little sick of tittle-tattle, and almost as sick of only-in-Dubai stories – the lion cub somebody spotted in a neighbour's garden, the guy deported for flipping somebody the finger in traffic, the tipsy girl at the Oil Barons' Golf Tournament who couldn't get a taxi home and drove down Sheikh Zayed Road in a golf cart. But what else are we to talk about? Dubai is where we are.

I don't feel too bad about imposing on Ollie. This is completely to his credit. He always makes me feel that my turning up and putting a large male foot on his lap is the greatest thing that could happen to him. He won't accept a single dirham from me, which makes me uneasy until I remember that a sine qua non of real friendship is a happy freedom from cost-benefit considerations. That said, I don't think I should completely banish from my mind the fact that I played a role in Ollie's success, namely bringing him the corns and chronically ingrowing toenails of Sandro Batros. The introduction had such a triumphant outcome that Sandro would not stop boasting that he had discovered the world's number-one foot guy, which led to Ollie being picked up by Fabulosity, which led to Ollie developing a worldwide client roster of luxurious multimillionaires. The rest is chiropodial history.

> *Sandro – I'm not one to attach importance to small tokens of appreciation, yet even I find it remarkable that you have not once expressed gratitude for, or even acknowledgment of, my role in procuring for you the services of Oliver Christakos. This leads me to wonder if there are any circumstances that would lead you to feel, let alone give voice to, simple human thankfulness.*

> *Hi Sandro – One more thing. You may be tempted to act on one of your many capricious and baseless threats to fire me. So be it. Cookies crumble. But please bear in mind that (1) Oliver holds your happiness in his hands; (2) he is my best friend.*

54

In accordance with our routine, I was first put in the care of one of Ollie's very pretty assistants. She led me to the Human Touch™ massage chair and pressed the buttons that set into motion the marvellous robotic devices, contained within the upholstery, whose actions are designed to approximate the touch of a highly skilful human massage therapist. (I have come to know this particular chair well and like it very much – and I speak as something of an amateur of such chairs and as the owner of a Pasha Royale X400™, perhaps the most 'intelligent' chaise de massage in the world. I always feel a tiny, absurd pang of infidelity about giving myself to a massage chair other than my Pasha.) After a fifteen-minute Human Touch™ rubdown, I soaked my feet. Then Ollie showed up in the very white, very medical jacket he wears at work.

He gave me a rapid pedicure. 'You're in pretty good nick, actually,' he remarked, and I wondered if he meant that I was pushing my luck, dropping in on him with healthy feet. But rather than showing me the door, Ollie asked if I would mind if he tried out a new treatment. He produced a small paintbrush and began to coat my skin (from toes to knees) with green enzymic goo. He looked more scientific than ever. He explained to me that an enzyme was a catalyst of chemical reactions, then explained what a catalyst was, then exactly described which enzymes he was using and which particular catalysis they were promoting. This excess of information was so soothing I nearly fell asleep. Little wonder: I'd been lulled into a soporific feeling of all going well in the world, of clever men and women in unseen laboratories toiling and tinkering and steadily solving our most disastrous mysteries, of benign systems gaining in efficiency, of our species progressively attaining a technical dimension of consciousness, of a deep and hitherto undisclosed algorithm of optimal human endeavour coming at last within the grasp of the good-doing intelligences of corporations and universities and governments and NGOs, of mankind's most resilient intellectual/moral/economic foes being routed forever and the blockheads and bashibazouks and baboons running for the hills once and for all.

Ollie said, 'Oh yeah, listen to this.'

To paraphrase him: A friend of a friend, an Iranian, goes to Dubai International Airport. It's his intention to fly home for a funeral. After he passes through security, the Iranian realizes that his return visa is not in order. What to do? He cannot go back through passport control into Dubai, and he cannot fly to Bandar Abbas for fear of not being allowed to return. The Iranian decides to stay where he is, in the huge duty-free area known as Concourse 1, until his travel documentation is put right. (I'm familiar with Concourse 1, even though these days I'm a Terminal 3 man and we have our own, I think better, concourse.) Unfortunately, this takes longer than anticipated. A week passes, then another. Still he is stuck in no-man's-land. His predicament comes to the notice of the mutual friend. The mutual friend is worried. He asks Ollie to check in on the marooned Iranian next time he flies out, maybe buy the poor guy a drink and a bite to eat. You bet, says Ollie.

Ollie said, 'So we meet in the Irish Village. I buy him a Coke and a beef pie, which he just gobbles up. He doesn't say anything. He's just eating and chugging down the Coke. I'm thinking he doesn't really speak English. He's just wolfing everything down. Then he burps – I mean, it's this really loud, kind of contented burp – and starts to tell me about his new life. Mate, you wouldn't believe it.'

'Let me guess,' I said. 'He's happy as a clam.'

Ollie looked at me with respect. 'Correct. He's a pig in shit. I'm completely wasting my time feeling sorry for him. He's the toast of the town. He knows everybody. They all love him.' Ollie put down his green-tipped spatula. 'You should have seen him, strolling around and waving to everyone. The cock of the fucking walk. Duty-free? How about just free? Free newspapers, free magazines, free food, free access to a health club, free internet, free everything. OK, the concourse is crowded, it's a shithole – but basically it's a mall. I mean, a mall is exactly where he'd like to be if he wasn't in the airport.'

I was laughing hard. Ollie had nailed it. Dubai's undeclared mission is to make itself indistinguishable from its airport. 'Where does he sleep?'

'Oh, he's found a nice little spot over by one of the gates. He's got himself a sleeping mat and a sleeping bag and, mate, he couldn't be more comfortable. He looked very well fucking rested when I saw him, I can tell you.' Ollie was hunched above my feet, doing the last touchups. 'Why wouldn't he? He's got nothing to worry about. He doesn't have to worry about work' – the Iranian had some middling finance job – 'because they're keeping his job open until the paperwork goes through. And he doesn't have to worry about his family because his salary's still coming in.'

'He's totally off the hook,' I said.

'Home fucking free,' Ollie said. He squinted and frowned at my green limbs as if he'd just finished the *Starry Night*.

I said, 'I had an interesting visitor yesterday evening.' It wasn't often that I was the one with news.

'Oh yeah?' Ollie said. 'Who's that?'

'Mrs Ted Wilson,' I said. 'She dropped by. She told me her husband was missing. Vanished.'

Ollie grinned – as if the advantage had somehow passed to him. He said, 'Which one?'

I told him I was talking about the wife of the Ted Wilson who was the Man from Atlantis.

Still the grinner, Ollie said, 'I know that. I'm asking you which Mrs Wilson you're talking about.'

I didn't understand.

'Now this is just what I'm hearing,' Ollie said. 'I'm not saying anything. I'm just passing on what I'm hearing.'

'I don't want to know,' I said.

'What I'm told,' Ollie unstoppably said, 'is there are two Mrs Wilsons. There's Mrs Wilson number one, who lives back in the States: your Mrs Wilson; and there's Mrs Wilson number two, who lives here.'

Yep, I didn't want to hear that.

B ut what were my options? Quickly seal Ollie's lips with duct tape? Stuff my ears with wads of cotton wool I kept handy for just such an eventuality?

It might be said I have only myself to blame: I opened my big mouth about Mrs Ted Wilson: I brought the multiple Mrs Wilsons on myself. But it is in the nature of a mouth to open, especially among friends. Or am I supposed to avoid Ollie? Why not withdraw completely from society while I'm at it? And why stop there? Why not withdraw from anatomy, too? Who needs a mouth? Who needs ears?

This isn't to say that we're totally helpless and that there's no defending the boundary between the here and the there. That's not my case at all. But there is a limit, if you will, to the fortifications one can build: there is the problem of force majeure. Here's an example. This summer, I have as an office intern Alain Batros, Sandro's fifteen-year-old son. I've never wanted an intern and, were I to want one, I should certainly not want Alain. However, there's nothing to be done about it. I must accept my instructions. The fortifications fail. Force majeure.

The kid's hours are 11 a.m. to 4 p.m., Monday–Friday. He sits in a chair at a little desk facing the wall, usually with his head resting in cupped hands, which he thinks conceals his closed eyes. From time to time he makes a groan. This is to be expected. He has the task of perusing unavoidably stale and contextless documents and double-checking the calculations they contain. It is without doubt an ultra-boring assignment, but unfortunately I am not operating a fairground. I have been instructed by the kid's own father that he is not to have access to a computer or electronic devices of any kind and that a spell of drudgery is exactly what he needs. Alain goes to boarding school in England (where things are not going well for him, is my impression) and usually spends his holidays in Beirut, where the Batros family (notwithstanding complicated taxational assertions to the contrary) most actually resides; but, in the words of Sandro, 'the time for fun and games is over'. The boy has been sentenced to passing the hottest months of the year in Dubai in the Jumeira family compound – Fort Batros, as I call it. 'I want him to have work experience,' Sandro has explained over the phone. 'I want him to learn what work means. Learn that work means work. It doesn't mean play. If it meant play, if it meant fucking around, they wouldn't call it work. See what I'm saying? Work is called work because it's work.'

'Yes, I think I follow you.'

'That's what you're going to teach him – what work is. What it is to get your ass into work and work your ass off. Do boring shit and do it all day long. He has to learn. He has to learn willpower. The boy's got no willpower,' Sandro says, lightly gasping. 'You're going to teach him willpower.'

It doesn't end there.

> *Eddie – This idea of making Alain's allowance contingent upon his achieving a certain weight loss strikes me as bordering on the unkind. Is there any way you could talk to your brother? Surely there must be a better way to proceed. In any case, I fail to see how my responsibilities extend to this sort of thing. Must I be involved?*

Eddie would of course never talk to Sandro about Alain. My phantom inquiry's phantom answer is: Yes, I must be involved.

59

The awful business is broken down, like the steps of an execution, into small, intrinsically blameless parts. Every Monday and Thursday, Ali accompanies Alain to the corporate bathroom and invites him to step into a stall, undress to his undershorts, and step on the scale. Ali sees the boy's feet step on the scale and sees the indicator jerk well past the 100-kg marker. He records the final measurement and e-mails me the number. I enter the new datum on a spreadsheet that reckons what allowance, if any, Alain will receive that week. The formula is Sandro's (i.e., his accountants'): essentially, Alain's weekly allowance depends on the progress he has made towards his weekly weight-loss target. It falls to me to communicate to the boy the result of this appalling computation, which always produces the same result: zero allowance. I discharge this burden by placing on his desk, during his lunch break, an envelope containing a Calculation Note and a Progress Graph. The Progress Graph charts Alain's progress towards the 90-kg weight target his father has set for him. If and when he achieves this target, he will receive the keys to an Alfa Romeo 1750 Spider Veloce that sits in a garage on the Isle of Man. Why the Isle of Man? Because its residents are permitted to drive at the early age of sixteen – a tantalization that will, it is hoped, induce the fifteen-year-old to achieve his weight target ASAP. (The USA, with its minimum driving age of 14–16, was not an option. Alain's portfolio of nationalities – the kid is a citizen of Lebanon, Ireland, France, the United Kingdom, and St Kitts and Nevis – does not yet include the American one.) Sandro has instructed me to buy an apartment on the Isle of Man with a view to creating (false) residency credentials for his son, who, it's safe to say, has no clue where the Isle of Man is. I am happy to take care of the property transaction, but I will not be party to any deception of the Manx authorities. I haven't made an issue of this with Sandro because the issue is moot: the kid has actually been gaining weight, and I would be amazed if he gets down to ninety kilos any time soon. Of course, it's not my job to be either amazed or unamazed. I am not this kid's overseer or Dutch uncle. It isn't for me to counsel him that drinking a giant beaker of Coca-Cola every lunchtime runs counter to his dietary objectives, or to root for him, or to lie awake at night wondering what will become of him and how things could be made better for this large, soft child whose circumstances give one not the slightest basis for hoping against hope that somehow he will acquire the wherewithal to care and be cared for, which is surely the great purpose and the basic meaning of growing up.

Still, it's in everybody's interests that the internship goes smoothly and productively, and to this end I've introduced the little big guy to Sudoku. The puzzles come in paperbacks and therefore do not offend against the no-computer rule; neither do they break the no-fun-and-games rule because they offer a brain workout that's certainly better than meaningless number-crunching. To make things even more exciting, I've introduced Alain to the Martial Arts Sudoku series, which has White Belt puzzles for beginners, and so on, up to Black Belt for real experts. When I call him over to my desk and explain how Sudoku works, he seems uninterested. But not much time passes before he tosses the White Belt book onto my desk and says, 'Too easy.' 'Wow, that's pretty fast,' I say. I have the next book ready for him and not without ceremony remove it from a desk drawer and deliver it into his possession. I say, 'Check out the *frontispiece*.' (I feel it will do the kid good to hear the word 'frontispiece', even if I am not exactly sure what 'frontispiece' means. I like to slip him the odd ten-dollar word, like 'litigious' and 'iconoclastic' and 'intricate'. They might come in useful.) I show him the plate that, in anticipation of this moment, I've pre-glued onto what I think may be the 'frontispiece' of this book. The plate reads,

Alain Batros is hereby admitted to the rank of Sudoku Green Belt.

The kid neither acknowledges the honour nor disdains it. He returns to his seat, assumes his slouch, and sullenly flicks through the pages of new puzzles. For what it's worth, sullenness strikes me as a logical, healthy and correct stance for Alain. But whether he is sullen or sunny – or in good or bad health, or succeeding or failing – is something I refuse to be dragged into. Once I have satisfied myself that he is for the time being safe and self-sufficient, I am entitled to view him as factically as possible, that is, view him as being on a par with the other occurrences – pencils, microbes, light streams, sounds, galaxies, etc. – out of which arise the accidental phenomena of this room and my consciousness of it. The kid becomes just part of the givens. That he may be overweight or fear the dark or have trouble making friends or enjoy watching basketball is not my concern and cannot be made so by Sandro placing him in the same room as me and counting on this obligatory mutual vicinity to make me act in loco parentis or in loco amicus or otherwise wear some unwarranted caretaking hat. I am obliged to accept the son's presence as my intern and to be a decent and reasonable temporary boss; but I am not obligated to accept and will not accept any responsibility for his greater welfare. Any occasional act of kindness I may choose to do for the kid is of a strictly private nature and between him and me and does not as it were constitute any kind of waiver or abandonment of my right to dwell within the aforementioned limits of obligation.

In order to strengthen and give helpful physical expression to these limits, I have instructed Ali to arrange for a partition to be placed between me and Alain – to, in effect, enclose me in my own room-within-a-room. That way the kid and I won't have to spend the day feeling under the other's surveillance.

# Chipping Barnet Library
Tel: 020 8359 4040
Email: chipping.barnet.library
@barnet.gov.uk

## Borrowed Items 31/05/2017 12:17
### XXXXXXXXX5978

| Item Title | Due Date |
| --- | --- |
| * Uncatalogued item. | 18/10/2017 |
| * The Lewis man | 18/10/2017 |
| * Prague fatale | 18/10/2017 |
| * The black country | 18/10/2017 |
| Spy games | 18/10/2017 |

### Amount Outstanding: £1.00

* Indicates items borrowed today
Thank you for using this unit

Although he may be an inept teenager, I would be crazy to lose sight of the fact that he is a Batros and in a position to blab about me. This will not have escaped him. Children are natural snitches and squealers and accusers. This is because adults are natural policers, prosecutors, fact-finders, judgers, punishers, torturers, hangers, electrocuters, gravediggers, and defamers of the dead.

The kid is flipping to the back of the puzzle book, where the solutions are set out.

'Hey,' I say. 'You can't do that.'

He slouches some more. Evidently he is stuck.

'Let me see that,' I say, and there is a loud squawk of chair legs as he gets up. I take a look at the puzzle. 'Mm,' I say. 'Not easy.' I'm not lying. It isn't an easy problem; and the fact is, I'm only a Brown Belt, and just barely. A lot of Brown Belt puzzles stump me, and too often I am faced with the choice of making a guess or abandoning the puzzle. Guessing is out of the question, of course, since that would defeat the point. The trouble is, not finishing the puzzle also defeats the point.

(I am in awe of Sudoku Martial Arts Black Belts. I would love to meet one of these logical warriors and find out how he or she does it – how, in particular, s/he masters the challenge of bifurcation. Bifurcation is called for when the path to the solution fatefully forks and it is no longer possible to induce whether numerical path A or B is the correct one. (Maybe it would be clearer to think of it as a 'symbolic' path, since the nine Sudoku numbers are not mathematical objects and function only as representations of nine unique things.) At my skill level, the player/martial artist has no option but randomly to choose one of the two paths and provisionally follow it in the hope that the guess will turn out to be correct. This process of tentative exploration is the hard part, because (assuming you don't cheat by lightly pencilling numbers into the puzzle with an eraser-tipped pencil) it is far from easy to keep aloft in one's

63

mind the multiplying number-scenarios produced by one's progress. If the provisional path proves to be a dead end, the player must backtrack all the way to the fork in the road (bifurcation is sometimes called 'Ariadne's thread') and take the alternative path – which could itself bifurcate, down the road. I have never met a Black Belt and find it hard to believe that actual Black Belts are out there, in the real world.)

Before I disclose the solution to his problem, I say to Alain, 'This here is the wall in the puzzle. You've hit the wall. And beyond this wall, there's probably going to be another wall. That's why you play Sudoku in the first place – to *scale* the walls.' ('Scale': a sneakily high-value verb for the kid.) 'I'm going to give you a little bit of help this time, but next time you're going to do it yourself.' Throughout this little pep talk he looks into space with an expression of vacancy I completely respect. He thinks I am very, very lame, and he is right. Still, we must go on. I show him a way to figure out his next move. He catches on and rapidly fills out a few more boxes. 'OK,' I say, 'now we're cooking with gas.' As he makes to leave, I say, 'Hold on there, mister.' I get scissors. I cut out the solutions pages and toss them into the trash. 'We won't be needing these. Our *prowess* renders them *superfluous*.'

And he drags himself back to his seat ten feet away from mine and I begin again to boil with rage that I have had taken from me a workspace that by rights should be mine alone and in which I should be entitled to put up my feet and pick my nose if I want to and live my life on my own fucking terms.

*Eddie – I want to go back to the last responsive thing you said to me. You'll recall this was back in November: I asked for your help with the Luxembourg thing, which as you know put me in an untenable position. The gist of your response was: 'If you don't like it, you're always free to leave.' Out of shock, I said nothing at the time;*

*and also, to be honest, out of some idea that you were right. But let me now say: 'Always free to leave?' You know as well as I do, it's not that simple. And suppose I were 'free' (I take it you mean 'at liberty') to leave – well, you were likewise 'free' to help me out, and your freedom (liberty) preceded mine, and the cost to you of exercising your freedom would have been much smaller than the cost to me of exercising mine. So let's not kid ourselves. You were the chooser, not I, and you chose to strong-arm me to the maximum degree permitted by your bargaining position. Eddie, that's not amicable.*

Writing mental mail eats up time and energy. An hour passes before I have worded the foregoing to my (relative) content-ment and I'm able to think about attending to my real work and my number-one priority, which is drafting my personal disclaimers. I lack attentiveness, though. I am too worn out and bothered. Normally I would take forty winks but God damn it I cannot on account of the stoolie in the corner.

The day after my pedicure, Ollie called to say that 'the diving community' was putting together a 'search and rescue party' for Ted Wilson. Ollie said, 'I guess they're asking us to go out and look for him. Leave no man behind and all that.'

Of course the correct response to this ridiculous idea would have been to ridicule it. But no – I was flattered to have been identified as a significant member of the 'diving community' and to have been handpicked for this special operation, I who had not pulled on a set of fins in over a year. I solemnly agreed to 'report' at 0430 the next morning at the Spinneys in Jumeira and from there head out to Oman in what was subsequently referred to, surely erroneously, as a 'rolling thunder' convoy.

I arrived at Spinneys in my silver-grey Autobiography just

as Paolo Weiss was arriving in his silver-grey Autobiography. I recognized a few other faces/cars. Dionisi Ottomanelli was there in his Jaguar XJ220, as was the Ferrari F430 of Jesper and Ingrid Poulsen. Keith Botha's Bentley Arnage T was unmistakable, even in the dark. We stood around in the parking lot with the restlessness of men and women on a mission. If anyone was a close friend of Ted Wilson, they didn't say so. Jesper Poulsen disclosed that he had once asked Wilson what drove him to dive. 'He said, "Because nobody can phone me underwater." ' This drew a laugh of assent. Trevor Winters, the diving-school owner and the chief instigator, planner and leader of our venture, conducted the briefing. He reminded us that Ted Wilson's 'diving transport' was his Mazda MX-5 Miata Sport automatic, and that the first sign of his whereabouts could well take the form of this vehicle. There was no need for Trevor to mention that the peninsular waters are practically unlimited and that the likelihood of any one of us finding the Man from Atlantis, or what remained of him, in the ocean, was very slight. For this reason, perhaps, nobody made mention of it, although Keith Botha did ask whether, in view of the troubling passage of time since Ted Wilson had last been seen – it had been a week – our outing should be 'downgraded' from an 'S & R' operation to a 'search' operation. Trevor said, 'Keith, I'd like us to go out there today with a little hope in our hearts. But you're right. We have to be ready for the worst.'

It was a sombre and burdened and exhilarated group of coffee-drinking, scuba-qualified automobilists that set forth from Spinneys at 0500 on the dot, and we must have offered an inexplicable spectacle as we moved in the morning-night through Dubai and Sharjah in a slow-moving, tailgating, fifteen-strong procession of, inter alia, C- and CLC-Class Mercedes-Benzes, Porsches Cayman and Cayenne and Carrera, a 1 series BMW, two Audi A3 Sportbacks, and a Nissan GT-R. The undertaking was governed by a mighty mood of adventure. Certainly, and speaking for myself, it was that very rare occasion when one's fictitiousness feels euphorically correct. I was no less animated and purposeful than if I'd been setting out to look for Red Rackham's treasure; and, as I travelled through the nocturnal cities, it was as if an existential transfer or translation had taken effect and it was the case without counterfactuality that I was an aquanaut and the cabin of the Autobiography, dark except for the dashboard's fire of needles and numerals, was that of a submersible passing between batholiths and brilliant upright reefs; and it was the equally real case, as the convoy turned east onto the E88 and quickened through the desert, that the moon gave the slip to a constabulary of moon-brightened clouds. Usually I find dawns disgusting: up in the Hajar Mountains, the appearance at the ocean's edge of yellow and apricot hues provoked a happy sense of daybreak I had not felt since, it may be, I was a just-qualified attorney and in the first purr of Midtown Tunnel traffic I walked to work through empty, wintry Murray Hill, and the overnight snow, cleanly banked on every sidewalk, loomed for me as the cliffs of Dover once loomed for English seafarers. What a home the world was! What a drama! It didn't matter that my part was that of the lemon hurrying to its juicer. I still had the verve, after twelve-hour days, for an office romance with the Beautiful Jennifer Horschel.

(That was the name applied to her by certain wistful male co-workers. In secret fact, Jenn's legal name was simply 'Jenn'. This monosyllable, whose dwarfism I found only endearing, was one of the things Jenn held against her parents even as she accepted that in this instance they had not sought to injure or handicap or short-change her but merely to give her a nice name. To make Jenn feel better, I let her in on my most embarrassing secret: my first given name. This unutterable word had been written on my birth certificate in honour of a Swiss great-uncle. From high school onwards, I disclosed its existence only under bureaucratic duress, when filling out forms. Jenn said,

'You have a secret name? What is it?' Very vulnerably, I told her – which is to say, wrote it down on a piece of paper. She stifled a shriek. 'Oh my God,' she said. 'You poor, poor thing.' (Not long after, a busybody in the law firm's HR department saw fit to exhume this forename 'as a matter of good order'. Ridiculously, my professional name thereafter began with the initial 'X.'. 'It'll make you stand out,' the busybody said. 'It'll give you an X factor.' How right he proved to be.) My revelation did make Jenn feel better, but her hatred of her own name was not lessened. I believe that having a stunted or halved name must in her mind have symbolized the improvidence of her chaotic upbringing in and around the Lehigh Valley, Pennsylvania, which left her unsuffixed in some broader sense and certainly did not equip her with the familial support enjoyed by so many of her peers at Dartmouth (to which she transferred from Penn State) and at law school in Georgetown, evidently few of whom had to combine their studies with crappy jobs or needed to make room in their lodgings for a half-sister fleeing a violent boyfriend or, for several weeks, another half-sister released on parole from Lehigh County Prison. When I met Jenn, she was holed up in a doorman building on Second Avenue, up by the Queensboro Bridge. She was twenty-six – one year younger than me but (as a result of three wavering semesters I spent at grad school) one year my senior at the firm. Her seniority wasn't just chronological. Jenn seemed unnaturally more experienced than me, able somehow to see things more quickly, as if an all-seeing tipster whispered in her ear. I guess she saw a lot, growing up – more than I saw in Zurich or Connecticut. We were both in Corporate – I in insolvency and restructuring, she in securities. She was regarded as a young superstar. We got to know each other in the cafeteria, late at night. At first we talked about the partners, those improbable fascinators; but as we continued to meet, Jenn offered a monologue, amusing and ethnological in tone, about the dark difficulty that was her youth. Combining the mentalities of the case-worker, the confidant, and the one who has a crush, I listened to her in a state of moral and romantic excitement; I even thought of taking notes, so importantly communicative seemed her disclosures of the Horschel clan's fuckups and tribulations, the like of which I had never come across except on TV and which left me, in relation to Jenn, with an edgeless feeling of duty. I somehow came to believe that this very lovely and intelligent and in all respects admirable person was gravely in need of help and, by fantastic good luck, this added up to a need for me. When Jenn and her Conran sofa moved into my rent-stabilized one-bedroom (in August 1998), it gave me great pleasure to write letters to her parents and siblings to the effect that she was now under my protection, that her days of housing and bailing out and bankrolling Horschels were over, that any communication with her would have to come through me, and that anyone who tried to interfere in her affairs would have to deal with yours truly. I described myself as Jenn's 'partner'. There was no question of our getting married because Jenn's parents had gone through six marriages between them and as a consequence their daughter feared the blessed estate. I, too, feared the blessed estate, even though my parents married only once. Work sanctified our union. We were always working. When I try to think of times Jenn and I were actually in the same room and happy to be there, I think of those early days when she would bring home work and I would spend hours at her side, helping to draft client letters and notes of advice. My contribution was chiefly linguistic; Jenn, the much better attorney, contributed the analysis. She made partner at thirty; I never did, and in due course moved sideways, into private client work. At our tête-à-tête dinner to celebrate her elevation, Jenn said that she would have a baby when she was thirty-four. That should give me enough time to establish myself, she said. Very good, I said, interiorly running to keep up. What about buying an apartment? she asked. I told her that I liked the rent-stabilized one-bedroom and that the financial logic of surrendering the rent-stabilized lease in favour of property ownership was unclear. OK, Jenn said, contentedly galloping on. But we'll get a bigger place after the baby, OK? OK, I said.

(Wrongfully, I withheld from her my developing interest in room theory. For example, how many more rooms did two persons in occupation of a one-bedroom need in circumstances where (i) the two persons were almost never simultaneously in the one-bedroom; (ii) on the rare occasion that the two persons were simultaneously in the one-bedroom, almost always one or both of them was asleep and therefore unconscious; (iii) on the still rarer occasion that the two persons were simultaneously in the one-bedroom and simultaneously conscious, almost always one person was in the bedroom and the other was in the bathroom or the living room? (A footnote: when we quarrelled, which wasn't often, we would be in the same room. After a while, I'd tire of the quarrel, and I'd exit the room and go to the other room, in order to be by myself there. Jenn would follow me in, in order to continue saying things, and eventually I would leave that room and go back to first room, and again she would follow me, and finally I'd have to go to the bathroom and lock the door, and still she would come after me, standing by the door and following me into the bathroom vocally, as it were. That happened consistently, which is interesting, because when we were not disputatious an opposite dynamic was typically in effect, namely, that if I entered the same room as Jenn, she would quite soon leave that room, as if the point of an apartment was to ensure that its occupants lived apart from one another. (This partly explains my resistance to moving to a larger place and thereby enabling our mutual dodging, whereas it was my hope that one day we would enjoy being in the same room together. It wasn't right to keep this motive secret. The right thing would have been to mention to Jenn that I resented all the dodging, and let her know where I stood, emotionally, even if my previous attempts at this kind of communication had not been productive, very possibly because of my own inadequacies as an emotions-communicator. (As it happens, my wrongdoing in this specific instance – i.e., resisting a move to a larger place for reasons kept secret – turned out to be consequentially good, because we were spared a conflict about how to dispose of a jointly owned property. To that extent, all's well that ends well.))))

So there it was: we had agreed on a plan. When Jenn turned thirty-three, we made the premeditated reproductive effort; sexual intercourse became focused and timeous. After six months, Jenn elected to receive fertility treatment. This necessitated that she self-administer certain drugs. The drugs made her depressed and anxious and paranoid for a week of each month – an especially disconcerting turn for her, because she naturally tended towards emotional efficiency. These painful symptoms bothered her for three consecutive months. During the third, something bad happened at work the details of which Jenn would not reveal but which involved, I gathered, strange behaviour attributable to her artificial biochemical state. Soon afterwards, she said that she didn't want to take any more fertility drugs. I said, OK, we'll do without them, and Jenn said, No. I can't do it any more. She was very upset, as far as I could tell, or perhaps very relieved, or both. There can be little doubt that her family background complicated for her the issue of children, among others. I said, OK, let's think about it again in a little while, OK, love? and she said, OK. We said no more about it. Then Jenn turned thirty-five and said she wanted to try again. It was now or never, she said. She said that there were no two ways about it, we had to find a bigger apartment, with more rooms. It was financially ridiculous not to, apart from anything else. I said, OK, even though by this point I had lost my cameral idealism and room-wise was on the same

71

page as Jenn, i.e., my interest in our being in the same room together had waned. To quote an old, possibly wise, legal colleague: There comes a point when there comes a point.)

At Dibba were dhows and inflatable speedboats loaded with diving equipment. Our group disbanded in teams of two. Some headed for Lima Rock, some to Octopus Rock, some to the Khor Mala Caves, some to Ras Qaisah, others elsewhere. Ollie and I were assigned the Ras Lima headland. The decision had been made to cover the well-known dive spots, even though Ted Wilson had become a legend precisely for his avoidance of these sites, which furthermore attracted so much scuba and snorkelling traffic that it was hard to believe that a findable diver in distress would not already have turned up. It wasn't until our boat was in the water that I began to feel preposterous. Ollie and I looked like Dumb and Dumber in our yellow flippers and matching short-sleeved O'Neill neoprene shirts.

I said, 'So what's the plan, exactly?'

He made a grimace. 'Let's get on with it.'

We toppled ass backward into the Gulf of Oman.

Everything beyond ten metres was lemonade murk. I was tense; I had forgotten about the unlimited expectancy that is a feeling of being in the sea.

Ollie went along a shallow trough. I followed. We had dived this site before, and soon I recognized a grove of lavender coral. On we went, through enigmatic marine vales. The blue-and-white-striped fish were out and about, as were the small black triangular dawdlers, as were, in a disorderly shoal, the innumerable now-glossy, now-dull colourless guys that are the pen pushers of the reefs. My Fish Identification Course did not cover these little fellows, and in fact the whole enterprise of human discernment, of passing what is sensed through the sieve of what is known, is more or less annulled underwater. Perhaps for this reason, I've never been able to dive without loneliness – and never could have gone into the water like Ted

Wilson, without human corroboration. Always I would need to sense, close by, friendly foot fins idling in the deep. And yet while looking for Ted Wilson's body, if that's what we were doing, I hardly felt companioned by my intermittently effervescent old buddy. We were present as searchers, not sightseers, and I felt a terrific pressure of intentionality. The sunbeams in vertical schools, the alien phyla, one's unnatural litheness – I was used to submitting without thought to these marvels and to their incalculable *Welt*. Very few human ideas survive in this implacably sovereign element; one finds oneself in a world devoid not only of air but of symbols, which are of course a kind of air. There are moments when even the sunniest diver has forced on him or her certain dark items of knowledge, among them, if I may extrapolate from my own diver's experience of being simultaneously a vessel and a passenger, that one is a biological room in which one is the detainee. None other than Cousteau, as I learned from watching his *Odyssey*, understood that a corollary of his oceanographic adventures was the contemplation, inevitably gloomy, of the processes of decomposition and disappearance that finally govern organic life and, for that matter, the lives of civilizations, ancient traces of which are apparently plentiful in the depths of the Mediterranean Sea in the form of coins and urns and ruins. None of this is to propose a special category of submerged truth; but there is no point in denying that diving changes things.

We came to a drop-off and went down.

Right away we saw a leopard shark, at rest on the white sand. On another day, I would have been overjoyed. Convulsively, I kicked away from the animal, from the abominable sound of my breathing, from the inertness of everything. I have to think this was provoked by the fraudulence of my situation; but in any case, panic displaced all notions except that of surfacing. I signalled to Ollie. We went up without delay.

'I can't do it,' I said, gasping. 'I'm not breathing right.'

Ollie said, 'OK. Let's get on the boat.'

I haven't fully recovered from this freak-out, which one might more precisely describe as a traumatic episode of extra- or supramural apprehension. A few months ago, I had reason to spend a discounted but still very expensive night in the Neptune Suite of the Atlantis Palm. The special feature of the Neptune Suite (aside from the two complimentary Dolphin Encounters with dolphins supposedly flown in from the Solomon Islands) is the huge blue water-window that gives on to the Atlantis's famous Lost Chambers aquarium and promises the experience of 'exploring the mysterious ruins of Atlantis'. My companion asked if the curtains might be left open overnight. Sure, I said. I got into bed and switched off the lights. The incandescence of the aquarium flooded the room, which now was subsumed by the thalassic realm and, so it felt to me, teemed with silent pelagic beings. 'This so cool,' my companion said. I smiled at her and hid my face under the bedclothes. Eventually I peeked out and, in the hope of overcoming my terror, forced myself to watch the approach of eels, sharks and other fishes. A small ray scooted up the window with its white underside against the glass – charming little spook, from one point of view, monster of otherness from another. I was in the latter camp. For hours I lay in an insomniacal agony of submersion that ended only when a pair of frogmen, each in a cloud of fish, swam towards us and began to wipe the glass.

The speedboat operator gave us tea. 'I say we head back,' Ollie said. 'This isn't working out.'

Dibba was hot, hot, hot. It was July, easily over forty degrees Celsius. Waiting around for the other divers was not an option. Later we heard that Trevor Winters, who was far from being a bad guy and not long afterwards was himself the subject of one of those Dubai evaporations, thanked everyone for their efforts and distributed commemorative T-shirts bearing the words TED WILSON POSSE.

By the time I got back to The Situation, I was wiped out. I took a cold (i.e., lukewarm) shower, dressed to my underclothes, and watched a jet skier fooling around in the lagoon. Then I climbed into my Pasha Royale X400™ massage chair and programmed a twenty-minute Full Body Integrated Shiatsu Massage, Intense mode. I selected Ambient Classics (the Pasha has built-in speakers) and pressed Start Bodywork. The chair and I began to tremble.

The Pasha remains my go-to comforter. I'm not sure how I would cope without it. Arguably this reveals something inadequate about me, but what is a private dwelling if not a redoubt against the tyranny of adequacy? And what's wrong with having a favourite chair? What difference does it make if its components include motors and rollers and air bags? Are these to be distinguished, analytically, from casters and springs and cushions? So what if one's chair produces physically pleasant vibrations and frictions? Or is an uncomfortable chair better than a comfortable one? Bottom line: the Pasha hurts nobody. It's not as if it's stuffed with minuscule underlings coerced into massaging me.

About nine minutes and fifteen seconds into a twenty-minute Full Body Shiatsu, the Pasha's heavy-duty twin rollers – Cagney and Lacey, I call them – get serious and rumble up the S-track and start the 'Deep Tissue Knead' action on the muscles that surround my upper spine. Here, I invariably open my eyes and look out the windows. It is soothing to look out the windows in combination with a Pasha massage, especially if there's an active construction site in view. I have become an aficionado of this species of vista. Admittedly, this has a compulsory aspect: I have yet to live in a Dubai apartment that does not give on to a scene of buildings being built. There has never been a time, in fact, when the stupendous and beautiful Burj Dubai/Khalifa itself has not been in sight from one window or another. The slow theatre of its years-long rising, its growing little by little taller and more slender until finally it achieved its last sheen and height, so that a person in almost any populated part of the emirate now has the option of looking up and contemplating nothing less than a wonder of the world – this excitement has been and continues to be a must-see part of the Dubai experience, a great theme of which has been the turning inside-out of the optical fictions for which the desert sands have been notorious from the earliest ages. I still think about the afternoon when, at a spot not far from the wilds allocated to now moribund Dubailand, I stopped the Autobiography and got out into the heat and wind to take in, without the mediation of the windshield, Dubai's little row of towers, visible as if adrift, miles away across the level desert. The city could not have more resembled a fata morgana – and that was the whole idea. If I might psychologize, the reliance on the mirage/wonder equation, which of course has an etymological basis, is not just a marketing ploy: it is a secret revenge on the mirage itself, and only one facet of the Dubaian counterattack on the natural. The crimes of nature against man, in this part of the world, are not restricted to the immemorial mockery of the visual sense. The slightest effort of reflection must yield an awareness of the suffering and lowliness that these barren and desolate sands have without cease inflicted on their human inhabitants; and it cannot be a surprise, now that the shoe is on the other foot, that the transformation of this place is characterized by attempts at domination directed not only against the heat and dust but, as is evident from the natives' somewhat irrational hostility to solar energy and their unusual dedication to the artificial settlement of marine areas, against the very sun and the very sea. This is what happens when you fuck with people for a long time. They fuck with you back.

There are some who would raise an eyebrow at my

favourable aesthetic assessment of the Burj. I'd invite them to come here and see the unprecedented perpendicular for themselves, but first of all to put away ideas formed in advance about this country, the brand of which, it's fair to say, places unusual reliance on the *Guinness Book of World Records* and in particular the sections of that book for children that are concerned with the breaking of records having to do with immensities. Unless I'm mistaken, in addition to the world's tallest artificial structure, our many Officially Amazing feats/features include the longest driverless metro, the tallest hotel, the largest gold ring, the most floors in a building, the building with the largest floor space, the biggest mall, and, I read somewhere, the most nationalities washing their hands at once. Even this last exploit (undertaken to mark Global Handwashing Day, and not, as the pre-judger might think, a mindless stunt) suggests to me that there remains intact in this small country a joyful, properly childlike sense of the lofty. Excelsior!

The construction process is interesting and sometimes gorgeous. I can't pretend to understand what I'm looking at, but nor can I deny the spectacular pleasure I get from tall rebars standing in thickets in concrete, or from the short-lived orange plastic mesh that is like orange peel, or from the patterns made by construction lanterns shining in exposed concrete interiors. Most compelling of all are the tower cranes. The Dubai skyline is unimaginable to me without their masts and jibs and guy lines. Each of these marvels would impress Eiffel himself and stirs one as much as any spire or minaret. If I had my way, they would remain permanently in place, in great numbers. A Dubai that is not under continuing construction would make less sense. I'm pretty sure that nobody is looking forward to the day when everything has been built and all that remains is the business of being in the buildings.

Let me add: I'm not blind to the jobsite labourers, South Asian men who are most conspicuous in the earlier stages of site-work and in whom, from the high-up and distant vantage point from which I inevitably observe them, one might take an almost entomological interest as they crisscross and here and there swarm, seemingly one and the same in their colour-coded corporate uniforms. I emphasize the qualifiers 'almost' and 'seemingly'. I'm aware that I'm looking at individual persons. I have taken steps to inform myself about the oppressive and predicamental working conditions, not to say near-enslavement, to which many of them are subject from day one. (Or even before day one: many are instructed, so I've heard, to don the abovementioned corporate attire in their country of origin so that they travel to and arrive in Dubai already colour-coded.) I also know enough to not give weight to the emotion of solidarity by which I experience, from inside my chilled apartment, a one-sided connection to these men, who are in the blazing hot outdoors. I'll simply say this: I have run the numbers, and I'm satisfied that I have given the situation of the foreign labour corps, and my relation to it, an appropriate measure of consideration and action.

(I don't want to dwell on this or pat myself on the back (if back-patting is what's called for, which I'm not saying it is). I will only, quickly, say:

1. The subjection of persons to unjust, harsh and otherwise wrongful treatment constitutes mistreatment of persons.
2. Labourers in Dubai are mistreated.
3. The problem of mistreatment is widespread.
3.1 Mistreatment is not confined to labourers in Dubai.
4. The concept of personhood is a valid basis for an ethics.
5. The personhood of all persons is equal.
5.1 Locality of a person is an invalid basis for preferring the personhood of one person to that of another.

5.2     A corollary of personhood is the freedom from mistreatment.

5.3     A corollary of an ethics of personhood is a practicable duty to promote all freedoms that are corollaries of personhood.

5.3.1   A practicable duty is a duty to take action that is reasonably practicable.

5.3.1.1 What is reasonably practicable depends on the facts of the case.

5.4     I ought to take practicable action to stop or reduce the mistreatment of persons.

5.4.1   In doing as I ought pursuant to 5.4, I ought not to act for the benefit of labourers in Dubai in preference to acting for the benefit of persons located elsewhere on the basis of my and the labourers' coincidental locality in Dubai.

5.4.1.1 I cannot establish a basis alternative to the basis referred to at 5.4.1 for acting preferentially as aforesaid for the benefit of labourers in Dubai.

6.      There exist organizations that take action to prevent, halt or reduce the mistreatment of persons ('organizations').

6.1     An organization may be effective.

6.2     It is practicable for me to identify effective organizations.

6.3     The effectiveness of an organization relates to the continuing receipt by the organization of donations from the public.

7.      It is impracticable for me to directly prevent, stop or reduce the mistreatment of persons.

8.      It is practicable for me to donate to effective organizations.

9.      A donation by me to effective organizations will have the effect of promoting the freedom of persons from mistreatment.

10.    A donation by me to effective organizations is a doing of
       my duty as described at 5.4 if the donation is commen-
       surate with what it is practicable for me to donate.


(Or something to that effect. I'm sure this reasoning is full
of holes. If I were to show it to professionals, they would fall
around laughing. Let them. I'm not trying to move the world-
historical philosophical needle here. I'm trying to figure out
how to do the right thing, and last I heard that wasn't something
you needed a Ph.D. to do.)

Human Rights First (HRF) and Human Rights Watch (HRW)
are nonprofit, nonpartisan, independent and reputable international advocacy and action organizations with global reaches.
They are effective organizations. In my first year in Dubai,
after I had had the chance to consider matters, I set up and
activated automatic bank transfers of 18.5 per cent of my gross
monthly salary to HRF and 18.5 per cent to HRW. (These are
US-tax-deductible charitable contributions, of course, but
that's between me and the IRS, and by the by. (I arrive at the
37 per cent number by calculating the maximum donation
that's consistent with my making reasonable and prudent provision for my long-term comfort and solvency. A monthly cash-
in-hand of six thousand USD, net of taxes and mortgage
payments, strikes me as reasonable and prudent for these
purposes. (Note: the Autobiography is a corporate car, owned
and paid for by Batros Family Office (Dubai) Ltd.))) I cheated
a little by asking HRW to allocate my donations to the struggle
for migrant workers' rights in the Gulf states, but only if in
HRW's judgment this would be appropriate. HRW confirmed
this was appropriate, thanked me, and did as I asked. I admit
that I'm uneasy about maybe not doing the right or valid
thing with this allocation, the self-serving purpose of which
is to make it easier for me to walk around Dubai without
feeling too guilty. I can live with that uneasiness, which is

not as bad as the alternative uneasiness. While far from saying that one can purchase rectitude or that I've now got some kind of get-out-of-jail card, I do feel I'm acquitting myself well enough so as not to have to lower my eyes to the ground when I meet someone.

(One last point: because I accept as a given that Dubai labourers are very badly treated, I don't owe it to the labourers to take steps to find out about exactly what kind of mistreatment they suffer from. Knowing those details would make no actionable difference to me. By contrast, HRW and HRF must go into the details, since that is their job, and what they find out is knowledge that can be imputed to me, that is, whatever they know, I know, even if I don't actually know what they know. It sounds counterintuitive, until one bears in mind the concept of outsourcing.))

On the afternoon of the Ted Wilson mission, I drew little relief from looking out the window. From the Pasha, I could see the Astrominium site (as it then was). All work on that mighty tower-to-be had just stopped. The sight of the huge abandoned pit was demoralizing. When the Full Body Shiatsu came to an end, I did not move. I lay limp in the Zero Gravity position, dreading the empty and shameful hours and days and weeks and years ahead. Normally I'm tolerant of my lot, but sometimes I am gloomy and cannot bear it and I question the rationality and desirability of sticking around in person for a further (all things being equal) three or four decades, and I find it calming that I have no dependants of any kind and am always at liberty to hang myself. The gloom passes, and gives way to the more searching notion that one's conduct is, by definition, a leading of the way, and we are all conductors, and not even the man without dependants is an island, and one's body is not one's own. It follows that to put oneself to death would offer a dispiriting example and one ought to not do it; one ought to biologically persist. Even though it thankfully remains the case that almost no one in Dubai – or elsewhere, at this point, I believe – really gives a shit what I do, I am still bound to try to do as little damage as I reasonably can. This mainly involves lying low. From the moment I arrived in this country, I have deliberately tried to be by myself inside my apartment as often and for as long as is consistent with not turning into an oddball.

I'll say one more thing about no man being an island: it isn't the whole story. I'm of course referring to one's inner Robinson and the inward island on which he must be marooned.

My face skin felt dry. I got out of the Pasha and found my moisturizing sunscreen. I used (and still use) a brand named 'hope'. Maybe this is because tubes of 'hope' display the following statement:

> **philosophy**: what was
> is not what will be. let
> hope light your path in
> life's journey, and it will
> set you free.

My phone shuddered. Mila! The text of her text:

How are you?

What timing!

Mila I met back in my early Dubai days, on a night I got drunk at the Hyatt Regency Premiere Club bar. I had never calculatingly spoken to a hooker before, so the encounter was nerve-racking as well as pleasant; as I say, I was drunk, and

Mila was and is very good at being kind and delighted, and very much presents on the *fille de joie* end of the sex-pro spectrum. We talked about Minsk, her hometown. We established that the Danube fails to flow through Minsk, fails indeed to flow through Belarus. With a pen and a paper napkin, Mila plotted for my benefit the whereabouts of her cryptic coastless country. Belarus is surrounded by Latvia, Russia, Ukraine, Poland and Lithuania.

An unpredicted result of befriending Mila and Mila's friends is that I've become really quite curious and knowledgeable about the layout of Russia and the post-Soviet states. I not only know the difference between Kazakhstan and Uzbekistan but have on my map Omsk and Bishkek and Yerevan and Perm and Poltava and Ternopil. This isn't to say that I'm interested in these ladies' circumstances. Absolutely the last thing I want to get into with them is their backstory. But I've always been interested in geography; and often, after she has left, I will Google the place a given girl says she's from and I will learn a little about the world. My investigations are mainly photographic. I have contemplated the smokestacks of Magnitogorsk and the poplars of Gharm. A gas station in burned grassland; a municipality approached through a wood of silver birches; a window among thousands in a sovietic housing complex – these are the icons of personal desolation with which I have come to associate the women I pay to have sex with, and sometimes it requires an effort of reasoning on my part to resist emotions connecting them to Rapunzel and Andromeda and the Little Mermaid and to remind myself, first, that the women Mila introduces me to are members of a special class, namely tourists who choose to fund their vacation or other financial objectives by engaging in a night or two of remunerated sexual-social activity, and are not sex slaves trafficked by criminal gangs; and second, that it would be ridiculously grandiose and/or patronizing of me to think that it falls to me to 'save' these women from their choices and/or from those circumstances that may, to one degree or another, have left them with imperfect options, for it must be recognized that prostitution of any kind is a far from ideal line of work and that, put in possession of a magic wand, like anyone of ordinary sensitivity I would see no reason not to wave out of existence those things that lead a person to become a sexual servant or reluctant equal-footing erotic contractor. Unfortunately, I am not a wizard. I am a john, and cannot escape the john paradigm. This does not mean I cannot do good. I can: a john can do good. He can meet the (regrettable but pre-existing and by him uncorrectable) on-the-spot needs of the woman whose company he pays for. This entails making as generous a bargain as he is reasonably able to make; keeping his side of the bargain (by which he is bound not only by terms of payment but by terms of courtesy and respect); and abiding by the etiquette that serves all parties well. This last requirement means making no personal promises or demands; refraining from embarrassing the other or snooping around into her undisclosed motives; and offering nothing less than full face-value acceptance of her self-presentation as a good-time girl light-heartedly making an extra buck.

Of that first night with Mila, strangely it is not the night itself I remember most happily (and I do remember it happily) but the morning after. I woke up with a woman who seemed pleased to be in a room with me. True, Mila headed out at the first drone of the imams (she was disguised in an abaya, which was logical but astounding); but she was also all smiles, and gave me her phone number, and uttered emphatic words of satisfaction. Apparently the night had been a great success for her, too. Apparently Mila's interests and mine not only were not in conflict, they were in identity. Apparently she and I had injured no third entity, animal or mineral, and our dealings had produced neither an increase nor a decrease in the total sum of human hope. Apparently it was a win-win-draw-draw.

(In my book, the win-win-win ideal, valuable advance though it is on the mere win-win, does not go far enough. It seems unsatisfactory to restrict the stakeholders in a given transaction to the two transactors plus the inescapable third party, to wit, the planetary/global lot. There is a fourth, admittedly subjective and conceptually vague interest at stake, namely the effect of the transaction in terms of the human race's susceptibility to downfall or glory. And I suspect, uselessly and a little awfully, that by definition there must be a further, fifth plane of moral reality, beyond our animal comprehension, involving interests that transcend even the destinies of our planet and of the human soul. I do not mean the divine or the universal as such. Nor am I mystically hinting at some cosmic good news. If only I were!)

In my victoriousness, I actually laughed out loud. The funny part wasn't just that the me-and-Jenn deal, when it was extant, had always felt like a draw-lose-draw-lose. It was that during all those years of trying to do the right thing with and by and for Jenn, I never felt in the right. Always I sensed, close by, the doghouse. Not that I blamed her for this. Even as I understood the doghouse as an outbuilding of the phony coupledom for which surely both of us were responsible, it was clearly a doghouse built by me, with my name on it. Chronic self-misrepresentation and inner absenteeism are inconsistent with the performance of the duties of a loving partner. They make a wrongdoer of one, and it must be the exceptional wrongdoer who does not of his or her own volition inhabit a place of fault and penalty. But when I look back on that doghouse, I see that my sense of it has grown foggier. For example, it occurs to me that a doghouse implies a dog, and a dog implies a master. The identity of the dog is clear enough – I was the dog. But who was the master? Not Jenn, surely. The role would have been too burdensome: a dog must be taken for walks, etc. So who, then?

It was during those doghouse days, as it happens, that I went through a phase of being in a sort of love with Matilda, the grey, breathless, arthritic pit-bull mutt who lived immediately downstairs from Jenn and me and could sometimes be heard howling. When Matilda's owners were out of town it was my job to feed her and take her to the dog run at Madison Square Park and sometimes even spend the night with her, at her place. I was not a zombie with Matilda, who for her part was purely Matilda. When the neighbours moved away, I missed her; it was painful to walk doglessly past the dog run. I suggested to Jenn that we might want to have a four-legged friend of our own. 'I'm being serious,' I said.

Jenn was sitting up in bed, laptop open, leafing through work papers: A4 lever-arch binders surrounded her. She put down the binder. We had never discussed the question of pets before. There was a look of interest on her face. It was exciting – to connect to her like this.

'I don't want to live with a dog,' she said. She picked up her binder.

Jenn was not being unkind. Far from it. She was honestly ascertaining her wants and communicating them economically and clearly. It was her form of considerateness, and I received it as such, and I still view it as such. Another way to state the matter would be: she was being Jenn. This was enormously consequential. Since I had made a binding commitment to Jenn the implied condition of which was to be with *Jenn*, i.e., the person characterized above all by Jenn-ness, it followed that, (i) if Jenn was being Jenn, then (ii) I had no good grounds for complaint about those actions of hers which, though they might provide grounds for complaint if they were the actions of another, were essentially instances of her being herself. Jenn understood this. When I said, 'Why not?' in response to her saying she did not want a dog, she, evidently anguished by my persistence, said, 'I'm not interested in dogs. I'm not a dog person. You know that. What do you want from me?' There was no good answer to this question, which of course had not been asked in order to solicit an answer but to make point (ii) above. But for some reason I decided to hear her literally, and I blurted, kind of jokily and experimentally, 'How about a little bit of attention?' She, Jenn, looked at me. 'You want my attention? I'll give you my attention.' It was a menace, obviously, and it scared me – rightly so, as subsequent events showed. So I said nothing more about it, and not only out of fear. Her threat had silently expressed a valid accusation: I was a zombie fraud and not speaking in good faith and deep down did not want Jenn's attention and had no good reason to ask for it. Therefore, even though she'd menaced me with the intention of cowing me, there was legitimacy in her stance; and on the question of the dog, she also had right on her side, because I was in effect asking her to be other than who she was, which was a non-doglover. I let it drop – slunk off to my doghouse, which of course also operated as a shelter. Though sometimes I did fantasize about Jenn coming home from the office to discover that I had punched two holes in my torso and impaled myself on the rings of a man-sized binder.

I continue to think it would be lovely to have a dog. I sometimes imagine this faithful, pleasantly malodorous hound – saved by me from the municipal killer – snoozing happily at my feet, or leaping to greet me on my return to The Situation. As a basis for action, the fantasy is problematic. I could handle the emirate's pet-owning regulations, pursuant to which dogs must without fail be microchipped and be annually re-registered and wear collar discs issued by the authorities. So be it. But The Situation (I discovered too late) is a no-dog building. Even if I sold up – not possible, unless I'm prepared to take a 40 or 50 or, God forbid, 60 per cent hit – and found somewhere dog-friendly, I would still be confronted with the rules that prohibit the walking of dogs in all public parks and on all beaches; and of course there is no question of a dog setting foot in a mall or even on Marina Walk (where often I take an evening amble and – though I am the opposite of a sailor and in fact loathe boats and regard boating, with its never-ending mopping and knotting and bucketing, as a dangerous, disagreeable form of cleaning house – I enjoy reveries in which I commandeer one of the more modest Marina vessels and weigh anchor in the dead of night and make a life as a lone salt who knows every cay and current and for whom happiness is a matter of cigarettes, stars and something to drink). Where the public presence of dogs is permitted, it is on condition that they are kept on a leash. There are stories of dogs running free on a beach near Jebel Ali, and I've heard about sandy waste areas on the outskirts of the city where unleashed dogs are unofficially tolerated. The fact remains that man's best friend, in this country, is practically an outlaw. I find it all somewhat disheartening.

I'm aware that a cat is a viable option. I draw the line at cats.

Mila very rarely personally fucks me these days. Only when one of her associates no-shows does she sometimes step in, whereupon she kindly encourages me to imagine that we are old flames stuck in a romance that will not die, try as we might to extinguish it. Our much more usual arrangement is that Mila books a room at the Unique (where she has her contacts) in the name of the person who that night will entertain G. Pardew; I pay her an upfront fee of five hundred USD (out of which sum she compensates her friend/associate) plus the cost of the room; and, after the event, I pay her in cash for room service and any overnight guest fee. Unless something has gone awry, I add a tip, also paid to Mila on trust, since my strong preference is not to have to think about money when I'm with my companion. (Something goes awry, in this context, if my companion is not nice. I'm not told in advance who Mila has set me up with – 'Surprise better,' as Mila says – and I am very flexible about the physical type of the lady in question and have never turned my nose up at anyone on arbitrary and demeaning grounds such as not liking this or that about her natural appearance, about which she can do little, although I might afterwards express some private opinion to Mila. But niceness is a must. I cannot not have niceness.) It comes to about a thousand USD a pop, about twice a month. It's both a luxury and a benign circulation or trickle-down of my wealth. I'd happily increase the frequency, but Mila's network operates by word of mouth, and it cannot astonish that her supply of dependable holidaymaking part-time hot women of the night is erratic.

I took a nap and woke up in the early evening. Then I re-showered and shaved so as to be Pardew-like and presentable. I was all set for an enjoyable evening: after the morning's search and rescue debacle, I felt I deserved it. I stepped into the elevator and ran into Mrs Ted Wilson.

I could not have been more shocked if it had been Dracula. I think I let out a small yelp of fright. The doors shut quickly. There was no getting out. It was me and her and the decorative mock hieroglyphs. I must believe that she found it as terrifying as I did, for she turned towards the corner of the car and stood with her face almost touching the stainless steel. Not a word was spoken. When the elevator reached the lobby, she ran away as if from a danger.

My companion that night was a merry Kyrgyz. She had a sweet Chinese face and was very talkative, even though she spoke no English. I saw that she'd already finished most of a bottle of room-service Veuve Clicquot, which, in the live-and-let-live, do-unto-others, let's-not-sweat-the-small-stuff spirit of these occasions, was absolutely fine by me. It was certainly no fault of hers that I was not able to relax. I was too shaken up by the encounter in the elevator. I found it intolerable that I could no longer go about in my own building without fear or favour, that I had to watch my step, duck and dive, keep myself to myself, accept a fate as a Quasimodo. I had to take action. *Dear Mrs Wilson*, I conceptually wrote while the Kyrgyz sucked my cock,

> *Allow me to communicate my regret about the unfortu-nate outcome of your recent visit to my apartment. Please understand that it was an exceptional and most unchar-acteristic occurrence. I am most assuredly a non-violent person. I cannot offer you an explanation of my conduct without burdening you with the long story of my personal history and the idiosyncratic sensitivities that are mine to bear. I would merely ask you to accept that I am aware that things got the better of me, and that you suffered as a consequence. Also, with great tentativeness and with a view only to your edification, I would humbly suggest that you inquire into your own possible contribution to what happened. It is not my place to say anything about this, and in any case I have nothing to say. Yours etc.*

Not for the first time, I felt the lack, in English, of letter closings available to the French. How fitting it would have been to end with

> *Je reste à votre disposition pour toute précision complé-mentaire et je vous prie d'agréer toute l'expression de ma très haute considération.*

I pulled away from the Kyrgyz. 'Please excuse me for a moment,' I said. I got out my phone and e-mailed Mrs Ted Wilson,

> Nice running into you today. May I buy you a coffee? I have information regarding Ted that may be of interest to you.

M rs Ted Wilson did not get back to me. I sent her a follow-up e-mail (which also got no reply) letting her know that in any case I would be at Al Nassma café, on Level One of the Mall of the Emirates, at 11 a.m. on Friday. Dubai Mall, which is newer, has more buzz and glitz than the Mall of the Emirates, but I have a soft spot for the latter's staid, almost déclassé vibe, which is most pronounced in the textiles and home furnishings section, where Al Nassma is to be found. Al Nassma specializes in chocolate made with camel's milk. Camel-milk chocolate not only tastes good but works as an icebreaker and talking point.

I arrived early, carrying a copy of *Philanthropy*, the magazine for philanthropists. I am not strictly a philanthropist, but I am an officer of the Batros Foundation and try to keep up with what's going on in the giving industry. It must be confessed, I was hoping the publication would make me look good, or at least philanthropic, in the eyes of Mrs Ted Wilson.

I don't think it's very wrong of me to dwell with a little pride on my part in the founding of the Batros Foundation.

Very early into my new job, I noticed that my e-mail inbox was the terminus of chaotic requests for alms, handouts, loans, donations, etc., received by the family. Sandro was the chief forwarder of these requests. He might add,

> pls do something for this man his mother was my mother's friend

or

> $3,000????

or

> tell him to screw himself.

I had (and have) no authority to make ad hoc payouts from the Batros Family Office (Dubai) Ltd account. When I formally requested, on Sandro's behalf, the consent of Eddie and Georges to the withdrawal of small charitable sums from the GEAs, I got no reply. No doubt they figured Sandro could easily make the payments from his own funds. Yet it seemed to me that there had to be a way lawfully and conveniently to give effect to the Batroses' benevolent intentions. I advised that the family consider setting up a private foundation, with clearly defined purposes and powers and criteria, as an effective and potentially tax-efficient vehicle for their giving. There was no answer. Some weeks later, I got a call from *le père* Batros.

This was a surprise and a big deal. It was Georges Batros who'd transformed the family business, a venerable if smallish shipping agency with offices in Beirut, Tripoli and Latakia, into the vast international concern known and trading as Entreprises Batros. The story of his commercial adventures was told in his self-published ghostwritten memoir, *La vie est belle*, in which he described as a series of very lucky breaks his successful forays into one market after another (marine-insurance agenting; automobile insurance for developing countries; exportation and distribution of generic pharmaceutical products to French-speaking Africa). Perhaps his biggest coup was Banque Batros S.A.L., a specialist in custodian services for Middle Eastern and West African clients founded in 1984: in 1996, he sold the bank (Batros interest: 32 per cent) hook, line and sinker to an American consortium for 440 million USD. The memoir did not mention it, but the family's real-estate portfolio has grown in value (if my back-of-an-envelope calculations are correct) by at least 160 million USD since the mid-Eighties; and now Eddie is making new fortunes, notably by betting big on agricultural holding companies in Argentina and Brazil. I have no reliable way to estimate the total value of Batros assets, but I would guess that it's not less than half a billion USD. (If the financial crisis had a negative effect on the family's wealth, I have not heard about it.) I cannot be any more specific. I'm not really sure where all the money comes from and what it all comes to.

Georges, a little fellow who looks like Charles Aznavour, gave me a signed copy of *La vie est belle* at our very brief first meeting. This took place on his fuck-off yacht, the *Giselle*. Named for his deceased mother, it was moored in Beirut harbour most of the year and, according to Eddie, was where Georges now spent most of his time, playing cards and shooting the shit with his crew and old pals. My dedication read, *Bonne chance, fiston*.

'*Fiston, écoute bien*,' he said when he called me in Dubai.

I did as instructed. The next morning I packed a bag, got into the Batros Gulfstream 100 ('*l'autobus*', in the family slang), and flew to Antalya, Turkey. From there I took a two-hour taxi ride to Finike, a small coastal town. The *Giselle*, too big for the marina, was anchored well offshore. A crewmember collected me in a rubber dinghy, incidentally trying to break the world water-speed record. Waiting at the top of the boarding ladder was Georges Batros. He wore a naval peaked cap, shorts, and no shirt. 'OK, *yallah*,' he said to the captain. To me he said, 'Welcome aboard,' and he kissed me on both cheeks.

Somebody took my bag, somebody took me to the dining deck, somebody made me a gin and tonic. I didn't want a gin and tonic, but what the hell. It was good to have got out of the desert, and I'd never been on a private cruise or visited this part of the ancient world. The yacht, or ship, slipped past aquamarine inlets and between small islands where wild olive trees grew out of grey and white rocks. The littoral mountains, precipitous and forested, were beautiful. A cool breeze blew. I inhabited the World of Rolex.

And yet I was jumpy. Why? Because I am not a total dope. I wasn't going to fall into the trap of equating beautiful surroundings with a beautiful state of affairs. When, in Beirut, Eddie introduced me to his father, he said, 'You're going to like him. He's mellowed a lot since the old days.' People who are said to have 'mellowed' always make me nervous. Meanwhile I had already figured out that to even begin to understand the Batros family you had to understand the money. The Batros sons are highly remunerated (salaries, bonuses, stock options, employment benefits) but many of their largest capital assets – houses, boats, lump sums from the GEAs, interest-free loans, etc. – have essentially remained in the gift of their father, who is the majority shareholder of Batros Holdings Ltd (incorporated in the DIFC), which in turn wholly owns the Batros subsidiaries, of which there are more than fifty, which in turn own who knows how many sub-subsidiaries. Georges still controls most of the money, is what it comes down to.

He joined me. He had undressed and wore only a white towel, around his waist. He unknotted the towel and draped it over the seat of his chair. Now he was naked. A pharmacologistical young woman ('*Une lesbienne*,' Georges later whispered) began to shampoo his hair. Most of the ultra-HNW individuals I've met are idiosyncratically demanding, and everyone is familiar with the larger-than-life, I-make-my-own-rules display of power, and I understand from Ollie that gratuitous domestic nudity is prevalent among the rich and famous as a kind of very authoritative informality. But even though I had willingly entered into the company of Georges Batros and maybe 'on some level' had sought him out, I began to feel that my situation was objectionable as well as precarious. I had no idea how long I was expected to stay on this boat or why I'd been summoned. The *Giselle*, I knew, was making its annual odyssey from Beirut to Saint-Jean-Cap-Ferrat, where Mme Batros (née Alice Rourke, in Mullingar, Ireland) was already summering in the Villa Batros, a magnificent clifftop mansion with a private jetty. Where was I supposed to get off? Piraeus? Portofino? Surely there is more than a trace of false imprisonment about hospitality from which there is no escape.

Georges got to his feet and took a shower. The female crew-member trained a high-powered hose on him as though he were on fire. He thoroughly lathered himself, dick and balls especially, and rinsed his hair and hopped around in the water jet. He kept chatting to me, even as the crewmember towelled him down. There was something faintly villainous about his showiness. He reminded me of those clever murderers who for a while run rings around Lieutenant Columbo.

'And how is your old friend Mr Trompe?' Georges, taking his seat, said. He was still in the buff, though now he wore his commodore's cap.

'Fine – I guess,' I said. 'I don't really know him.'

'Come, you're being modest,' Georges said. 'Weren't you invited to his wedding? At Palm Beach?'

This was correct – up to a point. Godfrey Pardew was the invitee, on account of the good work he had done for Donald Trump and especially Donald's father, Fred, in the realm of wills, trusts, divorces, prenuptial agreements and other sensitive matters. But Godfrey had declared himself 'regrettably unable' to fly down to Florida, and at the last minute he notified the Trump people that I (plus one, Jenn) would be attending on behalf of the firm in the stead of Mr and Mrs Pardew. The wedding was a lot of fun, as it happens, and I shared certain amusing details with Eddie on the night of our reunion at Asia de Cuba. That was a highly consequential anecdote, as things turned out, because it was my connection to Donald Trump that prompted Sandro to approve my appointment.

I'm not sure what Eddie told him, but out of the blue Sandro flew to New York, bought me dinner at the Rainbow Room, and (making zero mention of the London fiasco) questioned me for over an hour about that magical night at Mar-A-Lago. I was able to tell him what it was like to stand next to Shaquille

O'Neal, and to listen to Billy Joel playing the piano six feet away, and to take a leak with the great Trump in the adjoining urinal. Sandro was deeply moved. He confided that it was his dream to take part in *The Apprentice*, the Trump TV show in which job-seeking contestants compete for the approval of the magnate and are each 'fired' by him, save one – the apprentice. Sandro was in his late forties and presumably more qualified for the role of master than apprentice, so I was a little surprised. I began to understand his ambition to earn Trump's blessing only after it became clear that Georges neither trusted nor esteemed Sandro, and restricted his role to that of running the Dubai holding company – a titular job – and chiefly expected of him, his older son, that he spend enough time in Dubai so as to serve as a human data point for technical legal purposes. When Sandro asked me about getting on Trump's TV show, I told him I would see what I could do. This I duly did. I could do nothing.

'I went as a representative of my law firm,' I said to Georges. 'I'm not close to the Trump family.'

'Ah, this was not my impression,' Georges said. Then he was telling me all about the crewing arrangements – two Norwegians (captain, chief engineer), a Greek chef, and five others from ethnically prestigious parts of Western Europe. Their uniform consisted of white Lacoste shirts, white sailing shorts with the *Giselle* monogram, and classic blue-and-white boat shoes. They all wore the same sunglasses. Uniformity aside, they might have been gung-ho young bankers on holiday. Georges said, 'These people are the best in the world.'

I said something like, 'Yeah, they look like they're really stoked.'

He called out to one of the deck hands. 'Giancarlo!' The fellow came bounding over. Georges said something to him in Italian. Presently the boat dropped anchor. I heard splashes: Giancarlo and two others had plunged into the sea. They swam to the shore, climbed over the tricky rocks, and made their way up the hill to where a herd of goats was feeding on bushes. There was no sign of a goatherd. Giancarlo turned towards us and waved. He gestured at a black goat, and Georges gave him a double thumbs-up. The three men jumped on the black goat and wrestled it to the ground and instantly roped its legs. I might have been watching a rodeo. Giancarlo slit the animal's throat. They held it down while it kicked and bled out. This lasted for some time. Giancarlo towed the carcass back, trailing a messy red stream. The three men stood on the deck wet and bloody. They held up the dead goat. 'Bravo, bravo,' Georges Batros said, applauding. Everyone applauded, me included.

'You see?' he said to me. 'This is the quality of these men.'

'Unbelievable. Wow,' I said. There seemed no point in raising the issue of compensation for the owner of the goat.

A short while later, the chef arrived with a serving dish. 'The liver,' Georges said. 'Fresh, fresh.' He cut a piece off the red mass, squeezed lemon juice over it, and began to eat. 'Fantastic,' he said. 'Take some. There is nothing healthier.' I accepted a piece, against my will. I did not want to put a part of the goat inside me.

Georges said, 'This idea you have, to have a foundation, this is a good idea.'

It took a second or two to figure out what he was talking about.

'Tell me,' Georges said. He was very fastidious with his white napkin and was taking a long time to clean his mouth and wipe his hands. His huge helping of raw liver was suddenly gone, as if by prestidigitation. 'Who do you think we should help?'

'Whoever you want to help,' I said. 'It's your money.' I added, for some stupid reason, 'You have the honour of deciding.'

'Honour?' He laughed. 'This is not my area of expertise. I would like you to decide.'

'Uh, I'm no expert, either,' I said. 'It was just a suggestion. I just thought it might be a good idea. From the Batros standpoint. I mean, it's my impression that you get a lot of requests for help.'

'This is very true,' Georges said. 'A lot of people ask us for money.' He pointed at my chest. 'Tigers. Maybe we should help the tigers. They are very noble. I remember seeing them in Las Vegas. Poor Mr Roy, that was the tragedy of tragedies. Or was it Mr Siegfried? My question is, do you think we can save the tigers? How would we do it? How much money would it take? The problem is the Chinese,' he said. 'They eat tigers. I believe they will eat anything. Dogs, of course. They love the meat of the dog. It is not just the Chinese. The Indonesians, too. Let me tell you a story. I was in Indonesia once, in Sumatra. A savage place. I had to go up into the hills to speak to a big man. On the way up there, my driver is looking, looking, like this.' Georges gripped an invisible steering wheel and peered from side to side. 'Then' – he turned the wheel – '*boum*. We hit something. The driver gets out. He goes into the street. He picks up the dead dog by the legs and throws it in the back of the truck, like this. He says to me, We will give the dog to the big man. And this is what happened. The big man cooked the dog, and we ate it. Eating dogs isn't so stupid, in my opinion. In Switzerland they eat dog sausages, and I cannot say the Swiss are stupid. Cold, yes. Avaricious, yes. Stupid, no. But eating tigers for medicine? Very stupid. Maybe this should be our focus, the fight against stupidity. It's a very serious problem. There is a lot of stupidity in the world. It does much harm. You must understand this very well, coming from the United States.'

'I – yes,' I said. I was more taken aback by his comment on the Swiss, which on one view amounted to a comment on my mother.

'The people of China work very hard, but still they are stupid,' Georges Batros said. 'Our problem is, they are' – he searched for the English word – '*nombreux*.'

'Numerous.' I was wondering why he'd decided to have the conversation in English. In Beirut, we'd spoken in French.

'Exactly. They are numerous. There are more than one billion Chinese, *si je ne me trompe pas*. Also one billion Indians, and many of them are stupid, and again the tiger suffers. I am not sure where to begin. What do you suggest?'

'I don't know,' I said. 'Perhaps you could –'

'What are your arrangements?' Georges said.

I didn't know what he meant.

Georges said, 'What arrangements have you made to help others? That would be very good to know. I could follow your example.'

'I'm not sure that would be instructive,' I said. I smiled humbly. 'Our situations are not comparable,' I said. 'Unfortunately, I'm not in a position –'

'Yes, yes, yes – I understand. But you make good money. Eddie has taken care of you. You are in a position to help others, even if only a little. It would be a guide, an inspiration, to hear about your personal efforts.'

He was trying to push me around. I declined the top-up an attendant was offering me. To Georges, I said, 'My arrangements are my business, with respect.' (I had no arrangements at that time. I had only recently arrived in Dubai. I had not yet put in place my automatic transfers to HRF and HRW.)

'But what I give to charity, what I do with my money – that's your business?'

'I think there's been a misunderstanding, Mr Batros. I don't have an opinion about this. I was just trying to be useful as the family officer.'

'I like you,' Georges stated. 'You're Eddie's old friend. And Sandro trusts you. This is a point in your favour, because my sons can't agree about anything. So let me explain something to you. You have one function. You know what this function is? It is to make sure nobody steals. This is your function.'

Various ripostes came to mind ex post facto, but at that moment I said, 'Absolutely. Understood.' If Georges wanted to flex his biceps, put me in my place, show me who was boss, ream me out – whatever, sticks and stones. Fundamentally, spiritually, he had no standing. All I was interested in was keeping my job and getting the fuck off the yacht.

So it came about. Somebody took away my glass, somebody gave me my bag, somebody ushered me to the dinghy. Georges was at the top of the boarding ladder, waving. 'Please give my regards to Mr Trompe,' he called out. I was quickly transported to the nearest coastal village. I made a deal with a villager and was driven to Antalya. The *autobus* was long gone. I flew back commercial, via Istanbul. A week later, I was informed that the Batros Foundation had been incorporated in Dubai and that the board of directors had appointed me to the (pro bono and essentially honorary) office of Treasurer.

The Batros family endowed the Foundation with forty million USD. I signed the GEA authorization myself – an unforgettable, vertiginous moment. Almost four years later, the Foundation (through sub-charities and in cooperation with partner donors) supports medical clinics in Abidjan, Libreville, Tunis and Kinshasa. These projects are going very well, judging from the brochures and the websites, which feature photographs of very-happy-looking Africans. I have no involvement in the operational side, which is carried on by a mainly Lebanese team based in International Humanitarian City, over by Business Bay. The team reports directly to Georges but copies me in on about fifteen e-mails a day, few of which I am in a position to make much sense of. I do, as Treasurer, have power to authorize payments from the Foundation accounts, which in theory I oversee. This power enables me to ensure that the Foundation makes miscellaneous donations authorized by the Batros directors. To date I've received authorizations from Alice Batros, in support of CARI (working for Irish victims of childhood sexual abuse), and from Sandro, in support of Operation Smile (surgical repair of facial deformities in children) and the Heritage Foundation (development and dissemination of right-wing ideas). I have given the relevant instructions to the Batros Foundation employees and followed up personally. The donors can be sure that their benefaction has been effective.

It has never been explained to me by what process Georges Batros decided to green-light the Foundation. I believe I played an instigative role, even if this has never been recognized by any Batros. When I question the worth of my life, it comforts me to think that but for my instrumentality in this matter, a significant number of humans would probably be living less healthy, less happy, less worthwhile lives. One might say that this unforeseen good contains nothing less than the hidden meaning of my move to Dubai.

My dealings with the Batros family are confidential, and I'm not one to toot my own horn, so there was no question of sharing any of this with Mrs Ted Wilson at Al Nassma – if, that is, she showed up. I drank a cappuccino; I drank a second. As I watched one person after another who wasn't Mrs Wilson walk into the café, I passed into an awareness of another person – the one waiting for the arrival of Mrs Ted Wilson. What was he doing? Who did he think he was? Was it really his plan to inform Mrs Ted Wilson of an unverified rumour that there was a second Mrs Ted Wilson? As if she hadn't heard it already? As if he had some kind of standing in the matter? As if he was an Extraordinary Gentleman? As if she was really going to meet up for a coffee with an unstable lentil-thrower who didn't even know her husband? And then what – take a romantic stroll in the mall? Fall, for no reason, for a supererogatory weirdo? LOL.

I rolled up my *Philanthropy* and went to the office.

Speaking of which, who should drop by today but Sandro. He enters unannounced and catches me and his son working on a Green Belt Sudoku problem.

'What's this?' he says, picking up the puzzle book. Before anyone can reply, he lets go of the book and advances to my side of the new partition and with a great sigh takes a seat in my chair. Sandro must have the mistaken idea that the partition creates an acoustic barrier, because he says loudly, 'We need to talk.'

I pause him with a raised hand, which I suspect irritates him. I go to the kid. 'Why don't you sit at Ali's desk for a while.' The kid picks up his chair and follows me out. Ali gets up and offers the kid his own chair, behind the desk. I veto that. Ali must sit in his chair and the kid must sit in his chair.

Sandro is fiddling with my mouse and looking aggrieved. He tells me, 'I'm not happy with my doctors.'

'Which ones?' I say. Sandro's healthcare profile is complex. There's an orthopaedist in Lausanne for his bad knees, a pulmonologist in London for his bad breathing, and a cardiologist in New York for his bad heart. In Dubai, he retains physicians who provide 24/7/365 concierge medical services to a very small clientele. (The Batros family has its own in-house emergency room in both the Dubai and Beirut compounds. Each has an X-ray machine, CT scanner, blood-analysis facilities, ultrasound equipment, etc. The *Giselle* has an ER cabin, albeit a relatively rudimentary one. (Sandro's yacht, the *Mireille*, has no special cabin, but does have a defibrillator. (Eddie has no yacht.)))

'Lieberman,' Sandro says. Lieberman is the Park Avenue cardiologist. 'He's got me wearing this for the next couple of weeks.' To my dismay Sandro lifts his Notre Dame T-shirt (Notre Dame is his alma mater, though he never graduated). Even as I avert my eyes, I see that wiring has been taped to his breast tissue. 'It's a monitor. This way they can follow my heartbeat second to second.'

'OK, that makes sense,' I say. Sandro suffers from cardiac dysrhythmia.

'Yeah, but get this,' he says. 'The results show up in India. There's a computer in India watched by Indian guys. They see something, they call New York. I mean, what the WTF? Indian guys? I'm putting my life in the hands of Indian guys in India?'

'I'm sure they're highly qualified.'

'Yeah? I'm sure they're highly fucking minimum wage.'

I make a big show of getting out a piece of paper and taking a note.

Sandro sighs and heavily swivels. 'So . . . ?' He bobs his head towards the door, in the direction of his son. 'How's it going?'

'OK, I guess,' I say. I decide to try my luck, carefully. 'I have to tell you, Sandro, I'm not sure this is the most productive set-up. And this thing with weighing him . . .'

Sandro says, 'Tell me this: you got kids?' Another swivel, a big roomy one that surely puts my chair under huge strain. 'I didn't think so. However . . . Point taken. We've got to make this work. I think the answer is, you should take him under your wing.'

I am very, very silent. I am William the Silent and Harpo Marx and Justice Thomas.

He is saying, 'You're telling me it's not super-productive. OK – so make it productive. You're a smart guy – teach him something. He's a got a bunch of summer homework he needs to do. Help him with that. His mother isn't exactly the professor of brain surgery type.'

I'm not going to get sidetracked into a consideration of Mireille Batros, an exceedingly complicated person. 'Sandro –'

'You're going to teach him some values,' Sandro says. 'What's right and what's wrong. This is going to be your top priority.'

'Sandro, there's no way I –'

He begins to weep. 'I can't do this by myself any more.'

Here we go again. *Krokodilstränen*. *Les larmes de crocodile*. The human tear, once a great currency, is now worthless everywhere.

He says, 'You know our ATM machine?'

I do know. At Fort Batros, the family has an HSBC ATM for its exclusive use.

Sandro tells me that Alain underhandedly borrowed his ATM card, somehow figured out the PIN, and attempted to withdraw money. They caught him red-handed, the numbskull, because he couldn't quickly work out which way to insert the card.

'Oh dear,' I say. 'That's unfortunate.'

Sandro relates that he and Mireille cross-examined their son for an hour, made various threats, inflicted various penalties, and still he refused to say how he'd got hold of the card or the PIN, or how much he was planning to withdraw and for what purpose. Mireille's participation in this questioning is ironic, because Mireille's own debit and credit cards have been taken away from her on account of her alleged inability to control her spending.

'We got nothing out of him,' Sandro says. 'Not a word.'

I'm impressed with the kid. He didn't crack.

'I want you to find out what's going on,' Sandro says.

'How am I supposed to do that?'

Sandro points a thumb at himself. 'Bad cop.' He points an index finger at me. 'Good cop. Make friends with him. Make him feel like it's safe to talk to you.'

The demand is so absurd and unenforceable that it doesn't occur to me to object.

'You'll make it work,' Sandro says. He somehow raises himself out of my chair. 'We all set with Bryan Adams?'

'You mean Bryan Ferry,' I say. 'Yes, we –'

Customer ID: **********6136

## Items that you have renewed

Title: The dog
ID: 30131045190532
Due: **10 April 2022**

Total items: 1
Account balance: £0.00
20/03/2022 11:21
Checked out: 2
Overdue: 0
Hold requests: 0
Ready for collection: 0

## Items that you already have on loan

Title: What Alice knew
ID: 30131055454117
Due: **10 April 2022**

'I mean Bryan Adams. What am I going to do with Bryan Ferry? Mireille loves Bryan Adams.'

'You asked me to book Bryan Ferry. You didn't ask me to book Bryan Adams.'

'Bryan Adams. I told you to book fucking Bryan Adams. You booked Bryan Ferry?'

'I booked who you asked me to book.'

Sandro points at me again. He's always pointing. 'Now you're fucking with my sex life.' He goes to the door, where, in a cheesy move, he turns to face me darkly. 'Do not fuck with me on this. You got nine days to get Bryan Adams.'

*Exeunt* Sandro and all of his bullshit. Re-enter the kid and all of his.

I'm so angry, I can't even mental-mail.

'I'm stepping out,' I announce to Ali and Alain and, for all I know, Allah.

There is still a problem, however: where to go once I have stepped out. It is an old problem: the problem of the exit. If it is a difficult thing to leave a room, it is still more difficult to find the room's alternative.

My office is in the DIFC, which I consider to be a beautiful place to do business and to be human in Dubai. The semi-autonomous Dubai International Financial Centre, with its regulatory structures that remove it from the emirate's archaic justice system, is not just a financial free zone. It is also an architecturally free-floating environment. In contrast to almost any other place in Dubai, substantial amenities are offered to the person who wishes to be an outdoor pedestrian. Here are broad grey plazas and pools with charcoal or dove grey water. There are green lawns, and blue-grey-brown footbridges, and cafés with silver chairs, and cool grey-brown breezeways and charcoal-grey sculptures. The beautiful office buildings are grey and grey-blue and silver-grey. Grey-brown doves go about near the dove grey pools and beautiful women go coolly across the plazas in dark jackets over white or blue shirts, and the men on the plazas have charcoal or silver hair and blue shirts and dark suits or beautiful white robes. These harmonies and consistencies of tone and demeanour are nothing other than indicia of an agreement in feeling between all of us who partake in and of this polity, namely that, in essence and in potential, ours is a zone of win-win-win flows of money and ideas and humans, and that somewhere in our processes and practices, as we sense in our bones and sometimes almost sniff in the air, are the omens of that future community of cooperative productivity, that financial nationhood, of which all of us here more or less unconsciously dream.

My difficulty, at this moment, is that I cannot feel at one with the people who coolly go across the plazas, who after all have the intention of going into the interiors of the grey buildings, i.e., into rooms, whereas I am going out of my building with no intention of going into another building. I would even say that the harmoniousness of these people and their surroundings depends on the viability of the indoors as a place for those outdoors to go to, because after all there isn't much that can be accomplished by walking between buildings. In other words, I feel anomalous as I go across the plaza, and very hot; also, it is unsustainable to keep going across plazas. I must go back indoors, into a room. And here is a room: The Empty Quarter, one of our DIFC art galleries. I go in.

The exhibition is titled:

The Worst Journey in the World
Captain Scott's Antarctic Expedition 1910–1913
The Photographs of Herbert Ponting

I'm not a big art fan. Even so, I would have to be a very strange person to be uninterested in these photographs.

Because I'm broadly familiar with the story of Captain Scott and know that gloom and doom lies ahead, I start with *An Emperor Penguin*. Upright haughty bird! Good chap! The resemblance to the Ruler is startling. (If another expat were present, I might share this impression with him/her, sotto voce, and we'd have a nice little laugh. However, I have The Empty Quarter to myself.)

*The* Terra Nova *held up in the Pack, Dec. 13th, 1910.*

The good ship runs afoul of the ice. Yes, I can see how that would happen. To judge from Mr Ponting's astounding black-and-white images, this sphere of land-ice and sea-ice and air-ice, so-called Antarctica, is barely a place at all but, rather, an enormous and enormously weird natural activity, so that the spectacle of this doughty, three-masted silhouette trying to get somewhere seems multiply fallacious, as if an attempt were being made to sail a shadow into a hubbub, audible only in the form of coldness, emanating from sources that are not a whereabouts.

Ah, here are the huskies.

Each has its own portrait. Husky Tresor, Husky Wolk, Husky Vida. They have pensive, trusting faces. This makes one sad, inevitably.

And here are the humans.

*C.S. Wright on return from the barrier, Jan. 1912.*

*Portrait of B. Day on return from the barrier, Dec. 21st, 1911.*

These men are clearly in shock. What happened to them? What is the 'barrier'?

There's a book of writing for sale, *The Worst Journey in the*

*World*, by Apsley Cherry-Garrard. This is a fine name for an explorer. However, the book is enclosed in cling wrap and I cannot leaf through it. I must go back to the photographs on the walls.

*Capt. Scott, Apr. 13th, 1911.*

The great/flawed man himself, with one foot on a sled. The face is emotionally ajar, and discloses a slippery modern soul – self-absorbed, ambivalent, newly metaphysically brave. It's a face you see a lot. Walk into any DIFC office and you'll spot a Bob Scott.

*Portrait of C.H. Meares on his return from the barrier, Jan. 1912.*

Again the barrier? They had to keep making the men go there?

*Portrait of Dimitri on return from the barrier, Jan. 29th, 1912.*

It is much too much for me. Out I go.

I t must have been a day or two after my non-meeting with Mrs Ted Wilson that I ran into Brett Hutchinson in a DIFC parking lot and accepted his invitation to Friday brunch. I felt like I had to. A few months before, I'd loaned Brett twenty thousand AED. As soon as he'd been fired, his bank accounts had been automatically frozen in accordance with the local law, and the guy was up to his neck in liabilities and tied to the UAE for personal reasons and unable to make a run for it. Talk about being in a tough spot. Now that he was bravely back on his feet and relatively liquid (he'd repaid me fifteen thousand

AED and promised the balance in short order), he wanted to signal his gratitude and reclaim some lost acre of honour. It must be said, I didn't know Brett that well. I loaned him the money because he approached me as one American to another. I had misgivings about whether shared nationality was a valid reason for assisting co-national A rather than alter-national B, particularly where B's needs might be as great as, indeed greater than, those of A; yet I said yes to Brett without hesitation. It was striking how, when the shit hit the fan and people suddenly if temporarily found themselves in the same tight corner, loyalties of country were rediscovered in the matter of asking for help and giving it. Which isn't to say that there was an abrupt territorial reorganization of moral feelings; there were many who were kind without reference to kindredness, and in this sense may be said to have admirably rescued the language of goodness from its primal dirt. I might add that I feel more cleanly American than ever. Leaving the USA has resulted in a purification of nationality. By this I mean that my relationship to the US Constitution is no longer subject to distortion by residence and I am more appreciative than ever of the great ideals that make the United States special. I pay my federal taxes to the last dime, and, without in any way devaluing citizenship to a business of cash registers, I can assert that I am well in the black with my country.

Anyhow, Brett was a proud man from Little Rock. If he needed to buy me brunch to look himself in the eye, I wasn't going to stand in his way, even if the thought of another all-you-can-eat-and-drink Friday afternoon shindig was basically worrying. It didn't help that the event had as its stated theme, 'F*** the F****** Financial Crisis'.

The venue for the brunch was the subject of debate between a dozen or so of the brunchers. Some were in favour of the One & Only, others Al Qasr, others the Park Hyatt, others the Fairmont, others The Address (in Downtown Dubai, not The Address Dubai Marina). I would guess that two hundred messages went into circulation. The initial volley straightforwardly considered the hotels' relative merits (in the matters of value for money, lobsters, cigar-availability, ambiance, house champagne brands, etc.); but this give-and-take quickly frayed into off-topic threads, the most popular of which, this being Dubai, inevitably concerned the question of service. To be fair, I suppose it's theoretically possible that the affluent expat population largely consists of people who arrived with bees already in their bonnets about the performance of waiters, lackeys and help. But most of us here would shamefacedly agree that something about the local gradient eventually means that pretty much everyone who's white and/or well-to-do slides into bossiness and haughtiness in relation to pretty much everyone who's not white and not well-to-do. According to some commentators, our domineering cadre is essentially drawn from the same stock of provincial, socially second- or third-tier Europeans who, in the days of empire, populated the lesser despotic positions – policemen, clerks, overseers – and it's far from surprising, therefore, that members of what was once the taskmaster or slave-driver class should be given to pushing people around and looking down their lower-middle- or middle-middle-class noses at their supposed social and/or racial inferiors. Maybe this holds some truth; there's no denying I've seen repellently *de haut en bas* behaviour here from men and women about whom it might in all neutrality be said that in their own homeland they might not be widely perceived as having the socio-economic status to as it were plausibly claim for themselves a relative superiority. I have to wonder, though, if the negative critique of these individuals is a function of the critics' care for the well-being of the dominated persons or if it is, rather, self-serving viciousness and snobbery about persons who the critics feel have no entitlement of their own to viciousness and snobbery, a feeling that's detestable on the

110

intellectual level among others, since, unless I have been thoroughly misinformed, the so-called top or upper or upper-middle societal tiers cannot be said to have brought glory on themselves, whether historically or contemporarily, in the matter of the kindly or just treatment of less powerful others, e.g., serfs, peasants, defenceless foreign populations. It's ugly, however you look at it. It's not uplifting or entertaining to read, as I did on the aforementioned thread about the imbecilities of the servant classes,

> I got one. Our cleaning lady whose from Indonesia and a very nice young lady, put away some books with the spines facing INSIDE.

> Think I can beat that. I was at Starbucks yesterday and the Indian gentleman waiter tried to 'tidy away' the newspaper I was reading. He had no idea that the whole point of sitting down was to read the newspaper. He didn't know what reading a newspaper was!

> Try explaining that L socks go with R socks! Never works. They always think L goes with L because it looks the same. Drives me potty.

Normally, I would never think of intervening. On this occasion, I don't know why, I was prompted to write, it must be said hesitantly,

> I think that here in Dubai, there's a widespread confusion of the notions of service and servility. Restaurant/hotel service focuses on fawning and obsequiousness rather than efficiency. The question is whether this is due to the customer expectations (i.e., we demand servility), or inexperienced management, or both. We

111

know that it cannot only be due to the imported culture of the staff, because Indian waiters who work in New York, London, etc., are highly competent and resourceful. Ditto cabdrivers. Btw, has anyone noticed how disenchanted the taxi drivers here are, compared with those in New York, say? What is our role in this, I wonder?

Nobody responded to my wonderment, either online or at Yalumba, the restaurant at Le Méridien where the brunch was, in due course, held.

I turned up on the late side, at 2 p.m. Brett and his two English co-hosts had booked a huge banqueting table for thirty, and surrounding our table were other tables at which other champagne brunches were taking place, and there was a very happy, very loud, restaurant-wide brouhaha to which my table was contributing its fair share of laughing and yelling. A majority of heads wore pointy bright party hats. Not wanting to be a Buzz Killington, I put on a gleaming red fez.

Brett aside, I recognized only a few faces at my table, and only faintly. Brett seemed a little confused, or distracted, when I greeted him, and it took some rearranging of chairs to make room for me. I wandered Yalumba's famous buffets. They were wasted on me: I don't see anything great about crab displays or giant vats of macaroni and cheese, etc. Still, when in Dubai; and boiled potatoes, garlic mussels and a T-bone steak found their way onto my plate. At the table, I accepted red wine, and champagne from a salmanazar of Laurent-Perrier that happy aproned waiters wheeled around on a mobile ice-bed, courtesy of someone somewhere in the restaurant. Who was my benefactor? It seemed wrong to accept the drink without some sign of thanks (even though I was entirely satisfied by my red wine and had no selfish wish to drink champagne). In the end, I decided to raise my glass of bubbly to a table of generous-looking French dudes wearing berets, and they raised their glasses back, though it remained unclear if this was to acknowledge my gratitude or simply to return my friendly gesture.

The chief excitement in my section of the table was provided by the presence of a Scotsman named Jimmy. Jimmy was that very rare bird – the new arrival in Dubai. Here was a chink of economic light! Here might be the recovery's first swallow! Our joy was lessened by his revelation that his was not an open-market hiring but, in point of fact, a UAE government job – a six-month contract to work on supplementary procurement issues connected to the Metro construction. Never mind, he was a fresh face, and he gave older Dubai hands the chance to once more indulge in what may be our most indestructible conversational trope, that is, tutoring the newcomer to the Emirates about the outlandish legal hazards he or she faces in the areas of buying and consuming alcohol, gambling, having sex, driving, drunk driving, using recreational drugs, incurring debt, and so on and so forth, with illustrative cautionary tales whose invariable moral is that, contrary to its accommodating and modern appearance, for the non-national the emirate is a vast booby-trap of medieval judicial perils, and Johnny Foreigner must especially take great care when interacting with local citizens (who constitute only 10 per cent or so of the population) because de facto there is one law for Abdul Emirati and another for Johnny Foreigner, so that, for example, if Johnny is involved in an automobile collision with Abdul, responsibility for damage caused will in practice not be determined in accordance with familiar qualitative assessments of the acts and omissions of the parties involved but in accordance with considerations of identity, the local concept (supposedly alien to the person accustomed to Romano-Judeo-Christian jurisprudence) being that the applicability of the duty of care (known to some as the neighbour principle) is subject to modification by the nationalitative interrelation of the involved parties. I.e., it's not what you *do*, it's who you *are* vis-à-vis the person who does unto you or unto whom you do.

Jimmy was asked about his first impressions. 'I love the huge posters of the Sheikh you see everywhere,' he said. 'I wouldn't mind getting hold of one. I could make a fortune on eBay.'

A fork was waved in Jimmy's direction. 'That sort of hipster irony doesn't go down very well here.'

'Yeah,' someone said. Making quotation fingers, this person added, 'He's not "The Ruler", he's the fucking Ruler.'

The fork-waver warned Jimmy, 'You want to watch it. They don't have a sense of humour about that sort of thing. Just so you know.'

'They like to be ruled. It settles them down. I'm not against it, to be honest. Not in England, of course, but here.'

'He's a good bloke, Sheikh Mo. He's done a lot of good for his people.'

Jimmy: 'Is it true he's got a private jet just for his falcons?'

'Yes. So they say.'

'And he's got cheetahs, too.'

'No, he doesn't. That's total rubbish.'

The cheetah guy threw his party hat at the rubbisher, who in turn threw his napkin at the cheetah guy. There was a brief storm of things being thrown. Bread rolls flew from one end of the table to the other, to shouts of approval.

When things calmed down, somebody said, 'They say he's after getting married again.'

'That's what I heard, too. Sheikha number four.'

'Could be number five, for all we know.'

Jimmy: 'Why's it so hush-hush?'

Somebody began to air a theory (which I paraphrase and, to be honest, save from disjointedness) to the effect that the Ruler's overt power depended on an inner zone of secrecy for secrecy's sake, and this centrum of inexplicability (which deprived outsiders of data relating even to royal matrimonial and domestic arrangements) tacitly communicated the existence of broader political arrangements by which entitlement to significant information was made the subject of concentric separations, with the Ruler at the centre and the populace distributed more or less at the perimeter; etc., etc., with the inevitable reference to the Wizard of Oz.

To my left was a kind-looking blonde in her thirties. She must have been as restless as I was, because she said, 'Hello, I'm Samantha. What's your name?' She was drinking a cocktail involving champagne and Rémy Martin. The neighbouring table gave a hilarious roar as I answered her, and we both smiled, because it was good to have so many relaxed and happy souls assembled in one room, and at that moment, in fact, the music came on and a kicking conga line instantly formed and people from every corner of Yalumba joined in, laying hands on shoulders and waists and shuffling along singing the olé song and tooting on party blowers. Samantha said, 'Come on,' and I added myself to the shambling human concatenation, and I had fun, obviously because I was well on my way to getting loaded. It was a full five minutes before the music stopped and we all returned to our tables in the best of spirits.

Samantha told me she was heading home to England, to get a divorce and 'start all over again'.

'That must be very painful,' I said.

She suggested in a sensitive tone of voice that I might have gone through something similar, and I said, 'Perhaps I have.'

'Well, either you have or you haven't,' she said.

I laughed. Samantha seemed to be upset by this, which was the last thing I wanted, because I was really rooting for her, this spirited and good person, and I said, 'Sorry. I was just remembering something. My ex objected to me using that word – "perhaps".'

Samantha said, 'What do you mean, she objected?'

'She just didn't like it. It got on her nerves.'

'I suppose it depends on the context,' Samantha said with great pensiveness.

'Yes,' I agreed.

The Perhapsburg Empire – that used to be my unspoken nickname for the Jenn-me realm.

I said, 'And "henceforth". "Henceforth" really, really irritated her.'

Samantha giggled.

My theory, kept from Samantha, was that Jenn objected to this fancy (in her mind) vocabulary because it was (as she saw it) the tip of an iceberg of European haughtiness. I suspect she equated my Swiss ancestry with being looked down on from an alp. It sounds crazy, but I don't think she could quite accept, or understand, that an American could through no fault of his own know French (a language spoken by normal people all over the world), and that the whole thing wasn't just some kind of trick of one-upmanship designed to knock her back down into the Lehigh Valley.

The salmanazar! Three men hoisted the inexhaustible Brobdingnagian bottle and, not without anxiety, filled our glasses. Samantha was looking very appealing now, and I recognized that I was imagining myself alone with her and prospectively knowing the bliss of being with her, and it took a real effort to avail myself of the technique I've developed to protect myself and the woman in question at such moments, which is to fast-forward through the joyful scenes of carnality and closeness, valid imaginings though these may be, and slowly play in my cerebral cinema the moment when it's pain-pain and lose-lose-lose-lose and she's heartbroken and I'm boarding a boat to Tristan da Cunha.

Samantha declared, 'Henceforth I'm going to start saying "henceforth". Perhaps.' She laughed very hard, and her elbow dropped into a jumbo shrimp combo, and several of the jumbo shrimps sprang from the salad onto the table. A cheer went up.

'Bloody elbow,' Samantha said, wiping her arm with the tablecloth. 'Story of my life.' She laughed courageously.

I decided to not give voice to my deep, untrustworthy compassion.

Samantha told me that her husband, Gavin, had been unfaithful to her with a twenty-four-year-old he'd met while 'seal bashing' at Barasti. 'That's when he took up "scuba diving".' It was her turn to make air quotes. 'He'd tell me he was "scuba diving" with this friend from work, Ted, and then he'd be gone for the day. Very easy, really.'

Unthinkingly, I said, 'Ted? Not Ted Wilson?'

'You know him?' she said.

'Only very slightly,' I said, as if I were under accusation. 'He seems to have gone missing.'

'*Cherchez la femme*,' a bruncher interposed.

'*Cherchez la voiture*,' another said. 'I hear from a little bird that a very naughty little blue Mazda has been seen in some unlikely places.'

'Really? Where?' The topic had everyone's attention.

Our informant paused deliciously. 'Sharjah,' she said.

'Of course.'

'Of course what?'

'It's the perfect place to keep his floozy. Then the wife comes over from the States, and old Teddy says no thanks and does a runner. I bet you he's lying doggo there right now. He'll be back as soon as the missus flies home.'

I said, 'That doesn't make much –'

Samantha said, 'I wonder if he was in on it with Gavin.'

'Wouldn't surprise me. Scum collects.'

The fork-waver pointed at me. 'Hold on – weren't you in that search party?'

Everybody turned to examine me.

I said, 'I – yes. I was asked to take part, so I did.'

Samantha said disgustedly, 'You're a scuba diver too?'

'Not really,' I said. 'Not any more. I mean, I used to dive, sure. Yes. But never with Ted.'

'You must be a bit pissed off, mate, going to all that trouble while our Ted dips his wick in Sharjah.'

'Did he even really go diving? It was probably a cover, wasn't it?'

'He went diving all right.' There was laughter.

'Sounds to me like he's a psychopath,' someone said. 'I'm not saying he's going to murder anyone. I'm talking, you know, psychiatrically.'

More ha-ha-ha-ha.

'No, no, think about it,' the psychiatrist said. 'The fake-diver thing, the shag-pad in Sharjah, all the lying and cheating. The whole double-life thing. No conscience. No empathy for anyone else.'

'OK, here we go.' This bruncher was consulting his iPhone. '"Psychopathy Checklist".' When he started to read out the alleged characteristics of psychopaths, I removed my fez and left. I should have gone earlier, as soon as it became clear that the dignity, and in particular the privacy, of the Wilsons was going to be violated. Privacy is in many respects an indistinct ideal, but surely we can agree that there is such a thing as misappropriating another's biographical belongings.

I'd texted Ali an hour earlier. The stout fellow was waiting for me in the Méridien lobby. He drove me and the Autobiography home. Then he took a taxi back to his place or wherever it was he wished to go, Friday theoretically being his day of rest and liberty. I gave him taxi money, of course, and slipped him a hundred dirhams for good measure.

Of that group of brunchers, I would guess that less than half are still in Dubai. Evanescent conga!

Brett Hutchinson is one of those who went away, whether by choice or not I can't say. He has not stayed in touch, even though he still owes me five thousand AED. The day after the Yalumba event, he e-mailed me this:

> Hey bud. Great seeing you. I may be wrong, but I think
> you left without paying? Give me a buzz when you get
> a minute or just send me a check. Cheers.
> PS: Dh 700 a head inc. giant bottle of bubbly!

I like to think I try to be curious about others in the way I'd want those same others to be curious about me, namely in a way that is not alienated from the root meaning of curiosity: to care. I try to not be a busybody. I reject the idea that one can enter another life at no cost. I guard against the lowness of the detective. (When I first came out here, I would daily Google Jenn, then my old firm, then me. It was as fruitless as it was compulsive. I was like the dog with the empty bladder that nonetheless goes from tree to tree, stopping at each one to cock his leg in vain. Later, I went through a phase of Googling the Batroses, and, regardless of the search results, the outcome was the same: my degradation: my falling farther down the slope of Parnassus.) On the other hand, a measure of inquisitiveness is sometimes called for. If the petition 'Help!' reaches us, obviously we should want to look into it. I'm not arguing that the Wilsons cried out to me. But I did come away from Brett's brunch with the feeling that Ted Wilson, and Mrs Ted Wilson by association, had been run over in absentia. I don't know why such a little thing should have got to me. Every day, the immaterial ear of conscience – surely the organ that must distinguish a human being from the remainder of animals – receives other, louder calls.

Anyhow, I decided to Google Ted Wilson.

Predictably, Wilson had a LinkedIn page. I used to be LinkedIn, because my old law firm required it. Membership of LinkedIn or any self-revealing network is, however, incompatible with the sensitive and confidential nature of the family office job. It would be wrong if my 'profile' were visible to John and Jane Q. Public as a source of connectivity to, potentially, the Batroses. It's a relief that Googling my professional name these days produces next to nothing. This is because, virtually, I am legion. Anyone searching for me could easily get the impression that in the preceding twenty-four hours I have pitched victoriously in a high-school baseball game in Long Island; worked as a fire marshal in Idaho; jumped bail in Corsicana, Texas; and passed away in Maryland and Ireland and Australia. For all practical purposes, I am completely camouflaged by my name's commonness. If you look deeply into the image results and scroll past the pictures of scores of my namesakes, most of them on Mugshot.com, you can dig up a photograph of me from a long bygone corporate softball event in Central Park; but even there, the legend confuses me with a certain Graham Herold as we stand next to each other in a lineup of seven squinting softball players. As to why I find my online absence pleasing, I will only say that I also find pleasing my absence from the African wilds.

'Ted Wilson', another almost unsearchably ordinary name, became distinctive when qualified by the word 'Dubai'. In this way, I was able to find the LinkedIn page of 'Dr Ted Wilson'. It was informative. Wilson attended Reed College and obtained a Ph.D. in German economic history at the University of North Carolina at Chapel Hill. He held 'adjunct and visiting professorships, fellowships, and other faculty positions' at (chronologically) Duke, Emory, University of Hawaii at Manoa, Coventry University (United Kingdom), Lund University (Sweden), University of Illinois at Chicago, and finally the American University in Dubai, where he taught in the International Studies programme. In 2004, he joined his current employer, RCF ('Reality Creativity Futurity'), an Emirati-owned advertising, PR and branding (or, their website put it, 'Presence Management') agency. The 'Overview' stated:

Dr Wilson has taken his deep scholarly knowledge of the processes that give rise to the historic perception of nations, and applied it to the contemporary arena of country branding, public diplomacy, and reputational risk management. At RCF he has been instrumental in the successful development of Brand Dubai and other country brands. Dr Wilson's expertise at measuring, building, and managing Arabian Gulf national and commercial assets has been internationally acclaimed, with his team at RCF winning *BrandWeek*'s Best Emerging Market Story 2006 (for the 'Do You Really Know Dubai?' campaign), and also winning UAE Tourism's Most Valuable PR Campaign 2007 ('Hospitality of the Desert').

I visited RCF's site. Under the 'Our Team' tab, Ted Wilson was designated 'Team Leader, Country Branding Visions and Operations'. The photograph showed a smiling Wilson. Resting neatly on his forehead was a pair of round red spectacles. The caption asserted,

Ted is so ridiculously bright that at RCF we call him Two-Brains. User-friendly to the max, he is unsurpassed in his commitment to making Total Branding concepts a reality for our clients. When he's not burning the midnight oil, Ted enjoys scuba diving. 'I'm very lucky to have the best diving water in the world right on my doorstep,' he says.

I went further with my investigations, if that is the right word. It turned out that in addition to LinkedIn, Wilson had Friendster and Facebook and MySpace and Vimeo and Twitter accounts to his name and in each case had opted to make public the content of his pages, so that even I (who was then, and am now, a non-member of any such site) could freely and immediately access their content and, by implication, Wilson himself. I well understood that in Wilson's work circles, a certain trendy visibility was advantageous. Still, I was taken aback by the man's forwardness, which struck me as unbecoming as well as surprising. The surprise was of my own making: extrapolating from my sense of him as a furtive aquanaut and standoffish elevator rider, I had had in mind the conception of a lone wolf or lone ranger – by which I of course mean a man who keeps himself to himself, not a masked searcher for truth and justice. As for my judgment of unbecomingness, I quashed it right away, and not without guilt. I was the unbecoming one. I had no right to pass judgment on Wilson on the basis of some unexamined taste preference or, come to think of it, on any basis, especially as I knew very little about social networking services and their norms and could easily have been misdirecting at Wilson a more general horror founded on little more than my unfamiliarity with these virtual communities, whose character struck me as falling bafflingly between the stools of *Gesellschaft* and *Gemeinschaft*. If Wilson was innocuously and/or self-servingly into this sort of socializing, that was entirely up to him. *Laissez faire.* To each his own. Mind your own business. Judge not, that ye be not judged. *Honi soit qui mal y pense.* Take a look in the mirror. Turn the other cheek.

With hindsight – with retrospective knowledge of Wilson's complicated arrangements – it appears that I missed an important function of his web presence. There is no reason to believe that Wilson's incessant posting (he offered across his various platforms a not unusual mix of family and leisure photographs, day-to-day bulletins, whimsical observations, links to enthusiasms and amusements) wasn't genuine. I'm sure he got real satisfaction from his social networking activities, including the entirely understandable satisfaction of being (and being seen) at his most optimistic, interesting and well-behaved. But I think it becomes reasonable to theorize a further objective: Wilson was making a hiding place out of conspicuousness. The concealed space was created negatively, from his advertisement of a comprehensive or filled life, a life apparently without room for much else: where would such a man find the time to have a second life?

Facebook was Wilson's most important forum, and his use of other sites was relatively light. He had 264 Facebook friends, which back then seemed like a lot. These friends were located all over the world. His 'Wall' (which served not the enclosing and defensive function suggested by the noun but the contrary function of disclosure and welcome) saw much activity, with Wilson posting up to ten times daily and eliciting many Likes and messages. I must confess that I was quite moved. The gatherers at this Wall were clearly touched by the better angels of their nature. They were cheerful, funny and supportive. They deeply loved their children and their spouses, they cooked experimentally and generously, they read revisionist histories and challenging novels, they loved music and art and even dance. They were civil. They had grit. They cut each other slack, gladly granting one another the footing that, man or woman, black or white, Christian or Muslim, whether in Oslo or Dhaka or Windhoek, she/he was doing a good job, in trying conditions, of whatever it was he/she was trying to do. They shared educated and thoughtful insights into world politics and trustworthy links to pictures of cute dogs and new monkey species. They made common their feelings. They grew. They rooted for and bore sympathetic and useful witness to the others as, one by one, each made her or his way along life's rocky path, facing en route the loneliness, discouragement and pain that are the inevitable and persistent highwaymen of our ways. Ted Wilson, I was given to see, was a talented underwater photographer and a typeface buff. He loved listening to Gomez, Wilco, Nick Lowe, Squeeze, Fountains of Wayne and Brandi Carlile. He had watched *The Life Aquatic with Steve Zissou* 'at least fifty times', tearing up every time Bill Murray beheld the jaguar shark.

From the beginning, I'd been wary of Facebook and similar venues of connection, precisely out of a fear of the pyre of memories that awaits a match and, once lit, will set a blaze – of old friendships, old places, old desires – that would serve only to grieve me. But if *this* was how it worked – as a second chance, with new friends; as a rewriting of the record; as a festival of mutual absolution – I wanted some of it. I wanted to divulge my playlists and movie favourites, my moments of wit and hope and wry gloom. I wanted to become a sharer and a good egg and booster of morale, too. I wanted to friend Ted Wilson and his friends.

I couldn't friend him, though. He had disappeared. His Facebook account had been inactive for weeks. To be exact, there were no signs of activity by Ted Wilson. His friends continued to leave concerned and bewildered messages on his Wall. One of these, from someone who went by UnderservedDeserving, caught my eye:

> Teddy honey, please get in touch. Don't worry about anything. Whatever it is, we'll fix it. Just come back.

UnderservedDeserving, whose sex was evident, had been consistently leaving messages for Ted Wilson for at least two years. Many of these struck me as intimate and very nice. About an upcoming dive, UnderservedDeserving wrote,

> Be careful out there. x

About a photo of Ted posing poolside,

> Wow – hot! Must take a cold shower while watching a Dick Cheney video.

124

I wondered what Mrs Ted Wilson made of all this.

'UnderservedDeserving' had an institutional ring. I Googled it.

I'd guessed right – it was a small nonprofit with the mission of 'connecting national charities to economically and social neglected communities in Chicago'. The home page carried a photograph of its founder and managing director – Mrs Ted Wilson. Oh, right, I thought. Now I get it.

There's no such thing as 'to get' something. The inevitable consequence of resolving knotty unknown A is the creation of knotty unknown B, in this instance: What was the deal with this Facebook thing between Ted Wilson and his American wife (whom I cannot bring myself to call Mrs Ted Wilson I)? What was the deal with their marriage?

These questions arc unanswerable. Even if I'd been a confidant of both Wilsons and a professor of psychology to boot, there remains the problem of matrimonial mist. Who can say what goes on between couples beyond closed doors? Not even the couple behind the doors, if my experience is anything to go by. But without claiming a right to peep through a keyhole or to appoint myself adjudicator, and invoking only the human need to interpret, a need without which thought of any worth would not be possible, I will say that I was intrigued by the Wilsons' practice of communicating, not without intimacy, on publicly visible message boards. Always aware that I was taking the shaky and finally indefensible position of the conjecturer, always conscious of the importance of granting only a provisional and faltering status to whatever conclusions might offer themselves to me, I gave the matter some thought.

I surmised that the Wilsons Skyped from time to time; occasionally if rarely met in the flesh in Chicago; and supplemented their contacts on these message boards. I found this impressive. It suggested that, in spite of the distances of time and space by which they had divided and tested their pairing, they used whatever resources were available to generate the closeness and solicitude and playfulness that give substance to a marriage and make possible a distinction between a loving staying together on the one hand and, on the other hand, a pact whose principal aim, guided by considerations of perceived utility, is the sustenance of the marriage qua conjugal belonging, as if it were a piece of property or going concern in which the partners held a joint interest whose socio-economic and instrumental value was deemed by them to exceed a human being's potential for that brand of intimate feeling that draws together two persons for whom the good of the other is indivisible from their own good, which feeling transports us, I would suggest, as an incidence of itself and of the good-faith actions taken pursuant to it, away at long last from the natural violence and nothingism of the earliest dealings of *Homo sapiens* – a transportation that remains, I want to believe, the underexplored source of hope of any lasting sort. Ted and Mrs Wilson's commitment to Facebooking revealed adaptability and goodwill and mindfulness. How easy it would have been for them to give in to the difficulties of intercontinental human bonding and instead tend to the formalities of their situation, all the while, perhaps out of unconscious anger or a malign search for consolation by vengeance, increasingly associating themselves with the external forces insistent on the punishment and lowering in dignity of those who fail to sacrifice themselves to the perceived interest of the collective in controlling the doings of its members by imposing on the members stringent and potentially precipitous rules of conduct in the form of marital laws. It illuminated the foregoing to recall the night of our breakup, when Jenn said, 'You've murdered my marriage!' I was taken aback by every part of this statement – my characterization as the sole actor; the accusation of intentional killing; the 'my'. In the turbulence of the moment, I was able to voice only one point of incomprehension. 'What marriage?' I said. 'This marriage,' Jenn cried, making a waving gesture with

126

both arms. 'But we're not married,' I said. 'Of course we're married, you clown,' Jenn said. 'What do you think this is? A nine-year date?' She was right: there was no equitable difference between the coupledom we had and the one we would have had if, at some point, we'd spent half an hour at City Hall. To my surprise, Jenn didn't pursue this line of argument. This was logical, in hindsight, because she wasn't calling upon the analytical framework of marriage with the intention of gaining a better understanding of the nature of our rapport; rather, during this final, frightful argument, she was digging and putting down the conceptual foundation for subsequent extreme action by her the legitimacy of which in the eyes of the officious bystander, that spirit who cannot be placated yet must be, depended, first, on the transformation of the history of our private feelings and dealings into a thing (in the legal sense) from which Jenn might derive (quasi-) proprietorial/contractual rights; and second, on the licence customarily granted to persons claiming to enforce (quasi-) proprietorial/contractual rights and/or claiming to redress a violation of those rights as a justification for actions that would, in the absence of the licence, be viewed by the bystander as unruly and deplorable. It should be noted that the officious bystander/licensor invariably takes pleasure in watching such licensed hostilities, which offer the spectacle of the falling of two persons.

Going back to the Wilsons and the virtual meeting room they'd made for themselves, I was at first uneasy about the public nature of their chosen venue, as if they could only meet as part of a larger gathering and were one of those couples who are lifeless unless they're at a cocktail party. But when I paid attention to their actual comments, it was obvious they were basically just having fun and that if Ted Wilson's Wall was a kind of cocktail party, it would have been silly for them not to join in. There are many twosomes who seek out and enjoy the company of society, and being out-and-about from time to time is healthy for the one-on-one, and why should society, for these purposes, be limited to the physical? It occurred to me that I might be witnessing at first hand a historic psychic enlargement or exploration, that the quickening and tantalization felt by today's pioneering virtual communitarians was something like that of the early phenomenologists as they reconnoitred their dawning new dimension. These written interactions of Ted Wilson and Mrs Ted Wilson fortified my non-acceptance of the whispers about Ted Wilson's secret Dubai romance. This was incorrect of me: one should not entertain rumours about others, not even for the purpose of dismissing them, because to do otherwise is silently to accept the premise of the rumours, which is that people have a right to call balls and strikes about how other people lead their private lives. They don't. One should recognize and mistrust this judgmental propensity, belonging as it does to an animal whose so-called ethical sense comes not from above but from a primeval epoch of natural selection in which cooperative grouping resulted in better outcomes for individuals coping with a savage natural world. Five minutes of driving alone in the Dubai desert will bring home a forgotten zoological fact: solo survival is not and has never been humanly feasible. It has occurred to me that I should take young Alain Batros out to the Empty Quarter (the wilderness, not the art gallery) to dramatize for his benefit the lowly pragmatic origins of morality and to impress on him two things. *Uno*, it's a somewhat disagreeable reality that conscience, at root, is no more than a productive biological sensitivity to the reciprocity that is essential to our specific survival. The sense of fairness familiar to all societies has come to us from and because of the apish age of literal backscratching. *Due*, that a life in which an honest attempt is made to transcend the original quid pro quo is a life that has a shot at glory. The kid may not get it right away, but you never know.

What am I going to do about this boy?

'Bryan Adams sucks,' he tells me.

'He does?' I say. I'm startled by this declaration out of the blue, which may be the first entirely voluntary utterance he's made to me in the weeks he's been my intern. Nor is there a previous instance of his leaving his desk and standing at the entranceway of my part of the room. I beckon him in. 'How come?'

'His songs are so bad.'

That doesn't accord with my assessment of Bryan Adams, but hey. And I'm biased. Bryan Adams took on the Batros gig on a week's notice and at a considerable discount on his advertised minimum fee of one million USD. (Bryan Ferry's people were unhappy, understandably, but that was mediated by Fabulosity to everyone's relative satisfaction.) I wasn't at the Adams concert (not invited), but Sandro and Mireille are very pleased about how it went, I've heard (not from them).

*Hi Sandro – You're welcome.* De rien. *No trouble.* Nichts zu danken. *Any time.*

'What's so bad about them?' In an ideal world, Alain would have more complex critical skills.

'I don't know. Everything.'

(His *don't know* comes out as *døn't knøw*. For all his devotion to mumbling and drawling, the kid has this fancy English-Norwegian accent that must be, I guess, a payoff of his expensive schooling in England. (I like it just fine. (That said, I have a real soft spot for the habitual accent of Arab speakers of good English, in whose mouths the language, imbued with grave trills, can seem weighted with the sagacity of the East. (See Alec Guinness in *Lawrence of Arabia.*))))

I tilt my head respectfully. 'So who's good? Who should I be listening to?'

He shrugs. 'Slayer. Or maybe Dying Humanity.'

I decide against saying something that I would find funny but Alain wouldn't. 'Maybe I'll check them out,' I say. The kid's still hanging around, and I feel the touch of opportunity and duty. This outburst of musical opinion is the first sign of any knowledge on the boy's part. I know he's only just turned fifteen, but in the course of my minimal involvement in his summer assignments (as per Sandro's instructions), I've been astonished and re-astonished by just what a know-nothing he is. He can't point to Rome on the map. Somehow he has never heard of St Paul. He thinks 'the present tense' may have something to do with 'feeling worried'. I am giddily reminded that the human race refreshes itself in absolute ignorance and that without an enormous, never-ending labour of pedagogy, everything would go to hell.

I ask the kid to tell me more about Dying Humanity. He tells me they're from Germany.

'Where in Germany?' I say. He doesn't know. 'Let's look it up,' I say. 'Pull up a chair.' I figure this is without the ambit of the prohibition against the kid using a computer in the office.

Unfortunately, only German Wikipedia offers details of the band. Fortunately, I still have my childhood German. 'See this? It says they're from Annaberg-Buchholz.' He doesn't seem to care very much. 'Let's see where that is,' I say. Interesting: Annaberg-Buchholz is in the Erzgebirge – in English, the Ore Mountains, in the southeast of the country, by the Czech border. 'Wow, no wonder their music is so tough. These guys are from a tough area.'

'Tough how?'

'One thing at a time,' I say. I get him to look up 'ore'; then 'heavy industry'; then the Deutsche Demokratische Republik, which is as remote to him as the civilization of the Incas was to me; and this is how we continue for a full hour and a quarter, chancily hopping from one link to another until we end up, anticlimax, on the topic of Dallas, Texas. 'I've been to Dallas,'

130

I tell Alain. 'Don't go there. Not unless they're paying you well.' 'Why?' 'Why?' I'm closing the files we opened. 'Because life's too short. Avoid D-Town like the plague.'

As Alain takes his leave – he looks worn out, poor guy, and I have to say I'm pretty worn out myself – it occurs to me to say, 'Hold on there, Al.' I say, 'You know about the plague? About the Black Death?' He shakes his head. 'That's your home-work. Find out about the Black Death and write down ten interesting things about it. No, let's make that five things. We'll take a look at it tomorrow. You OK with that?'

He seems to be. He goes back to his desk. He knows as well as I do that it's noon, and at noon he must be weighed. To avoid the weighing is one reason I pop out, back to The Situation, for a couple of hours. Another reason is that I like to take a shit around midday, and I've made the executive decision that the round trip is well worth it. (It's definitely not the case that I'm snubbing the facilities available to all in my office building, which are first-rate.) I may be wrong, but I seem to do more shitting than ever. Certainly I often find myself thinking, when I take a seat: Again? Still, I'm not complaining. In there, in the bathroom, everything is out of your hands. Time out. Pax. And am I the only one to appreciate the sweet egality of it all? For a little while, you're no better or worse than anyone else. You're shooting par.

Or are you? Among the more embarrassing criticisms of the emirate is that it cannot deal, on a municipal level, with the huge and booming volume of digestive waste produced by its population. Much of the sewage is collected in septic tanks whose contents are moved to the treatment plant in fleets of trucks. Apparently the lines of trucks waiting to enter the plant are so long, and the waiting is so unendurable and/or cost-ineffective, that some truckers have resorted to illegally dumping their loads behind sand dunes and in the city's storm drains, the latter practice resulting in unfortunate incidents of faecal

131

stuff turning up in Dubai's otherwise tiptop swimming waters. I believe the situation is now under control, though incorrigible naysayers continue to attach a negative symbolic meaning to the issue. There's nothing I can do about it, in any case. The call of nature must be answered.

Today, as ever, it's a relief to withdraw to the privy and lock the door, even though the front door is locked and there's no one else around.

Or is there? By a startling olfactory or digestive coincidence, the smell I make is exactly the smell made by my father.

Done. But the midday intermission is not complete without a look-see at Project X.

Still nothing. The structure of mystery is unchanged. Is that pile of dirt fresh? How come nobody ever uses the portable toilet? Curiouser and curiouser.

It is reassuring to look over to my left, where, just beyond Privilege Bay, a construction project is indubitably in progress. Today, I see, prettily green truck-mounted cranes are on site and, taken together with the abundance of yellow hard hats and primrose-blue overalls, grant the scene a vernal air. Incredible, how they manage to work in that heat. Almost thirty floors have gone up of what will clearly be a nondescript residential proposition. Although situated across the water channel and so belonging to a discrete niche of the market, this tower will be our visual neighbour and, I fear, put at risk the distinctive silhouette of Privilege Bay. This is another reason, as if we needed one, why it is vital that Project X develops quickly into a top-dog building. As matters stand, we are in danger of suffering the fate of downtown Manhattan, whose skyline, as I recall, seems these days to be situated in Jersey City.

Which reminds me: the other day I received a nasty report. Apparently people have started to refer to The Situation and The Statement and The Aspiration as 'Tampax Towers', on account of the allegedly high number of female flight attendants who are said to live among us in shared accommodation, an arrangement seen by some as running counter to the Uncompromising Few and Pioneers of Luxury and Dreamers of New Dreams narratives. I don't share this perception. I have nothing but respect for the flight crews of Emirates, who can be rightly proud of their indispensable role in the great success of their corporation and specifically of the Emirates Experience for which the airline is uniquely and rightly world-famous. Any residential community would and should proudly welcome them. *Willkommen*, I therefore say. *Soyez les bienvenues.* Добро пожаловать!

(How clearly I remember my first exposure to this superior polyglot race, which is how these ethnically elusive women with smiling creaseless faces first struck me. They seemed indigenous to the skies. Uncannily Eurasian- or Afro-Asian- or Latin-Asian- or Eurafrican-looking specimens in red pillbox hats and white headscarves, they made me think of the calm interstellar travellers familiar to us from the Star Trek entertainment franchise. When it was announced that the 'team' of flight attendants between them spoke English, Arabic, French, Latvian, Russian, Malay, German and Tagalog, I fell into a state of admiration that has, if anything, only been deepened by the passage of time, which has of course seen a decline in the fortunes of almost all economic things Emirati and, unless I'm mistaken, has led to an adjustment in the profile of Emirates passengers, who these days would appear to be drawn largely from the same market the Dubaian migrant working-class is drawn from, a development, dare one say it, that puts into question the image of the airline as the transporter of choice of the voyaging elite: yet our indomitable multilingual female highfliers still go about their work as brightly as ever. One evening not that long ago, in circumstances that are beside the point, I found myself on the roof of The Situation's parking lot, which is located about fifty yards behind the residential proposition itself. I had an accidental view into the lower floors of The Situation, and I could not help seeing the young women in their illuminated apartments as they pedalled on exercise bikes and watched television and cooked dinner. How courageous they were! How young and adventurous! I must have been fascinated, because a good few minutes went by before I became conscious of myself as a voyeur cloaked in the dark of night; whereupon I left. I have since felt, and fought off, the urge to return to that roof and take another look. What is this urge? What would I be looking for? What could I possibly be hoping to see?)

All that said, no residential proposition should be dominated by any single class or demographic, and 'Tampax Towers' is not a value-adding moniker. For the good of all, the situation must be monitored with care.

It's as I'm turning my gaze away from Project X that out of the corner of my eye I see, or half-see, or imagine, a small dark dropping motion to my left. My guess is, a gull or other large bird. Bird life in the emirate is booming, by all accounts. Migrant birds pass through in great numbers. Tweeting and cooing may be heard every morning, in every neighbourhood. I've heard tell that, some decades ago, the Dubai authorities netted a large quantity of our feathered friends from around the Gulf region and released them in the city. This sounds apocryphal, but you never know. The abduction of an entire avian population is by no means beyond our Rulers.

My bowel movement is normally followed by an internet-fuelled episode of self-pleasuring. This coy verb comes to mind ironically, I'm sad to say. Although I'm not going to deny the element of sensational gratification, I register with dismay the growing difficulty I'm having in sticking to my goal of jerking off at least four or five times a week, without which I would be in danger of not extinguishing, or not keeping in check, the natural desire to copulate and then mate. Including my time with Jenn, I've spent over a decade going from one dirty website to another, and at this point, I'm running out of juice. I must acknowledge that, as an ultramarathoner of masturbation, my devotion to amateur or homemade pornography, which kept me going during the Jenn years, has in Dubai been swept away by the never-ending search for novel and effective stimulation. There isn't a porno twist, tweak or twang I haven't exhaustively gone into. Asian babes, MILFs, BBWs, celebrities, extremists, Africans, naturists, insertion specialists, acrobats, horny bosses, straponistas, Italians, mature lesbians, vintage sluts, cuties, horny boot wearers, randy yachtswomen, exhibitionists, busty teens, hairy cougars, anal queens, cum gobblers, wife-swappers, nerds, bottle-fuckers, beauties, strangers, bored natural house-wives, brunettes – I've been through all of these and many more. I don't like the way this is trending. Some months ago I went through a phase of jerking off to scenes of (grown-up and, I honestly believe, consenting and professional) women being penetrated by enormous dildos attached to what were called fucking machines. That was a grey area.

A week ago, I had an unambiguously very bad experience. What can I say? I was watching a woman and four men doing various things. It was all proceeding as one might expect, until one of the men punched the woman in the face, and then another pulled on her ponytail so that she could be punched again in the face, which she was, by the other men, and the female performer was crying and bleeding at the mouth and trying to not be punched, and in the blink of an eye the fake orgy had turned into a gang sexual assault – and yet I couldn't stop the movie, my hands were full, I was about to ejaculate, there was no stopping that, and even though I did turn my eyes away from the screen, I kept jerking off until I was done. Only then did I shut the laptop and quit the scene of the crime. Too late. I had already acted in concert with the sexual assaulters. It will be objected that the crime victim, as I believe her to be, was an actor, as were the other actors in the filmed events: they, too, were actors; I'd seen the *performance* of a crime. My retort:

Actors are in the first place persons. It cannot be forgotten that the phase of public pretending is preceded by an initial private phase of pretence in which the person assumes the part of actor. When I revisualize the video in question, I see that the female actor ceased to pretend to be an actor. She reverted to naturality with the first or second punch; and it seems clear that after that reversion she did not consent to being punched repeatedly in the face and to having sexual interaction, vaginal and oral and anal, with the men punching her. It follows that the female actor was not an actor pretending to be raped. She was a person being raped. This isn't automatically to incriminate the men as rapists; their relevant mental states are open to argument; one would need to hear from them. Me, I have heard from myself. I know what I did. I saw the rape happen and used my seeing of it for my own sexual benefit.

What am I supposed to do now? Turn myself in? To whom? Where are the authorities when you need them?

And I cannot jerk off any more because I'm afraid that, if I do, I will see the female person being punched and I will want to see that.

What do I do? I go back to work. I turn myself in to Alain and Ali.

Where is Ali, though? Not in the office. Only Alain is here, and he is in my chair, and on my computer. What the fuck.

'Excuse me?' I say.

The kid smoothly closes his windows and, if I'm not mistaken, clears his history. He says, 'I was finding out about Black Death,' and goes back to his desk and opens his Green Belt Sudoku book as if nothing has happened and it's all been my bad dream and not his bad.

I take the responsibility. I forgot to shut down the computer, and boys will be boys. Still, the kid and I need to talk.

'That's my computer, Alain. You need my permission to use it. You don't have my permission unless I say so.'

I get nothing back from him. He stares at the wall. Fair enough. I've said what needed to be said. Regarding exactly what he was doing on my computer, I'm not going to get into it with him, even though his explanation was brazenly false. He would deny falsity, and there would be a factual dispute and a battle of wills, and that's too much to ask of me. I'm not his parent. His parents are his parents.

Meanwhile, Ali has returned. I step out to talk to him and shut the door of the office so that he and I can talk beyond the earshot of the kid, who is inside my office.

'Everything OK?'

'Everything OK, boss,' Ali says.

'Listen, Ali, you can't leave the boy here by himself. You have to wait until I come back.'

'I went to the dry-cleaning,' Ali says.

The evidence, as if it were needed, is next to his desk: a dozen hanging shirts.

I say, 'Yes, that's good. Thank you. But next time, do me a favour, wait until I get back. We have to look after Alain. If there's a problem, you can always call me.' I can't understand why he has slipped up like this. It's not like him at all. The man is straight as an arrow.

'No problem, boss,' he says. 'What do you want me to do for this afternoon?'

'Let me see,' I say. 'Has the Range Rover been serviced?' He tells me he's already taken care of it. 'Very good,' I say. I'm racking my brains. The office is shipshape and I can't think of anything I might need from him in the way of errands or tasks. The truth is, I have the family office and my domestic arrangements in very good order; at this point, things pretty much run themselves. I can't think of anything for Ali to do. This is a problem, because Ali's raison d'être (in the work context; his other contexts are not visible to me) is the doing of things. I have toyed with the notion of a gentler, happier, less perplexing and more comic world in which Ali is not so much a factotum or office boy as a companionable sidekick, a world in which the infrastructure of injustice that supports the terms 'valet' and 'manservant' is marvellously absent or made harmless, and Ali unproblematically is a Jeeves or Passepartout to my Wooster or Fogg, and the two of us have adventures in which we extricate each other from amusing and diverting entanglements and difficulties, our solidarity sturdy and unstated, our needs always mild, and the evil of the day forever sufficient unto it. This ridiculous daydream is founded on Ali's extraordinary real-life consistency of deportment. He is never out of character, and his character is that of the rock. In over three years, he has never been noticeably joyful or miserable, irritated or pleased, obtuse or over-clever, obsequious or big for his boots. He is free of nuance: no cloud passes across the sun when Ali is around. If he has a *Binnenleben*, I am not privy to it. Ali's dignified two-dimensionality coheres in his garb, the shadow-less white dishdash and white headscarf which I've never seen him out of, even in winter, when other Emirati men turn to blue and brown fabrics in order to mix things up a little. There's a story, who knows if it's true, that at some point, maybe in the Seventies, the then Ruler essentially took control of the national wardrobe and instituted the dress code we see today, a sartorial initiative that, if it indeed occurred, had the effect of transforming a dusty, scruffy, jumbled-looking male popu-lace into the bespoke toothpaste-white strollers we see today, and whom we cannot help perceiving as emblematic substitutes for their homeland's hygienic new orderliness and coolness. It's a look that's working out for them, you'd have to say. I would love to wear a dishdash and headscarf myself, albeit for reasons of crypsis.

I've thought of something Ali can do. I toss him the keys to the Autobiography and tell him to go down to Project X and see if, by any chance, he can find out what's happening.

I'm still in a somewhat agitated state, however, and when I notice that there's a good-sized FedEx box on my desk, I rip open the box as if tearing a foe limb from limb. The box contains more boxes; a moment goes by before I understand: my stamps have arrived! My stamps!

(When was the last time I felt such joy? Easy: Christmas 1980, when Santa Claus, descending the chimney for me for the last time, brought with him a sky-blue Tigra seven-speed racer. (In the spring, Dad and I bicycled together on the shore of the Zürichsee. With the aid of an illustrated map we picked out, in a multitude of white-hatted Alps, Chammliberg and Schärhorn and the Tödi. (*Et pauvre Maman nous a attendu à la maison et à notre retour m'a fait une petite bise alcoolisée.*)))

Everything I ordered is present and correct. I'll admit it, I splurged. I've got myself:

- A metal high-quality date stamp (self-inking in black ink) with the custom text, BATROS FAMILY OFFICE (DUBAI) LTD.
- A chrome desktop embosser with a circular plate for embossing a mark of the Entreprises Batros logo (in which the curlicued E and B are entangled as if in a bathrobe monogram) and the circumscription BATROS FAMILY OFFICE (DUBAI) LTD.
- A gold desktop embosser with a rectangular plate. The EB logo comes with the custom text GENERAL EXPENDITURE TRUSTEE BATROS TRUST CO. LTD.
- A small circular wood-and-rubber stamp (text: FAMILY OFFICER, BATROS FAMILY OFFICE (DUBAI) LTD) with a stamp pad and a bottle of blue ink.

- A small triangular wood-and-rubber stamp (GENERAL EXPENDITURE TRUSTEE BATROS TRUST CO. LTD) with a stamp pad and a bottle of green ink.
- A large square wood-and-rubber stamp with a stamp pad and a bottle of red ink and the text SIGNED SUBJECT AND WITHOUT PREJUDICE TO TERMS AND CONDITIONS SET OUT AT WWW.BATROSFAMILYOFFICER.COM.
- A large rectangular wood-and-rubber stamp with a stamp pad with orange ink. Text: SIGNED SUBJECT AND WITHOUT PREJUDICE TO TERMS AND CONDITIONS SET OUT AT WWW.BATROSGEATRUST.COM.
- A 'rocker' ink blotter.
- A green leather desk pad (38" x 24").

I remove the leather desk pad from its wrapping. I put it on my desk in front of me. I place the embossers to my west, the stamp pads to the north, and the stamps to the east. I keep the ink bottles at hand: slowly, carefully, and not without alchemy, I imbue each stamp pad with its colour. Done.

I put away the ink bottles in my filing cabinet, which is always locked and which only I have the key to. The stamps and embossers will in due course also 'live' in the filing cabinet, in which the embossers will be kept in a further lockbox (again, only I have the key) and will be doubly under lock and key and doubly secure. Now I'm ready to start stamping and embossing. One thing at a time, however. Let's first of all give these guys a workout.

Before I shut the partition door, I want to make sure the kid is at his desk, doing Sudoku or something. He is.

I place a sheet of white typing paper on the leather pad. I get out the date stamp. I adjust the band by turning the oversize wheel: now it's set to today's date: 01 AUG 2011. OK, here we go. *Ke-thunk*. That sounded good and that felt good and that looks good: the black tattoo is very professional and very sharp. I am repelled by, and untrusting of, smudged or blurred documents. They are indistinct enough as it is, as it were.

I successively tint and then bang on paper the blue, the green, the red and the orange stamps. *Dumb. Dumb. Dumb. Dumb.* Very good.

The (superfluous, because the imprints are superb) handheld seesaw blotter? It is as fun as I suspected a handheld seesaw would be.

Last, and most, the big guys – the embossers. I have to stand up to grip the lever steadily. *Cramp*, the chrome one says. *Cramp*, repeats the gold one. Wow. OMG. O. M. G.

To be clear: centrally, my happiness isn't aesthetic or recreational. To be perhaps less clear: these two modes of pleasure are but the flowering branches of practicality's tree. What I'm saying is, my new office items are not bureaucratic toys. The point of the embossing is not to make a pretty design on paper but to make life harder for any scoundrels who might want to forge my signature. They will not be thrilled that there has been added, on top of my John Hancock, a further stratum of identification and authentication personal to me, i.e., my boss. The two smaller stamps add a third baffling stratum, and will be useful in various administrative situations. Most important of all, though, are the big bright stamps, which are not big and bright by accident. The red/orange texts they impress on a document serve to vividly qualify, I'd like to say helpfully elucidate, the scope and effect of the act constituted in the putting by me of my name to the document. The mechanism of qualification and elucidation is one that's now common in the world of legal dealings in writing: the reader is referred to a website that functions as an addendum or rider to the document in question, alternatively as a collateral contract between the referrer and the referee or, in the further alternative, in some way that I haven't yet figured out, as something that otherwise gives to the reference the legal effect I want, i.e., an effect protective of me. A nitpicking technical analysis isn't my priority. This is real-world stuff. I'm not going to get hung up on niceties.

With Ali's help, I've created two websites. They respectively set out the standard terms and conditions on which I sign off qua Family Officer or GEA Trustee. I have to say that writing those provisions was trickier than I'd anticipated. For example, it turns out that creating a website creates issues particular to the creation of a website. I had no option except to begin with a disclaimer about the website itself:

> No warranty or representation of any kind, implied, expressed, or statutory, including but not limited to warranties of non-infringement of third party rights, title, or freedom from computer virus or any other harmful or destructive electronic or Internetian agent, is given or made by the Trustee [or Family Officer] with respect to the contents of this website. The Trustee [etc.] does not accept any responsibility or liability for the accuracy, content, completeness, legality, or reliability of the information contained on this website or for any loss or damage of whatever nature (direct, indirect, consequential, or other) whether arising in contract, tort, or otherwise, which may result or follow from your use of (or inability to use) this website, or from your use of (or failure to use) the information on this site. No legal or other kind of advice is given on this website. The legal and other kinds of information on this website are 'as is'. You must not rely on the information on this website as an alternative to seeking and receiving legal advice from your attorney or other professional legal services provider.

That was the easy part – the preliminaries. I cannot exaggerate how testing I found it to draft the main matter, i.e., to state efficaciously that which I wanted to say. The problems I encountered – conceptual, verbal, juristic – were horribly comparable, in their stubborn, enigmatic vitality, to those poison-resistant super-rats that, we are told, threaten to defeat every hostility of modern science precisely because they, the super-rats, have been strengthened by scientific hostilities. I'm suggesting that every attempt I made to eliminate a textual vagueness or errancy or inadequacy of sense resulted only in the making of more, less eliminable problems of sense. It was as if the very project of making sense was being mocked; as if the words I typed on the word processor's white page, words of black letters, were not the symbols for which I'd mistaken them; as if, that is, each word, with its little lucifer of denotation, was in fact consubstantial with the darkness of uncommunication against which it supposedly was a counteractor; that is, the significance of a word lay not in its letter-by-letter symbolism but in its literal presence on the page, a presence that, though obvious, was a secret; that is, a word was exactly and covertly what it appeared to be, a letters-shaped blackness, which is to say, a kind of verbatim detail of the immovable, possibly entropic, and in any case finally annihilating, residual super-reality of blackness; so that every mark I made by pressing a key of my keyboard had a consequence opposite to the one I'd intended, namely, a decrease in the totality of light brought into the world and an increase in the totality of gloom. Or so it began to seem to me, after several months of futile refinements and do-overs, and a million miscarried meanings. I became so confused – so lost in a fantastic vigilance of ambiguity, obscurity and import – that one morning I sprang out of bed with a madman's idea of a breakthrough: I had been trying to kill, or cage, the rats of complexity. Wrong! Let the revolting fuckers multiply! Let them run wild! Let them turn on whoever dared to approach! And who were these approachers, anyway? The transactions I signed off on, to which my disclaimers applied, were between professional bargainers and strong-armers doing everything to maximize their own advantage. There were no vulnerable parties here – no minors, no uninformed consumers, no persons acting under duress or undue influence, no judicially recognized or protected weaklings. Nobody here was being forced or duped into doing anything he/she didn't or wouldn't want to do. Nobody was going into this thing with her/his eyes not open. In a weekend-long lingual-legal rage, I composed a heartless, fearless, terrifying work of negation that burdened every person save myself with every conceivable responsibility and loss and risk, that in every instance unfairly and unlimitedly and gratuitously and disproportionately favoured me at the expense of the world and, most repellently of all, that withheld the basic hospitality of writing: my disclaimer, as completed, was a graphic monstrosity, a cruelly rambling, almost agrammatical near-balderdash of baffling dependent clauses and ultra-boring, ultra-technical phraseology that enveloped the reader in a dingy, alien, almost unbreatheable word-atmosphere offering barely a vent of punctuation, indentation, or line-breakage. Put that in your pipe and smoke it! At the same time, I was mental-mailing. *Eddie – Remember when you told me (I paraphrase) that, by accepting the position of Family Officer, I was accepting the termination of a camaraderie that went back to our time on Lansdowne Road? You said something about hardball. So be it, my sometime amigo. Think of this as a brushback pitch.* At three in the morning, I went to bed. I was still brainstorming, however. It struck me with great power that romantic human dealings also might profit from the availability of standard terms and conditions – from articles of association, one might less forbiddingly say – spelling out the footing of A's entry into B's intimate company and the precepts A would wish to apply to the conduct of such intimacy. Why not? Were we not always being told that good communication is the be-all and end-all of successful emotional transactions? Ideally, B would have articles of association of her/his own: A and B could openly discuss, from the outset, the question of how to proceed jointly, and come to an agreement – or disagreement – that would save them a bunch of he said-she saids and who knows how much else of the havoc caused and powered by human misunderstanding or claims thereto. To those who would ask, Gee, do we really need to have a heavy-duty convention before we get to date someone? I would answer, (a) Take it from me, it beats the alternative; and (b) It could be made fun, in a screwball comedy kind of way. To repeat: why not? Users of dating sites freely expressed requirements about a prospective partner's intentions, not to mention stipulations about hobbies, height, ethnicity, smoking, looks, sexuality, etc. My idea was to go farther – go beyond the superficial pre-sorting of matchmaking, go beyond, especially, the (unspoken) mutual oaths on which (quasi-)marriages were founded and the apparatus of coercion by which the oaths were guaranteed. What this 'beyond' might involve, specifically, was for another day. I was tired as a workman. I went to bed.

Just as I was about to drop off, I had one last moonstricken rush of insight – that human articles of association, in their nobility like the great constitutional documents of the Age of Enlightenment, should promulgate a mission of human attachment surpassing of reciprocity. I could not understand this, my own thought, except in this respect: as I fell asleep, it seemed to me that I'd spied, like stout Cortez, a beautiful and unexplored ocean.

I woke up in daylight a few hours later. I looked again at my draft disclaimer. Filled with incredulous disgust, I deleted it. As for the 'articles of association': where had that folly come from? What was the matter with me?

Still, it was a constructive episode. In my post-delusional clarity, I found myself able to quickly produce the text that now appears on my websites. The text makes plain in straightforward terms that I'm signing papers as a mechanical agent; that my signature should for all substantive (as opposed to formal) purposes be treated as that of my principal (i.e., the relevant Batros(es)); that although I might be aware in very broad terms of the nature of the documents, I have no personal knowledge of their contents or any authority or expertise applicable to the contents; that I have accepted my mechanical agency on the basis of appropriate assurances received from my principal as to the lawfulness, efficacy, and adequacy of the papers I sign and the actions or outcomes connected to them; and that my principal, not I, bears all and any relevant responsibility and liability.

Is that too much to ask for? Is it so wrong? I might equally have ordered this stamp:

> PLEASE DON'T HURT ME BECAUSE
> I'M SIGNING THIS

I notified the Family Members in writing of the websites and of my intention to refer to them by stamps and bosses. There was no reply, which was logical. I was merely proposing to make explicit an unstated but well-understood state of affairs.

I've spent over an hour quite joyfully stamping and bossing – an activity that isn't without its physical demands – when Ali returns from his outing to Project X.

He gives me to understand that a few men were gathered at Project X but that on approaching he learned they were not connected to the inexplicable structure. They were gathered on the bank of Privilege Bay to rubberneck the construction site across the water.

'A man fell down from the building into the water,' Ali explains.

'What?' I say. 'Fell down? When?'

'Before I arrived. Maybe half an hour before. They were getting him out of the water.'

'What do you mean, getting him out? He died?'

'I believe he was dead,' Ali reports. He says, 'He jumped. It happens a lot. Every week it happens. Every week, always one or two of the men jump from the buildings.'

I saw the jumper from my apartment. The dropping thing I saw out of the corner of my eye at lunchtime – that was the jumper. Or was not. I did not really catch sight of that which was dropping. I glimpsed, I should say I think I glimpsed, a shadow-like movement, and whatever it was was gone as soon as I turned to look. It could have been anything. It could have been a bird; it could have been something inanimate. That cannot be ruled out. Nor can it be ruled out that it was nothing. Nothing can be ruled out.

Ali offers to go back to Privilege Bay tomorrow to pursue his investigation. I tell him there's no need. 'It's nearly three o'clock,' I say. 'Why don't you take Alain home now.'

To my amazement, Ali doesn't jump to it. He stays right where he is, motionless – except for his bearded mouth, which he is twisting into significant shapes. I'm about to give voice to my bemusement when the penny drops: he is signalling something in connection with the kid, who is sitting on the other side of the partition and no doubt overhearing our every word. 'There is a problem with the car,' Ali announces volubly. 'I need to show you.'

'Very well,' I say. 'Let's go take a look.' I lock my computer. I say to the kid, 'Al, sit tight for five minutes.'

Down in the entrance lobby, Ali and I find a quiet spot where two black leather chairs have been specially set aside for conversationalists. A certain kind of showy private confabulation is big in Dubai. Wherever you go, there always seems to be a pair of brazen conspirators in the corner.

Ali looks rattled, which is a first. Here is a glimpse of his third dimension. Here is a cloud. Uh-oh.

He says, 'Boss, Mr Alain is a big, big problem for me.'

He tells me that the kid has been shaking him down. On three occasions during the last ten days, Alain has asked Ali to give him five hundred dirhams. Ali gave him a hundred a couple of days ago, hoping that would put an end to it, but today, during my lunchtime absence, the boy repeated his demand. There's no need for Ali to spell out what lies behind the demand: he is a bidoon, and the kid is the son of the big boss. No doubt the kid is ticked off with Ali for weighing him, as if Ali were somehow at fault. They're a family of messenger-shooters and cat-kickers, the Batroses.

I can see that Ali is very nervous about having spoken about this at all. He is still afraid of the kid, and rightly so, because the kid is a kid and, because he is a kid, has no real clue that anybody other than him is a human being. I would guess that he barely knows that he, the kid, is a human being. Still, I'm shocked. I did not see this coming. I tell Ali not to worry. I take a bill for one hundred dirhams from my wallet and direct Ali to accept it as a reimbursement of the money screwed out of him. 'Thank you for telling me about this,' I say. Then I direct him to clock out.

Of course, I am anything but thankful. It would have been much better if Ali had ponied up for a couple of weeks or found some other way to not involve me until the kid was off my hands. Now, however, I am seized with knowledge of the facts. That's not good. A fact is where it all starts to go wrong. A fact is a knock on the door.

I chauffeur the young extortionist home. He has taken a seat in the back. I say nothing. He says nothing.

We pull up across the street from Fort Batros. A high white wall surrounds the property's several acres. Behind the wall one can see a sizeable cluster of palm trees and, aloft amid

148

the palms, a gaping three-metre satellite dish that would interest me very much if I were a pterodactyl looking for a nest.

'OK, see you tomorrow,' I say. In accordance with protocol, he doesn't move until two security guards have hastened over from the guardhouse and opened the passenger door. They escort him to the enormous metal double gates and lead him through the doorway that's built into one of the gates. One of the guards indicates with a wave that the kid is safely home. I don't doubt it. Fort Batros has a round-the-clock security presence and alarms and floodlights and various other defensive measures in part attributable, as I understand it, to the requirements of the kidnapping insurer. I have never been inside the property, which is managed by an Italian gentleman hired away from the Four Seasons Hotel Milano, but I have gone online and aerially surveyed it. In addition to the family villa, the grounds contain a tennis court and two swimming pools and outhouses and cabins: the expectable inferno.

This isn't to say that high walls and swimming pools and luxury cabanas are intrinsically bad; and I absolutely don't have anything against the ideal of the family home. As a matter of fact, sometimes I long for the experience of being made welcome by a family in its domain. I'm no Norman Rockwell, but I do believe in the existence of families that are not units of suffering and power. My own nuclear family was not one of these success stories, sadly for all concerned, and I'm forced to conclude that neither was the group comprising Jenn and me and, spectrally, our not-to-be child; but one can hardly fall from these particular disappointments into a general theoretical gloom about familial love or the special domestic comfort that a successful household can offer a visitor. The specialness, here, does not consist in giving a guy/girl the best chair and pouring him a glass of wine and lending him a sympathetic ear and generally bending towards her, indispensable though these things are; it consists, fundamentally, in exercising for the guest's benefit the power of shelter and exoneration that is the prerogative of the family in its residence, which constitutes (the family home, that is) a private enclave within larger, all-too-hostile dominions. At home – *chez soi* – one is a potentate; one may grant an outsider relief from the outside; and this must be what I yearn for.

It's possible that this old question – of the stranger and his reception – detains me because it detained none other than Ted Wilson. This was made apparent by his short advertising film for the Dubai Tourist Board, the award-winning *Hospitality of the Desert*. In the film, which I Googled without difficulty, a man in tattered Middle Eastern robes walks alone in the desert. It's a timeless scene, shot in black and white. He is in difficulty, this wanderer. The sun is in that mood we recognize as 'pitiless', and the sand formations have the undulating immenseness we associate with the phrase 'sea of sand'. The wanderer covers his face with his scarf and trudges on, up a dune. There is a second man in the desert: an unambiguous Arab in blazing white. He sees someone approaching. The Arab carefully watches this figure: there is something menacing about the slowly advancing silhouette. With a concise gesture, the Arab issues a wordless command to his servants, who have materialized along with goats and camels and a modest encampment of tents. Cut to a tent's shade: the sheikh – for that is who/what the Arab is – proffers the traveller a cup of water and, on a silver dish, dates and white cheese. That is the drama: the humility of the aristocratic host before the vagrant: the reversal of station. In a burst of colour and pop music, everything skips to present-day Dubai, where a family of ecstatic Western tourists checks into a hotel with the help of an Emirati guide/friend/host; whereupon we see the foreigners enjoying a series of stock touristic pleasures, the scenes punctuated by close-ups of the sagacious black-bearded face of the Emirati host/helper. Next, the tourists are waving goodbye to the Emirati at the airport; and then we're back in the timeless desert, where the traveller, in fresh clothes, heads out into the desert on a horse supplied to him. The sheikh wears a wise smile. The legend appears:

WELCOME TO DUBAI

I'm no expert, but I detect a difference between this ad and the others. I'm thinking of the little films brought to us by the 'Reaffirm Your Uniqueness' and 'The Prestige of Excellence' and 'Dubai: The Exception' campaigns. These obviously laughable and tawdry productions push without irony the idea that Dubai is where an elite of beautiful cosmopolitan tastemakers convenes in order to lead lives of extraordinary *luxe* and cachet and to buy and use and disport themselves in and with famous handbags, clothes, bathroom fittings, etc. We see men tossing car keys to smiling parking valets, and women emerging long-leggedly from sports cars, and childless couples in their late thirties getting together to drink champagne on yachts. The cheesier, the better, I say. There is a transparency of falsity in this absurd idea of a good-looking socio-economic *Weltklasse* that almost confers a kind of blamelessness on the falsifiers, whose misrepresentations are (no offence) not far removed from those offered by very young children caught red-handed, and may be regarded, even enjoyed, as good old-fashioned hogwash. Wilson's effort, by comparison, was sly. I'm not one to pick on a man or knock down the efforts of someone who's just doing his/her job, and in any case whatever I might think about any of this is subject to the universal rule that dooms to futility a private effort of vigilance and so won't make a difference to anything. Still, I'll allow myself a small say. 'Hospitality of the Desert' proposed to do battle with the (of course calamitous and disgusting) prejudices directed against

151

Arab/Muslim peoples (the terrorist-towelhead travesty) by offering an alternative mischaracterization, namely the whole wisdom of the desert-slash-ancient custodian of hospitality-slash-ethics thing. The latter is hardly on the same scale of wrongdoing as the cartoons it opposes, but it trawls the same swamp of plausibility; it calls forth fresh species of toads and snakes and slime. There is no high ground here, admittedly. There never is. Maybe the best that can be done, in terms of not making a bad situation worse, is to stick with the vivid fantasia of opulence, or, even better, to go back to the straight-forward before-and-after photographic montage that was once very popular here but now seems to be falling out of fashion, i.e., the juxtaposition of a 'before' photograph of the acreage of sand that Dubai until very recently was, and an 'after' photo-graph of the extraordinary city we now see. This captures something honourable and true, if you ask me.

No one will ask me, I can safely say; the question is deeply moot. So, too, is the more personal question of my own recep-tion by others, since it hasn't happened since I got here. That's right – for reasons that have, I hope, more to do with local custom than with what I'm (perceived to be) like, I have barely crossed the threshold of a private residence in Dubai. I haven't even been to Ollie's house, in Arabian Ranches. For that matter I have only once met Ollie's (English) wife Lynn, and that was the time I ran into the whole family in Dubai Mall. The term 'family' in this instance includes the live-in Filipina nanny (Winda? Wanda? Wilda?), who, on the occasion I'm thinking of, took complete care of the little boy, Charlie, so that Ollie and Lynn were at liberty to stroll around in a carefree manner and permit themselves a measure of public parental insouciance that would be unavailable to them back home in Australia/England or, if available, would not be totally free of stigma, there being in those places people who frown on the conspicu-ous assignment to an employee of responsibilities deemed to be proper to a mother and/or father, and there being for the time being in those countries a degree of social uneasiness about noticeable master–servant relations. Here in Dubai, there's nothing particularly unseemly or unusual about one's children and one's child-minders trailing behind one at the mall, especially since Emirati women amble at some distance behind their menfolk, often with the little ones. Nor is it suspect or *de mauvais goût* to have a residential domestic workforce: on the contrary, integral to the appeal of the expat experience is that the labour of mopping and dusting and washing and cooking that typically forms part of the *in patria* experience may, *ex patria*, be transferred at a low cost to others – the so-called help. What about their experience – the labour trans-ferees? This question, inherently valid, arises especially in the minds of the self-appointed inspectorate located overseas and to our northwest, where news agencies periodically run stories of women who have escaped from domestic service as if from slavery and reportedly are found desperately wandering the malls of Dubai without a penny to, I was going to say, their names, except that these escapees evidently are usually deprived by their employers of their passports and suffer from an official namelessness, not to mention denationalization. I completely accept the factual soundness of these stories. The imbalance of power that inevitably characterizes the employment by the relatively rich of persons radically relocated from poor parts of the world must perforce give rise to cases of mistreatment of the powerless. However, no consideration of this problem would be satisfactory without the paying of some attention to the trope by which it is publicized, namely the trope of the scandal. I am not such a theology ignoramus as to be unaware of the time-honoured sense of this word: a stumbling block on the true path of religious virtue or, in a different context, Christian faith. This is hardly applicable to the present case: the mistreatment of help in Dubai is hardly a shocking reverse in the sacred project of human goodness to which the scandalized bystander is committed. I say this not out of cynicism but out of a recognition that real-life scandalization is a delight, conferring as it does a wonderfully unpaid-for feeling of righteousness. So let's get it straight: most of the tut-tutting we hear is the sound of nothing other than opportunistic moral hedonism. And let's acknowledge that it would be wrongheaded to disregard the fact that a large number of low-net-worth workers in Dubai enjoy relatively satisfactory outcomes, the pertinent point of comparison being the outcomes they would have enjoyed but for their employment in Dubai. Ollie and Lynn retain an Ethiopian live-in housemaid whom I've never met or seen but who is most unlikely, knowing her employers as I do, to be a detainee. I think it may fairly be assumed that she's better off cleaning the nice house of nice people in Arabian Ranches than doing whatever she'd be doing in Addis Ababa, fine city though it may be.

Anyhow, we all walked over to Morelli's Gelato for ice cream. Lynn Christakos is very pretty, in the sporty, clean-cut way of a star golfer's girlfriend, and I found her good-natured and reasonable. She and I were in line at the counter, chatting away, when into the salon there stormed, I say without exaggeration, a group of black-robed and black-gloved and black-masked women. They came like a black wave through the tables, and for a second I thought they were coming to get me. I jumped to one side to let them pass. After they'd bought ice creams and surged away (having skipped the queue, pursuant to the relevant unwritten local rule), I said to Lynn, 'Jesus, they gave me a fright.'

Lynn laughed. 'They're only mums,' she said. 'Just imagine them with no clothes on.'

I forced out a culpable little laugh. More than once I've had pipedreams involving women precisely like these women (i.e., dressed in attire designed as a powerful antidote to nudity but

154

counterproductively causing in me precisely the effect of mentally undressing them), and I had the crazy thought that Lynn had X-ray powers that had opened a window onto my revolting inner life. 'Yeah, good idea, I might try that,' I said. Mildly risqué banter is not what I'm best at, which is a handicap in Dubai, where the nudge and the wink are vital social tools. According to Ollie, Lynn loves it here. In common with many expat mothers, however, she runs away from the summer heat and humidity and goes with the little boy (and, on a tourist visa, the Filipina nanny) to her parents' house in Lancashire, England, for a couple of months of rain. In her absence, Ollie gets bored. This is when he becomes a prankster.

There was the famous time when, under the impression that I was getting what Ollie had termed 'a really cutting-edge preventive ungual treatment', I unwittingly allowed one of Ollie's technicians to paint my toenails pink. When the lady technician removed the cucumber slices from my eyes and showed me her handiwork, I let out a shout of dismay that I immediately regretted because it seemed to upset the technician, who clearly was not in on the joke and plainly was worried that she'd done something wrong and was in big trouble. Ollie, of course, was laughing his head off.

This isn't my favourite side of him. Our friendship was made underwater, where the scope for dicking around is zero. Quite frankly, I don't share his taste for mischief and high jinks. One story he told about a night out in Moscow still haunts me. Evidently, Ollie emerged alone from a nightclub in the early hours. (What he was doing in a Moscow nightclub isn't for me to understand or misunderstand.) There was fresh snow on the streets, and the snow in combination with the hour's lateness and darkness had produced a vacant and hushed and newly ominous city – a city somehow connected to one's childhood, if I may gloss the story. Ollie phoned for his car. He was waiting on the sidewalk when along came a horse, pale and jingling and clouded; and in the saddle was a beautiful young woman wearing a fur coat and a fur Cossack's hat. As Ollie stood there, of course bewitched, a zooming BMW Z4 came down the street and, at a short distance beyond the horse, braked hard. The driver rolled down his window and leaned out to take a look at the horsewoman of mystery. As she drew level with the BMW, this man reached out of the car window and fired a pistol into the air. The horse skidded sideways, regained its balance, and bolted. The gunman sprang laughing out of the car, gun in hand. He hooted and slapped his thigh and jumped up and down as he watched the runaway going away with the woman hanging on for her life. Somehow she was not unseated; but the man slipped on ice and violently toppled backwards into the snow like a clown overthrown by a banana peel. This caused him to accidentally shoot. It didn't put an end to his joy. Laughing more loudly than ever, he kicked his legs in the air and helplessly rolled and rolled in the snow.

Let's acknowledge right away that Ollie played no part in what happened. He was an onlooker. What bothers me is that he didn't tell his story as if he'd found himself in the wrong place at the wrong time, which is what I take to be the standard reaction of the eyewitness to a dangerous crime. To hear it from Ollie, he'd lucked into an amazing show. I accept that almost every element of the incident – Moscow, a make-believe night, a horse, gunfire, the randomness at the heart of everything – places what he saw beyond the frontier of the normal and invites a corresponding displacement of sensitivities. But it's not obligatory to accept the invitation. I am the last person to propose an answer to the problem of determining what portion of the world may be treated as a pure amusement and what portion may not; I just know that I see nothing funny about a woman fighting for her life. And who can say if she succeeded? How do we know a car didn't run her down? Isn't it in any case certain that she was in terror? And even if one were to learn that she made it home safely and now viewed the episode as the most fun she ever had, Ollie's story still cannot be removed from the complication of schadenfreude.

Oh, lighten up, for fuck's sake, says a voice in my ear.

Fair enough. It's very possible I'm being oversensitive – that I'm like those thin-skinned smoke detectors that screech at the presence of the slightest cooking fume and, if life is to go on, must be shut down.

When our homes were warm even when air-conditioned and Lynn and son and nanny in due course migrated north, Ollie dragged me out for a drink at Buddha-Bar. It's in the Grosvenor House hotel, five minutes by taxi from The Situation, and so difficult for me to duck out of going to. The only time I'd been there, three sharp-looking anglophone businessmen, intently discussing what I took to be an important commercial opportunity, occupied the neighbouring table. When I eavesdropped, I learned that they were in a conversation about world travel in which they authoritatively misinformed one another about Minorca and Majorca. In this sense, I found Buddha-Bar unchanged. There was a supercar (a Lamborghini Gallardo) stationed at the hotel entrance; there was a velvet rope, to my mind an archaism of late-twentieth-century New York and its dream of VIPs and in-crowds; there was a pointlessly hushed ambiance; and, scattered in the calculated gloom, there was a clientele of very made-up and dressed-up older British tourists who looked as if they actually believed that they'd passed a test of selectness and, when I entered, stared intently at me as if I might turn out to be Hulk Hogan or Henry Kissinger.

And there was Ollie, signalling to me from a shadowy booth. A blonde woman was with him, and I realized right away that he'd sprung another one of his little surprises – a blind date. When I drew closer, I saw that my date wasn't as blind as I'd thought, indeed wasn't my date. She was Mrs Ted Wilson.

W hat happened next is inexplicably preceded, in my mind, by what happened one evening years ago, in Union Square, New York, when Jenn and I were walking home from the movies. We became separated in the crowd. I stopped on the busy sidewalk and turned with an extended left hand and said, I'm over here, darling, and reached for her. Instead of Jenn I found myself eye to eye with a beautiful dark-haired woman in her early thirties, herself holding the hand of a man not at all amused by the accidental offer to his girlfriend of another man's hand. The couple moved on; Jenn, I'm assuming, took my hand for a little while. Whatever the exact nature of our physical contact, I walked next to her in surreptitious anguish, because in that instant of misidentification a fantasy of distressing power and implication had been released – in which the dark-haired beauty drops the hand of her boyfriend and takes my hand with a smile, and together we stroll into a Union Square filled, as always on summer evenings, with young romancing couples, and we walk on through a steaming urban night, laughing and talking as everything and everyone converts into lights and vapour; and we, my dark-haired woman friend and I, jump into an old but reliable jalopy and drive out across George Washington Bridge, and drive and drive into the green deep of the continent, an adventure of gas-station snacks and motel sex and maxed-out credit cards, driving onward through forests and farmland until, on a remote highway that pursues a twisting river – in Montana, maybe, or Durango, or Manitoba – a small, solid town catches us, and we stop there, and we take refreshments in a friendly little coffee shop, and we spontane-ously begin our lives again for good there, among good neigh-bours. We befriend the lonely, pretty doctor and the gentle judge. We hold small, rewarding jobs, and we make two clever girls who hopscotch in the springtime. I have always wanted daughters. A chronicle of my awareness of my unhappiness would start with this banal, upsetting daydream, which, as I say, serves as a prologue to that moment in Buddha-Bar, when it was too late to make a run for it and there was nothing to be done except to stand there and wait for the unfortunate Mrs Ted Wilson to be, entirely reasonably, not nice to me.

Ollie made the introductions – and she didn't recognize me!

My first thought was that this was more trickery – that they had conferred about the lentil-throwing incident and decided that to leave me like this, in a suspenseful limbo of non-identification, would be a fitting comic punishment. Then, as the two of them continued with their discussion – I'd taken a seat next to Ollie and was sort of trying to hide behind him – it became clear that my presence wasn't a source of disturbance, or even of interest. This permitted me to conclude that, amazingly, who I was had not registered with Mrs Ted Wilson; and when I paid attention to what they were talking about and understood that Ollie was sympathizing with her about her traumatic discovery, apparently made only a day or two before, that the rumours were true and there was indeed a second, Dubai-based Mrs Ted Wilson (who was herself searching for Ted), I guessed that this Mrs Ted Wilson was in that state of perceptual impairment that I personally know to be a symptom of vital confusion and distress. In those first several months of the Jenn–me split, more than once I stepped off a subway train at a perfectly familiar station only to find myself at a loss as to where I was, a lostness referable in part to my temporary insanity, in part to the real-world derangement that had placed me not only in an unforeseen Lincoln Tunnel luxury rental but in a life populated by a new and unwelcome dramatis personae, chief among them oneself. I am certain that Mrs Ted Wilson must at some point that evening have asked herself, What am I doing here? Who the hell are these guys? How did it come to this?

I was meanwhile asking myself: How do I get out of here? By getting up and exiting Buddha-Bar, was the answer – and at most five minutes passed between my arrival at the table and (on the pretext of having to take a phone call) my departure. Outwardly, all was straightforward. Inwardly, things were complex. Among the thoughts and feelings that formed part, during those few minutes at Buddha-Bar, of the catastrophe known as my subjectivity, were: (1) I will be exposed. (2) What does [(1)] mean? What or who would be the content of the exposure? (3) Ollie and I are jackals feasting on another person's suffering. (4) What has Mrs Wilson done with her hair? She seems to have a Pre-Raphaelite thing going on. (5) If I stay, I'll have to walk Mrs Wilson home. And then . . . ? (6) Might I be a little in love with Mrs Wilson? (7) Wow, [(6)] is nuts. I'm really out of control. (8) Ollie is preying on Mrs Wilson *and* helping her. Whereas I'm keeping my nose clean and being of no use. Paradox. (9) I ought to give my full attention to Mrs Wilson in order to gain an understanding of her experience and offer her the empathy that is called for. Out of the question, as a practical matter. Must leave. (10) Who is Mrs Wilson, anyway? And who is Mrs Wilson II? (11) So is Ted Wilson alive or dead? (12) Buddha-Bar really, really is not my scene. (13) Is Ollie going to sleep with her? No. (14) Am I going to sleep with her? No. (15) I'd like to sleep with her/take her into my protection – it comes down to the same thing. Not. (16) She wouldn't want me, in any case. (17) I have to go. Now. (18) Those are nice breasts, as far as one can tell. You never know until you know. Nice shoulders, definitely. Augurs well re everything else – although again, no necessary correlation. (19) Oh shit, did she just catch me looking? (20) Go, now. *Go, Dog. Go!* (21) Night after night, Maman read that book to me. When we moved to the States, I found it embarrassing to call her that. Mom, she became. *Pardonne-moi, Maman.* (22) OK, that's it, now I'm going.

This is the kind of thing that passes for my moment-to-moment inner life. It's discouraging.

On the walk back to The Situation, I initiated the following exchange of texts with Ollie:

Can't do this. Pls convey my apologies.

?

Poor woman. Let her be.

??

He called me the next day. 'You all right? What were those texts about?'

I told him the whole set-up had made me feel uncomfortable. 'Uncomfortable?' 'Yeah, it did.' After quite a pause, he said, 'Fair enough, mate.' The conversation pretty much ended there. I could tell he was hurt/pissed off by what he deemed, not wrongly, to be my holier-than-him stance. Of course, this wasn't a subject for feelings-sharing. We handled the matter the way we handle all of our (very rare) disagreements: a week or two goes by, and then I phone him and ask to buy him lunch, and he assents. Or vice versa. I bought lunch, this time; we ate at the Lime Tree Café (the Jumeira branch); and no mention was made of our difference of opinion about the correctness of the evening out with Mrs Ted Wilson. That's what friends do: they forgive and forget. They let bygones be bygones. They move on.

It's in this forward-leaning spirit that I've written off, perhaps I should say written down, the irrecoverable opportunity costs of time and happiness attributable to the unhappy Jenn years. As for her aggressive behaviour in connection with the breakup, I don't blame her. Note that this isn't a case of forgiveness: I don't hold her responsible, period, on the grounds that during this difficult time she was not herself. I'm not asserting *crime passionel*: I assert that the 'Jenn' behaving badly was not Jenn.

This opens the question of who it was, exactly, who (lawfully but immorally) withdrew all the funds credited to our joint current and savings accounts (72,000.98 USD and 244,346.17 USD respectively (incidentally, Jenn's (much larger) salary, for a reason I must have forgotten, always went into an account in her sole name, whereas the money I earned went into our joint accounts and was used for our joint expenditures)) and left me with a net worth of 11,945.00 USD (the salary payment that I just managed to withdraw); who it was who took sole possession of the apartment and all of its furniture and threw into the garbage my family photographs, clothes, books (including my childhood books (including *Go, Dog. Go!*)); etc., etc. I take the view that these were the deeds of a not-Jenn, not Jenn, and that to a large extent I'm the Victor Frankenstein responsible for the bringing forth of the not- or un-Jenn who, as I realized too late and with an astonishment that has never quite left me, did not have my interests at heart. There remains the conundrum, in this analysis, of the whereabouts, during the time of wrongdoing, of Jenn herself, and of the nature of the relationship between submerged true Jenn and emergent false Jenn, in particular – persistent question –: How come true Jenn, when she resurfaced, as one must assume she in due course did, didn't make good the damage to me done in her absence by her malfeasant alter ego? I'm not suggesting that she was responsible for the actions of the other Jenn, but I do note that it would have been the easiest thing in the world, as a practicality, for her to reimburse me. The matter can be put this way: X, a good person, is subject to episodes of somnambulism. During one of these episodes she unconsciously takes possession of an envelope belonging to V, her friend. X wakes up and finds the envelope. It is marked 'V's Life Savings', and it contains one hundred thousand USD. V asks X for the return of the envelope. X – who is, incidentally, a rich woman with no financial obligations or ambitions that she cannot very easily

162

satisfy, whereas V is hard up – refuses. She keeps V's money. Question: Why would X, a good person, do this? Answer: I don't know. It's incomprehensible.

I can think of a few people who might say: Your hypothetical case, as stated, omits important facts. X's behaviour becomes highly explicable if you disclose that V was X's long-term partner and (in X's eyes) 'dumped' her and 'betrayed' her. Hell hath no fury like a woman scorned.

With respect, this misses the point. Never mind that plenty of 'scorned' women don't get into a fury; or get into a fury but don't want to destroy the 'scorner'; or want to destroy the scorner but don't, because it would be wrong. Never mind that the whole 'hell hath no fury' racket (historically justifiable, I'm theorizing, as a way of granting profoundly oppressed womankind some measure of power and justice and psychological ventilation in epochs marked by the prevalence of crudely retributive ideas) in this day and age represents a tacit prolongation of the supposedly discontinued treatment of women as persons with less-developed moral and rational faculties akin to those we associate with young children and (in the inoffensive technical sense) idiots, an act of gender condescension whose inherent unacceptability is moreover combined with an anachronistic dangerousness, by which I mean that the modern legal and social and economic power enjoyed by many women in Western societies (the female entitlement to which power is, I underline for the avoidance of doubt, of course absolutely beyond question or qualification and not for me or anyone else to allow or tolerate or oversee or bless), when exercised wrathfully pursuant to the outdated 'hell hath no fury' licence, is a dangerous weapon. To put it another way, it's one thing for a helplessly vulnerable quasi-servant to be madder than hell; it's something else if the infuriated party acting with impunity is a rich partner in a law firm who is practically one's domestic and professional ruler. But, as I say, never mind. It's all good.

My point is that the Jenn I lived with, or next to, though by no means a saint (why should she have been? I certainly wasn't), would not have done the things done by the non- or un-Jenn on the hellish fury basis. That's why I can't explain why she decided, in effect, to wear the latter's bloodstained shoes.

I don't want to be detained further by this stuff, because life's too short. YOLO. But one last item makes a demand on the attention. It will be noted that our famous maxim doesn't go, 'Hell hath no fury like a woman in a state of severe romantic disappointment.' Rather, it makes express reference to an action attributed to her (ex-)partner – the one who is deemed to have committed an act of 'scorning'. I have inputted 'scorn' in the Free Dictionary. To scorn someone means to treat that person with disdain or contempt; to mock. I have looked up 'disdain' in the Online Etymology Dictionary: it is negatively derived, as one might expect, from the Old French *deignier*, to deem worthy or fit, which in turn comes from the Latin *dignus*, worthy, proper, or fitting, which in turn is rooted (as is 'decent', I see) in the Proto-Indo-European (i.e., over-five-thousand-year-old) *dek*, to accept, receive, greet, be suitable. I've also looked up 'mock'. Though it obviously arrives immediately from *mocquer* (Old French), beyond that it is of uncertain origin (though there is a suggestion that the word may have to do with the Vulgar Latin *muccare*, to blow the nose (in a gesture of derision), which is itself the offspring of *mucus*, slime or snot). These investigations confirm that the evocation of the figure of the 'scorned woman' contains within it an automatic characterization of the male (or female: I am not aware that the 'hell hath' maxim is of only heterosexual application) as actively snotty, derisive and contemptuous. This blanket judgment, precisely because it is the nature of a judgment, in turn contains a grotesque rumour of the judicial – of a procedurally verified finding.

Was I a scorner? A looker-down? As I recall, this was a very lowly time for me, and I cannot think how I would have been able to look down on anyone, let alone high-up Jenn. Was I an oaf? Yes. Did I culpably cause damage? For sure. Did I fail her? Guilty as charged. It's all somewhat foggy at this point, but certain memories are clear. Jenn had bravely done her bit – taken the follicle-stimulating hormones, gone every second day to follicle-measuring appointments, and above all taken on the chin the emotional agony that the dismal saga of artificial fertilization inflicts. All that remained, in order to try to make the baby we agreed we would try to have, was for me to do my part. The IVF calendar had produced an insemination date on which I'd be travelling for work, and this meant that I had to produce a semen sample in advance: the fluid would be frozen and used in my absence. I duly took myself to the clinic, or facility, which was in the basement of a brownstone in the East Twenties or Thirties. It was a strange little place. A sadness of masturbators, as I will collectively name them, sat around on grey chairs, each waiting his turn. A human voice was heard only when someone had dealings with the cheerful nurse-like woman who sat at a desk behind an open hatch. She gave me a form that required me, as I recall, to be specific about the number of days I'd been 'abstinent'. I shamefully provided this and other information, and took a seat. The semen production took place in a separate area, the entrance to which was closed by a shut door. Once in a while, a guy went in and a guy came out. I did my best to not monitor the amount of time anybody took in there. Jenn texted,

Good luck.

A different nurse-like worker entered the waiting room. She called out a name that did not sound like a name at all. Everybody looked around. She tried again, with a different articulation. I realized she was trying to summon me, by my first, horrifying name. When I stood up, everyone looked at me with, I'm sure, a kind of revulsion. In I went. A short corridor gave on to the two chambers where masturbation happened. I entered one of these, on my own naturally, though I recall that I was nonetheless taken aback to find myself alone in this little room. There was a surprisingly cheap armchair – maybe I'd been half-expecting some kind of special custom-made jack-off lounger – a few worn pornographic magazines, and a tiny piece-of-shit non-flatscreen TV that must have been about twenty years old. Onan himself would have found the set-up a challenge. I studied the laminated instruction card and wrote my name on the receptacle label and stuck the label on the receptacle. I activated the shit TV. There was a scene of a male repetitively fucking some featureless moaning blonde. I hit Fast Forward. Now some other dude was banging a woman from behind while she gave his or her buddy head. I watched for a few more seconds, hoping for some contagious performance of desire on the part of the woman actor, because surely that is the core fantasy – that one is desired. I was already distracted about how much time this was taking. What was normal? Five minutes? Ten? The question of volume worried me, too: I wanted audio, but I didn't want it to be overheard by anyone. Fuck it, just do it, I said to myself. I dropped my pants and got started – standing up, because there was no way I was going to sit on that chair. A minute or two passed. My dick was inert as a sock. I turned off the TV and tried with closed eyes. When that didn't work, I turned off the light, which was a bad idea, because I needed to capture the ejaculate in the receptacle and I couldn't see a damn thing. I tried to relax; I breathed deeply; I recalled certain erotic triumphs of my youth; and I began to get a response. But every time I thought I might be getting close to producing something, the climactic sensation dissipated. I kept working at it. By the time I finally gave up, half an hour had passed, and the guys out there were surely wondering what the hell I was up to. 'I'm having a problem,' I said to the nurse, actually hanging my head. She looked at my information sheet. 'You live nearby, right?' I said I did. She said, 'Why don't you take the vessel home with you, honey, and then just bring it back here right away when you're done.'

Meanwhile, another text from Jenn:

Done?

I was done, all right – as of that moment. I walked to the rent-stabilized one-bedroom in a chill of nausea. I waited there. When she came through the door, I told her I needed to talk to her. She went off into the bedroom, and when eventually I went in there after her, she went back out into the living room. 'Could you please stop moving around?' I said. 'I want to say something.'

'I'm really, really tired.'

I was very clear in my mind what I wanted to say. I did not want to start a discussion. The time for discussion had come and gone. I made sure to use very plain sentences. I told her I'd tried and failed to produce a semen sample. I told her I did not intend to try again.

She said, 'You mean you're breaking up with me?' As usual, she'd gone straight to the pith.

I expressed no disagreement.

Next, I remember, she said, 'I need a drink.' Later she said, 'OK, this isn't happening. Let's just go to bed and see where we are tomorrow.' Later still, in tears, she said, 'You can't do this to me. I want a baby – you give me a baby! You owe me. You owe me my baby!' At some other point she said, 'You can't back out now. It's not right. It's not fair. What am I supposed to do? Start dating? Find someone else? I'm thirty-five years old!' She made further statements, including the statement that

I was the murderer of her marriage. She said, 'OK, look, just give me the sperm. I'll have the baby myself. I'll take care of the baby. I don't need you. I can do this. I'm strong.' And, 'I'm going to be a laughing stock.' And, 'You wait until I'm having fertility treatment, and then you quit? Oh, boy. It's like you've done this on purpose. Is that it? I'm right, aren't I? You've done this on purpose.' And, 'My God. You're a monster. A monster. A narcissistic psychopath. My God. That's it. That explains everything.' She tore off her clothes and bent over and spread her ass cheeks, and said, 'Fuck me! Go on! Fuck me! Can you do that? Get your cock out like a man! You fucking asshole! You coward! You had to wait until now? What's the matter? You don't like pussy? You fucking psychopathic asshole.' This was when she went for me, when she was naked, lunging at me with a terrible scream and clawing at my crotch and face. I fended her off and ran to my usual retreat, the bathroom, and locked the door. Leave me alone, I said. Please leave me alone. She started to punch and kick the door, which she had never done before, and there was the terrifying new sound of wood splitting. 'Open up. Let me in, you coward,' she said. 'Be a man. Face up to what you've done.' I stayed where I was, leaning against the door, panting. A very long time went by, as I experienced it, in which I stayed in the bathroom and she stood at the door and screamed obscenities and threats. Then she began weeping loudly, and the barrier I'd rightly or wrongly put up to defend myself against her agony crumbled, and as she sobbed I opened the door, hoping maybe to be of some comfort or at least to bear witness to her pain, of which I was the cause. I'd opened the door no more than three inches when I felt the crash as she tried, with another terrible cry, to push her way into the bathroom. The sobbing had been a ruse. I was only just able to heave back and lock the door once more.

Then came a quiet. I could hear movements. There was a longer period of quiet. I didn't dare move. I was well aware that this was a perilous situation – one of those moments of extremity when, the statistics show, the otherwise nonviolent can kill or seriously injure. I heard the front door shut. I waited. After a few minutes, I turned off the bathroom light and saw no light coming through at the door's edges. She had left the apartment and hit the light switches on her way out, as was her habit. I opened the door. My intention was to pack a suitcase right away and get out.

I saw her sitting on the sofa in the darkness. I shouted with fright. 'Sit down,' she said. 'I want you to listen. You owe it to me.' I didn't sit down, but I listened. She had put on clothes. The lights were still off. She said, 'Sit down, please.' I did. She turned on the lights. She began to speak in a monologue. Now and then I tried to say something and wasn't able to, because she kept talking so as not to permit an interruption. The gist of what she said was that I had a choice to make. I could choose to be a good man or choose to be a bad man. If I wanted to be a good man, a man of substance, a serious man, I would stay the course. If I wanted to be a small man, a scrap of a man, a nothing man, I would leave. These were the two paths. There was no third way. Either I would be a man who had stood by his life-partner and made a family with her and lived a valuable and serious life, or I would be a man who would have nothing to show for himself but the ruination of another human being. Trying to speak, I made it as far as '–', because Jenn did not relent. I could, Jenn said, choose to be a real man, an honourable man, or a mediocre, second-rate man. That was the nature of the election I faced: this, or that. It was a fateful moment, she said. The determination that was mine to make was a determination as to whether I wanted to be a whole person or a broken and scattered person. If I chose the path of wrong, I would never be able to piece myself together again. I would be a broken man, without integrity. That was how life worked. You made choices, and your choices had consequences.

For years it had been her understanding that my choice had already been made, namely to commit to a life with her and to start a family with her. Now I wanted to unchoose, or rechoose. You couldn't. There was no such thing. I had chosen, and she had placed reliance on my choice. She had set up her life on it. To now go back on that choice would be to break and scatter not only me but her, too. That was the reality. I held her fate in my hands.

'_'

She said she believed that I was good, not bad. She said she understood that I believed that I was unhappy. But I wasn't unhappy. My feelings of unhappiness were false. I did not understand this because there was a delusion at the centre of my life. It was my job to recognize and overcome this delusion. My superficial feelings of unhappiness masked deeper states of truth. In any case, being happy or unhappy did not consist in having feelings as I understood them, superficially. It consisted in the giving of oneself to someone else. The feelings associated with the giving, these were the feelings of true happiness. Because I was a good person, not a bad person, on reflection I would understand all of this. I would overcome my delusion. I would recover the sense of reality that I had lost. To live without reality would certainly have made me unhappy. My unhappiness was the unhappiness of someone who had lost his sense of reality.

Before or since, I've never felt what I felt as Jenn spoke to me in that room. I felt I was being interred from within. Each assertion she made was another shovelful. I couldn't breathe. My lungs were filling up. I couldn't take it. I got to my feet.

'No, you will not leave,' Jenn said. 'You will stay, darling. You will stay in this room with me until I'm finished. You have had your say . . .'

'_'

'. . . you have had your say, and now I am having my say.'

'_'

'Please sit down. Thank you.'

She resumed in the same calm tone. There was no saying anything. She would not halt or even hesitate in her talking, and her speech only quickened whenever I opened my mouth or gave some other sign of wanting to speak. She went on and on, irresistibly shovelling words into me, stopping every cavity of my being. I felt numb. I felt cold. I began to tremble. She was right. There were no options. There was no going. There was only staying. She was in the right. What I wanted put me in the wrong. I had to stay here with her. It was my duty to be in rooms I did not want to be in, to have a life I did not want to have, to have a life in which I would not be present. That was the effect of my duty. That was what was owed to her. I owed her an existence lacking the characteristics of being alive, a life as an apparatus of outcomes that were not mine. There was no alternative. It was my duty. I had to accept a posthumous life.

OK, I told her. OK, you're right. I understand. I will stay. Now please stop.

She went on. When I began to drop off, she said I could not. It was my duty to stay awake and to listen. She went on talking, until finally, finally, she had no more to say, and she left the room. I stayed in the room.

The next morning, we got dressed and went to work together. We parted company on the tenth floor of the office building, where I got out of the elevator and Jenn kept going up. I walked to my desk. Then I went to the emergency staircase and ran down fifteen floors. I left the building and got a taxi to the one-bedroom rent-stabilized apartment. All this happened automatically, or so it felt. I found the suitcase I'd been dreaming of and I stuffed it full of clothes and toiletries and personal documents. During the stuffing I became conscious of what I was doing and again became very frightened, maybe because

171

all my life I had been obedient and good, or had tried to be, and now was being bad, maybe because Jenn was more frightening than ever before. I found a hotel room, in Jersey City, close to the PATH train, and I went there directly from the one-bedroom and, once I had checked in under a false name and put up the Do Not Disturb sign and double-locked the door, I felt relatively safe, because apart from anything there was no way Jenn would want to set foot in Jersey City, which I knew she regarded as an extension of the Lehigh Valley, to which she had sworn she would never return. I was right. She didn't follow me into New Jersey. Three weeks later, I moved into the luxury rental by the Lincoln Tunnel.

Those are (in my recollection) the principal events of the breakup. I would argue that they do not disclose evidence of scorn on my part. They do disclose the destruction by me of Jenn. The facts definitely point towards that conclusion. Since I cannot be Jenn, I am not in a position to say how much damage I caused her. I can say that I do not ever again want to be in the situation of seeing someone in the amount of pain and upset suffered by Jenn that was visible to me – and definitely not in the position of again seeing such a person in such a state from the vantage point of the one who has inflicted the pain and done the upsetting (i.e., me). Hence my decision: never again. Never again me–woman.

This must be doable. It may be that most lives add up, in the end, to the sum of the mistakes that cannot be corrected. But I have to believe there's a way for the everyman (the masculine includes the feminine) to avoid the following epitaph:

HERE LIES [EVERYMAN].
ON BALANCE, HE DID HARM.

E asier said than done, the not doing of harm. Take the Alain/ Ali problem. To mention Alain's extortion to Sandro is to put Ali at risk. To let sleeping dogs lie for Ali's benefit is to put the kid at risk, since clearly he needs to learn to not extort. Whom do I hold harmless – Ali or Alain?

Here's what I've done: seeing as the kid's internship is for just one more week, I've told Ali to take the week off, on full pay. That puts a floor under the situation. In the meantime, I've taken the kid under my proactive supervision to see if I can exert a neutral-to-positive influence on him. It's only for a few days, after all. If, during this time, he chooses to talk to me about his behaviour vis-à-vis Ali, I will listen, and decide what to do next. Otherwise the subject is closed. What I don't want to happen is to find Ali or myself in the middle of a storm of accusations, counter-accusations, inquiries, blaming, etc. It seems improbable that that would end well.

The kid's job, this week, is to write a report for his school titled 'My Summer Holiday'. That is a really uninspiring assign-ment, in my opinion, but the kid's going to have to suck it up. I'll occupy myself stamping and embossing and signing docu-ments, answering/deleting e-mails, and trying to think of ways to pass the time without betraying my boredom and dread to the kid. I too have to suck it up, in short. The good news is that, however miserable I may feel, no one else has to pay for it. Not that I'm miserable as a rule – I'm doing pretty much OK, all things considered, and I'd like to think that, in spite of every-thing, in spite of all that I've renounced, I'm a manageably at large, happy-go-lucky type of guy. But I do have my ups and downs, especially in the office, where often there's a disjunction between being and doing – i.e., not enough work to keep me busy, but not so little work as to enable me to take the day off – and I can, especially if Sandro is pushing my buttons, get into an awful rage (when I'm as bad as the Incredible Hulk, with the difference that I become monstrously enfeebled and have to lie

173

down), and in these instances I'm again relieved that I'm single, because it means that only I am connected to my ill humour and unhappiness, and mine is the only parade that's rained on, and I'm not going home to yell at the wife and kids.

I did, once, furtively interview for another job. Ollie was the go-between. He told me there was another Lebanese family, maybe even richer than the Batroses, looking for a man like me. This happened last year, when I was having a particularly infuriating time of it with Sandro. The job interview was to take place at the personal quarters of the head of the family. I say 'personal quarters' because this location, which took up the entirety of floor twenty-five of perhaps the Marina's then most exclusive tower, was neither the office nor the home of the paterfamilias but, one gathered, a venue for his more heartfelt activities – he parked his cars there (in his sky garage), he bowled in his private bowling alley, and, according to a silly rumour, he kept a suite occupied by a pair of Kazakh mistresses. The appointment was scheduled for eleven o'clock. I arrived on time. It was noon before I was taken from the first reception area into a second reception area, from where, after another wait of exactly an hour, I was led by a woman with red perfect fingernails into a third room of reception. Each of these three stations was windowless and smaller than its predecessor and situated progressively deeper in the building's interior, so that I began to feel the uneasiness, admittedly rare, of the one who finds himself involuntarily caving. In the last room there was nothing of note but a glass table with a bowl of fruit. It was the fruit that came to preoccupy the other man in the room.

'Can we eat these, do you think?' he asked me easily, even though these were the first words between us. Evidently our shared occupancy of this empty room – five minutes earlier, he too had been escorted in – had created a relation. I guess it doesn't take much.

Under consideration was a stack of apples and grapes, the

whole perfectly wrapped in transparent plastic film. Apparently the film was the problem, because it gave rise to the question, at least in the mind of this individual, of whether we were looking at food to eat or at something else. The man leaned forward to take a closer look. He was sweating. He experimented with lifting part of the cling wrap, but seeing that he was about to disturb the integrity of this whole, he sat back. 'I didn't eat breakfast,' he said with a sorry laugh.

I laughed back, but I had myself been thrown into a mild crisis that was not about the ambiguity of the fruit object but about what to do in relation to this perplexing individual. Who was he? Obviously there was no right or wrong way forward in the matter of the fruit display, and clearly the considerate thing to do would be to tear off the cling wrap, help myself to a Granny Smith by way of example, and put the guy out of his inexplicable misery. But I refrained. This man was very possibly an applicant for the position I was after. It suited my purpose to have him starving and flustered.

After I'd thought about it some more, I got up, wished my rival well, and left. I couldn't take the job from him; I hadn't come all the way to Dubai to get into a mano-a-mano; and to tell the truth, after waiting around for a couple of hours I had a not-good feeling about this family/business. I went back to Batrosia.

There is one big hitch with the status quo: with Ali absent, I am the one who must weigh the kid.

'OK, Al, it's that time,' I say. 'Let's do this thing.'

'I don't want to. There's no point.'

The kid's right. I've seen the numbers. They don't add up to a Spider Veloce.

'Yeah, well,' I say, 'you got to do what you got to do.'

He is drooping forward on his desk as if an arrow were sticking out of his back. I have a strong urge to forget all about it and make up a number. That's a nonstarter. I can't conspire with the kid to create a fraudulent document.

175

'OK,' I say, 'how about you handle this yourself. I'll stay out of it.'

He swipes violently at the pens on his desk and they fly to the floor.

> *Yo Sandro – 'Man hands on misery to man./It deepens like a coastal shelf.' Read the poem, dude.*

I put the scale in front of Alain and pat him on the shoulder. I say, 'Hang in there.' I say, 'I know, it's a bummer,' and I go back to my desk. Later, he comes to me with a note on which he's written his weight. This slovenly rebellious scribble asks me to believe he's lost a couple of pounds over the weekend. Am I to gainsay him? Am I to eyeball the kid and look him up and down? Like fuck I am. I treat the data point as legit, and graph it.

This thing has put me in a bitter mood that isn't helped by the obligation, no longer avoidable, to face my correspondence. I have some paper mail today: junk mail and mail that, though not strictly junk, can also be tossed into the wastepaper basket in the corner. Shoot first, ask questions later, is my approach. For example, the last of this morning's paper basketballs purports to be a Joint Notice from the Dubai Financial Services Authority and the International Humanitarian City Authority, which informs me that I am expected at the FSA office on a certain date, in order to discuss unspecified 'compliance issues'. The term 'compliance' is an orange light, signalling as it does a glitch about some arcane local regulation. I crumple up the Joint Notice. Experience teaches, first, that nuisances often go away of their own accord; and second, that without proof of service, letters of a legal nature belong in the garbage. I shoot from downtown. Nothing but net.

My bitterness persists. When I deal with my electronic inbox, I'm more dismissive than I'd like to be.

Hi. Thx for this. No idea. Sorry.

L –, Your inquiry defeats me grammatically. Cheers.

I delete most of the e-mails en masse: I check a bunch of them and send them to the trash with one deadly click. That is a significant satisfaction. I'm busy checking away, when I see that I'm about to delete a personal message from an unexpected source – New York.

When I left the US, I passed on my new e-mail address to a select few, and then I guess I sort of sat back to wait and see who would write. Not many, was the answer. Discounting automatically generated mail (friending requests, etc.), we're talking about a few college buddies who've cc'd me in on some stuff, usually announcements about newborns and other accomplishments. I'm not criticizing anyone here, except possibly myself. I'm bad about writing e-mails, and I did suddenly and almost completely absent myself from my social circle (which was a pretty small one to begin with), you could even say went into hiding, and I understand that most of those who were my friends have entered that phase of healthy egoism associated with having a young family and trying really hard to not get fired and not jump off the Verrazano Bridge, and I don't participate in social media, and I have no first-person news to declare, so I cannot be thunderstruck that it has all gone quiet on the old-friend front. Yet I am thunderstruck, it seems.

The e-mail is from Bob Bell.

> Hi! Hope all is well in the land of black gold. Just doing
> a deal with some Saudis. Very nice people. Bob

I would never have predicted that Bob Bell would be the one to stay in touch, mainly because we were never really in touch to begin with. He was once a client of mine and, quite frankly, not an important one. I advised his company – he didn't own it, he worked for it – on a small restructuring matter, and I can't have met Bob, a small gentleman of my age who lives with his wife and daughter in Ronkonkoma, more than three times, including the one time we went out for a (business) drink, when he told me at length about his love of the Rangers. Bob Bell will drop me a line if something Arabian has caught his attention. This happens once or twice a year. I can only think that he is a believer in the value of networking. You know what? I'll take it.

I write back,

> All well here, Bob. Very good to hear from you. Let's hope the Rangers get it together for next season. Must have been a tough winter for you!

Although I'm grateful for the disembodied low-stakes amiability of Bob Bell, it's not salvation. I appreciate actual pals as much as the next man, and this is where Ollie Christakos comes in. I'm on affable terms with quite a few people here, but I'd be in a tight spot if my friendship with Ollie were perchance to end. When we met up at the Lime Tree, I wasn't just happy to see him but very glad to find that the Buddha-Bar/Mrs Ted Wilson misunderstanding was water under the bridge.

That said, his first words were, 'So, I suppose you'll be wanting to hear all about it.'

I laughed guiltily. He was right. I wanted him to spill the beans. Apparently, I didn't much care if he would be gossiping or slandering anyone or betraying confidences. I was interested. No doubt as a result of genetically successful instinctually nosy and pilfering ancestral primates, we itch to know, and the more disallowed the knowledge, the stronger the itch. It comes down, as maybe everything does, unfortunately, to getting an edge at the expense of the other guy. I well understood that I was taking a theftuous interest in the Wilsons' lives. Then again, it felt to me as if Ollie had information relevant to the mystery of the wreck of my own life.

Ollie told me that Mrs Ted Wilson had received confirmation from the authorities that her husband had bigamously married a Dubai resident of Filipino nationality and fathered a child with this second wife, who predictably claimed to have no knowledge of a pre-existing wife, and no knowledge whatsoever of what had happened to him, Ted Wilson, of whom there was still no sign. Mrs Ted Wilson had flown back to Chicago to seek a divorce.

I said, 'How sad.'

'Yes,' Ollie said.

We were drinking limeades in the shadow of the great canopies that stretch above the café courtyard and make it possible, if not necessarily pleasant, to sit outdoors in the summer heat. It's one of my favourite spots in Dubai. One could be in Los Angeles.

'What I'd like to know,' I said, 'is where he got the time. Half the day he's posting online, the other half he's diving, and on top of that he's working round the clock. And the guy's got two families? You've got to hand it to him.'

'Love makes time,' Ollie said.

'Yeah, I guess so,' I said.

His statement had sounded wise and maybe for this reason worn-out, and I didn't give it much thought. Yet Ollie's hypothesis has stuck with me, and I have to ask myself if he did not put his finger on something of great importance. My impression is that he spoke from the heart – the inmost island. Of the Ollie who is there, the Robinson Ollie, naturally I know next to nothing.

'Just imagine,' he said. 'Flying back on that plane alone. Talking to the kids about the father who's just not there any more. Bloody hell. It doesn't bear thinking about.'

Therefore we didn't bear it. A waitress from New Zealand took our orders. We ate lunch and had a few laughs.

At four o'clock, Alain's driver shows up. Before he is taken away, the kid enters my workspace, holding his summer assignment. He leaves it on my desk, as if I'm his teacher.

'Good job,' I tell him.

Alain's essay can wait till the morning. I'm done. I'm going to head home, take a shower, hit the Pasha, eat takeout Thai, jerk off, take a sleeping pill. Then it's lights out and sweet dreams, Charlie Brown.


N ot so fast.
       I discover, when I get back to The Situation, that because I no longer have it in me to look at porn, I no longer have it in me to jerk off. I'm going to assume that my erotic circuitry is capable of rebooting and that this impairment will sooner or later fix itself and before long I'll rejoin the ranks of men and women who self-touch in the time-honoured way, naturally and self-sufficiently. Until that happy day arrives, I'll have to make the best of it. This means texting Mila to ask if she or one of her friends might be able to meet up real soon for a drink, cough, cough.

Meanwhile it's still too early for bed, so it's back to my computer and my digital vagabondage. The true meaning of humiliation is to be discovered here, I suspect. To 'surf' even non-pornographically is to ride one two-foot wave of imbecility after another. Even if one refuses to 'drop in' on stories about The Real Bodies of Mothers or Ten Things You Need to Know Today or Yoga Poses You Can Do Without Leaving Your Bed, and one actually 'catches' a self-respecting attempt to inform, entertain, or enlighten – even in that eventuality, the readers' comments, by their inanity and mean-spiritedness, are almost certain to bring about one's 'wipeout'. I think it's the phenomenon of these commenters – who must be taken to represent the masses, a body from which nobody is excluded – in combination with my new intercontinental perspective, that has left me with a most unfortunate impression that my fatherland – inescapably, the United States of America – is, or has become, a strange, gigantically foolish place that sooner or later will be undone by the calamitous mental life of its population, whose bizarre domination by misconceptions is all too well incorporated by its representatives in Washington, DC. It didn't take long before I gave up trying to follow from the Emirates my countrywomen's (the feminine includes the masculine) political dramas. The election of Barack Obama was very interesting, but his presidency coincided from the outset with the *Finanzkrise* (and thereafter with the Great Recession/Lower Depression), and the opacity of the latter was superimposed on the former. The most pressing responsibility of citizenship, it seemed, was to quickly acquire competence in economic and financial theory, an onerous requirement made worse by the obvious cluelessness and/or bad faith of the governing or controlling theorizers, and, speaking for myself, by a strange feeling that even these would-be controllers or governors were ruled by an undetectable legislature whose existence could be deduced from the existence of overwhelming laws of money the content of which was unknown to, or beyond the control of, our overwhelmed ostensible governors or controllers. Who knows. It cannot end well; dolts thrive; one senses an eventual crash of crashes. The only chink of light is that my despair about human stupidity – a commonplace – is almost certainly itself stupid; and fortunately there are few signs that meta-fools like me have the power to direct the affairs of mankind.

The trouble with chinks of light is their connotation of a wall of darkness. Nowhere is the wall darker than at Ted Wilson's Wall. Unmodified since his total disappearance, it is still open to visits and messages from whom it may or may not concern. If ever I should suspect myself of undue optimism, I can visit this electronic relic and refresh my sense of the baseness of our natures. What can to this day be seen on

Wilson's Wall, which I shall name a disgrace, began with the return of Mrs Ted Wilson to Chicago and the attendant public confirmation of Ted Wilson's bigamy. Somebody posted,

You are such an asshole Ted.

This message, in and of itself not too bad, served as the as it were first sign of nightfall in a land of ghouls, and out of the dark came evil spirits, goblins, bogeys and bloodsuckers. Very quickly the Wall was covered with messages such as,

What whore are you fucking now Ted?

I've heard all about your love of underage fuck buddies, you rapist.

Hey Ted – terrific job abandoning three kids and two wives.

are you getting your new bitch to shit on you Ted? are you getting what you always wanted? are you happy now?

Psychopath.

douche

I hope you're dead you cheating piece of slime.

I'm sure he is dead. Suicide is the most selfish act in the world and he seems like a pretty selfish guy :(

There were many more. This vile aggression went on for months, and my bewilderment only grew as the vilification intensified and nobody did or said anything about it. Who were these people? Where were his friends or the people he had friended? Where was his well-wishing Facebook community? Was nobody thinking of Mrs Ted Wilson and her college-age children, who must have visited the Wall and witnessed the public stoning and gang shaming of their (late?) ex-husband/father? I remember worrying if there was something I could and should do, whether, specifically, I ought to join Facebook for the purpose of posting a message of my own, not only in order to come to Wilson's defence, if that is the right word, but to rescue myself from the culpable helplessness into which I had been dragooned by this turn of events. Yes, I felt as if violence was being done to me, who was unknown to these verbal thugs; I felt under attack. Under attack from what? From the peristalsis of circumstance, which forces one forward as a turd is forced. I remember thinking that I had to 'speak out', if not to effect change, if not to rebuff the hooligans, then at least to put on the record where I actually stood in the Wilson matter rather than where, against my will, I had been made to stand, i.e., to stand by.

(The record! I've always found it a hoot, this mythic tabula on which our deeds are inscribed and preserved. Where is this record? Who is the recorder? Who are the readers of the record? Egocentricity! Superstition! Anthropocentricity! (One understands the metaphysical origins of the error, of course, it being an almost unacceptable and unbelievable proposition that we exist in an adjudicatory emptiness, and arguably a definition of the human must refer to our distinguishing if babyish sense of (and/or need for) being kept under observation or lorded over. (The fantasy of the record is closely preceded, surely, by the fantasy of the forum – the ideal if invisible fact-finding or listening body to which one mutters one's arguments, sometimes audibly. I do it all the time. It's consternating, really.)) Yet here, it appeared, *was* a record: the eternal, ineffaceable webpage of a disused but still functional Facebook Wall.)

I resolved to do nothing – resolved to not 'speak out'. I couldn't work out what my speech would be, and I didn't want the mob to turn on me. I was cowed, it cannot be denied, and filled with the shame of the cowed one. In the time that has passed, my silence has continued, and my shame has deepened. It is open to me this very evening to join Facebook and say my piece on Wilson's Wall. I won't, though. It would rouse the virtual beast – a frightening creature, even if these days it gives off only an occasional hiss of poisonous nostril steam:

I know you're out there Ted. So do your children.

DON'T THINK YOU'VE BEEN FORGIVEN YOU TWO-TIMING MANIAC

In fairness, nothing I might post on the Wall would make a difference to the injustice done to Wilson. When Wilson disappeared, so did the very idea of Wilson's facts, and with them the very idea of justice. I'm not in possession of corrective new information, and, even if I were, it would be non-information, because the factual component of the case is the property of the accusers, who, by virtue of being the de facto fact-owners, have unlimited powers of assertion and denial and making shit up. This makes my blood boil, to be honest. Take the last-mentioned accusation: Ted Wilson is a 'two-timing maniac'. I don't take this to mean that he's insane – which, if true, would remove him from the realm of responsibility to the realm of illness – but to mean that he is a villain of the most conscience-less sort. Maybe he is; it's entirely possible; but there are other possibilities. Maybe something other than maniacal two-timing is going on. In order to investigate this – an investigation I insist on, it seems – we must ignore the frenzy of incrimination by which Wilson is already in the stocks, his face dripping with old tomatoes and rotten eggs. (Where do people find eggs that

184

are rotten? Do they keep them in store, in anticipation of the opportunity to throw them?) We must undertake our inquiry neutrally and methodically, beginning with the basic situation, a man and woman in a marriage, and with the basic acknowledgment that because marital relations are transacted in private, we cannot know what experiences they involve. We begin with a mystery, in short.

(It's a mystery that cannot be dispelled by a couple's self-presentation. I'd guess that nobody at the firm had an inkling about where the Jenn–me deal really stood, behind closed doors. I didn't go around leaking how I was doing (i.e., not well; the line between my being alive and my being dead had faded almost to the point of unimportance), and Jenn – well, she was outwardly sunny because inwardly she was, I believe, in the main OK with the outcomes produced by the her–me undertaking. I'm making no criticism at all here, just adverting to the fact that Jenn drew sustenance from stable-partnership products – a residence, financial pooling, professional assistance, social status, and, in due course, a reproductive and parenting cooperative – rather than from a partner qua partner. She wasn't really a great fan of the whole person-to-person *Liebe an sich* thing, if such a thing actually exists. (She was a wonderfully devoted and even emotional advocate for her clients, and a terrific colleague at work. (On the phone, I always knew when she was with workmates because she would speak to me in a considerate, upbeat tone that in all honesty I very rarely met with if we were talking privately, when she could be a little ratty, if I may say so. (This gave rise, in my mind, to one of those distinctions that seemed important for a while but which, over time, I've come to see as another low point in my personal history of thinking, namely the difference between rattiness *in rem* (innate rattiness, or rattiness towards the world) and rattiness *in personam* (rattiness towards a certain person). I held it against Jenn that she was quite capable of non-rattiness at work yet found it a challenge to not be ratty at home, when face-to-face with me. This wasn't fair to her, because she could well have been innately ratty while being, at work, pleasant *in personam*. Or, she could have been naturally pleasant but when at home made grumpy by me through no fault of her own. Even by my standards, this line of thinking is unusually futile.))))

So:

1. This was a geographically strange marriage. The Ted Wilsons had long lived in different countries, with no end in sight to their separation. That they opted for this arrangement does not diminish its strangeness. On the contrary, arguably. (It's as if an owner of a pair of socks decided to keep one sock at home and its match in the country. (We all know what eventually happens to pairs of socks: one of them disappears, or gets a hole in it, and they are separated permanently. (Although in my case the retained sock will often live on alone, and be mismatched with a leftover sock from a different pair.)))

2. This, the above, puts the marital case in the category of the exceptional: there is no need to spell out the implications of a couple living apart, at least to anyone who believes that, unlike cats, most of us are not solitary creatures with no need for close companionship.

3. We are concerned, then, with the case of a married person's inability to abide forever by promises whose presuppositions (of proximity and intimacy) have evaporated. If this inability is a flaw, very many of us are similarly flawed. It follows that the flaw is non-pathological.

4. Accordingly, one can hardly state with confidence, of either Mr or Mrs Ted Wilson, that it would have been maniacal or psychopathic of them, over the course of years of apartness, to seek from a third party the subject-matter of an

abstracted marital monopoly, i.e., the humanly essential flesh-and-blood tenderness that comprehends, but is not exhausted or defined by, sexual pleasure. (It pains me to say it, and I'm not suggesting anything, but we have no information as to whether Mrs Ted Wilson did or didn't herself take a lover or paramour, to use decorous language I associate with young ladies in the court of Louis XIV who've been entered into wedlock with a romantically unsuitable (much older) man in order to further extra-personal diplomatic/ financial objectives, and who are deemed to be entitled to a discreet liaison with a younger, more personally compatible gentleman. (Interestingly, men are not typically said to 'take a lover', and I'm not aware that our language provides them with an equivalent euphemism. This may be another anachronistic disjuncture, especially as it's no longer the case that a husband is permitted to sexually have his way with his wife whether or not she is agreeable. The spousal rapist no longer goes scot-free, in theory. (This may be the moment to mention what I think is an important prevalent confusion about the promise of fidelity, i.e., faithful monogamy. The essence of monogamy does not consist in abstention from third-party sexual relations but in the dedication of sexual activity to a single person. In other words, the wilfully sexually inactive spouse is not being monogamous: he/she is being celibate. Those who are in doubt as to the conjugal significance of celibacy are referred to its historic synonymity with the Latin source-word, *caelibatus*: 'state of being unmarried'. Properly understood, then, the intentional celibate, in his/her contravention of the vow of fidelity, is in the same boat of transgression as the intentional adulterer. (Maybe this is all by way of a prologue to a confession: Jenn and I 'cheated' (word beloved by the online barbarians) on each other. What little sex we had was clearly a disturbance of a celibate status quo rather than an enactment of a monogamous one. The most erotic episode of our last few years came when, tweezers in hand, I carefully removed a wasp's stinger from the sole of her foot and, in the weeks that followed, scratched the bite mark at her request. She practically swooned with toxical ecstasy. (Since I'm looking back, I have to rub my eyes and ask where we got the idea that it was somehow sensible and coherent and *reasonably practicable* to pay a woeful price of eternal intimate isolation in order to be 'with' each other. Likewise, who or what put it into the heads of the Wilsons that they could pull off an international union that wasn't actually a union? What are they teaching in schools these days? Which planet are we all on? (Nowadays the more unremarkable or self-evident something is, the harder and longer I'll be rubbing my eyes. That's not how it's supposed to work.))))))

5. OK, so Ted Wilson and Mrs Ted Wilson II (as she isn't, yet) are having a non-maniacal adulterous relationship. Then, she gets accidentally pregnant (it happens to the best of us) and she decides to keep the baby (again, by no means an outlandish decision). This gives rise to a problem. This is Dubai, remember, where it's illegal and unacceptable for an unmarried woman to be with child. So Wilson marries her – not for his sake but for her sake and the child's. He falls on the sword of bigamy. How do we feel about Ted Wilson now? (I'm not saying *tout comprendre, c'est tout pardonner*. I'm just asking the question. (To be clear, we don't know the facts. We'd need to see the certificates of marriage and birth and do the prurient math. But I'll bet that my scenario isn't far from what happened. It certainly cannot be ruled out.))

6. We have answered, in the negative, the charge that Ted Wilson, insofar as he had relations of a worldly and criminally matrimonial nature with a woman other than Mrs Ted Wilson, must necessarily have been a 'two-timing *maniac*'. I want to quickly go back to the question of *two-timing*. An overlooked

feature of the case against Wilson is the absence of any suggestion that he took action that was wrong *as such.* So far as one is aware, he led two 'good' lives – one with Mrs Ted Wilson, one with Mrs Ted Wilson II. (Debatably, until it all fell apart, he was twice as virtuous as the next guy, seeing as he was discharging the responsibilities and producing the good outcomes associated with meeting the needs of two women. (I'm just dipping my toe in water, here. I'm also asking if, as someone who is currently neither betraying anyone nor providing for anyone, i.e., as a zero-timer, I'm not actually worse than Ted Wilson.)) Wilson's wrongdoing lay in the simultaneity of his two lives. Again, no value judgment. I'm just putting out there that we begin to see a link between morality and chronology. The link becomes clearer if we remember that serial romantic involvement is not generally deplored, so that if Wilson had taken up with Mrs TW2 after his relationship with Mrs TW had ended, all would have been OK. The accusation of 'two-timing' is therefore more apt than the Wall accuser knew: Wilson's crime was essentially temporal. His *timing* was bad. (The rebutter will impatiently say: No, no, no, his crime was his dishonesty: he acted with wrongful secrecy, in breach of trust. The rebuttal has great force. I wonder, though, if it's dispositive. What if both the Mrs Ted Wilsons had expressly consented to their mutual husband having concurrent relationships in Dubai and Chicago: would this arrangement have met with general approval? I doubt it. Leaving aside the disapprobation excited by polygamy (which I can attest to, having heard the nasty comments made about Emirati families), it seems to me that the very doubleness of Wilson's life would be outrageous. Hold on – he gets two bites at the cherry? Correction – he gets *two cherries*? We're stuck with one life and he gets two? Unfair! We're stuck with the tyranny of the linear and he isn't? He gets a double helping and we

189

don't? He gets to take *both* forks in the road and we're stuck with the path not taken and the false consolation that alternativity is a spiritual splendour? Not on my watch, buddy. Not if I have anything to do with it. (As it happens, I see things differently. I think two lives would be unendurable and unnatural. Oneness may be hard – but twoness? It has a diabolical dimension, to my mind. How would you split yourself? How would you do justice to both your selves and to both your others? (Then again, there's Ollie's revolutionary conjecture: love makes time. (It certainly seems true that lovelessness shrinks time. Jenn and I always seemed squeezed. Always we were in agreement that certain practical things needed to be done right away. Always it was first things first. Always we were in the hurry that postpones the second thing, the good stuff, whatever that was supposed to be. (I now see that our idea of the good stuff wasn't having a good *time* together, or a good that was stuff-like, but having a good situation, i.e., the circumstance, rather than the substance, was the good, and vital to the good was the displacement of time and its replacement by activity. This was a category error, but what did we know? It was all new to us, every second of it. (There's your problem with experience, right there: it's inapplicable, going forward.)))))) (On one view, which I share, I was guilty too, and above all, of causing the most serious chronological damage: I failed to tell Jenn that I didn't want to have a baby with her *earlier*, so as to give her a reasonable period of time in which to mate with someone else. (I'm aware that I have a defence open to me, namely that Jenn specifically asserted that she didn't want a child. The defence doesn't hold up. There was always the chance she'd change her mind, and there was nothing to stop me from telling her that *come what may* I would not have a child with her because our quasi-marriage was a living death for me – surely a pretty significant piece of information that is absolutely one's obligation to

190

communicate to one's partner in a timely fashion. Jenn, I'm so sorry.))


M Y morning starts with a glitch: the office has not been cleaned overnight. I'm not going to complain to the building administration, because I'm guessing that the cleaning crew (whoever they are; they never swim into my ken; they are substantiated only by newly empty trash containers and a lemony after-smell) really don't need more shit in their lives; and, let's face it, we're only talking about carrying two small, light waste-paper baskets to the utility area in the hallway, tipping their contents into a larger container, and walking the baskets back to the office. Normally, Ali would take care of this without my even having to think about it; but he's on enforced leave. It isn't an ill wind, though: the chore is perfect for the kid.

I say to him, 'Hey, Alain, do me a favour. Can you take these out?' I'm standing by his desk, tendering the little baskets.

'I døn't think sø,' I hear him say.

This makes me curious. 'How come?' I say.

'How come what?' he says, so lethargically it comes out as a moan. I get it. His time here is coming to an end, and he feels he can experiment with insubordination and insolence. I'm just grateful he didn't have this thought earlier.

How come he doesn't think he should take out the trash? I answer.

'It's not my job,' he says.

Funny. As if the kid had a job. 'And whose job is it?'

The kid is sitting at his desk, face resting on one hand. He is contemplating his next move.

'Oh, fuck off,' he murmurs very quietly at the wall.

That's a bold play – a power play. He's pushing me into the corner of truculence. Or so he thinks. I still have my best move to come.

'Listen,' I say. 'You're hurting my feelings when you say something like that.' (I learned about this communication technique in the days when I searched online for expert emotional guidance. Apparently the vulnerable announcement of one's suffering will almost certainly give pause to one's interlocutor and awaken in him/her a measure of receptiveness to oneself that would certainly not be forthcoming if one proceeded the usual way, by complaint and criticism.)

The kid sniggers.

Now, that snigger bothers me. Vulgar abuse and childish f-bombs are water off a duck's back. But this snigger is directed at the very notion of fellow feeling.

I take out the trash myself. Then I retreat behind the partition. The kid and I stew in our respective juices.

> *I hope you're happy with your handiwork, Sandro. Your son is unresponsive to the most basic appeal to his humanity.*

> *S – You know what? Forget that last message. It's not my funeral.*

I fight off a bitter urge to take the brat into the bathroom and weigh him.

To cool off, I go online, onto the Dubai Police website. One of the more civilized aspects of the Dubaian way of doing things, in my opinion, is that cameras and radars, not traffic cops, control speeding. If you're electronically caught, you get an electronic ticket that you don't know about until you've checked the police website. I'm not against this system. It's true that there's something fundamentally unsettling about machine-based justice, but I prefer it to the delay, dishonour and terror inflicted by a flashing, squawking American patrol car. The street-parking situation here is crystal clear: either you feed a meter or you get a ticket. You are spared the cruel enigmas and triple meanings of the parking signs of midtown New York City, which rise like strange totems up the sign-poles and gave me great trouble during my stay in the Lincoln Tunnel luxury rental, when I leased a car to cheer myself up. Three times I got towed. I found out that the fleet of the police tow trucks was based a block away and those flatbed-driving fuckers would essentially fill their daily quota in the neighbourhood, where the lowest-hanging fruit in the city – tourists, commercial drivers, and me – was most densely concentrated. On the other hand, the car pound was right next door, and I won't say that it didn't occur to me to skip the whole parking and ticketing and towing production and drive directly to the pound and leave the car right there.

(Each time I went to the pound, I'd get a police document stamped REDEEMED. One day, looking more closely at this police-blue piece of paper, I noticed this notice:

!!! WARNING !!!
THE SCOFFLAW STATUS IS UNDETERMINED

What? I was maybe a scofflaw? I had that hanging over my head too? *Even though I wasn't a scofflaw?* I made phone calls. I mailed registered letters to the New York City Department of Finance with copy receipts of the parking fines I had paid. I sent faxes and e-mails. Several times over I demonstrated my innocence. It made no difference. There was never an official response. My scofflaw status remains to be determined.)

I see that I have no Dubai speeding tickets. Excellent. Phew. Since I'm logged in, I check on Sandro's status. This is one of those borderline responsibilities I've had to accept. I'd love to be able to dine out on stories of Sandro's motoring excesses, but of course that would be a breach of confidence and not even Ollie can be told about the roughly ten thousand USD worth of traffic violation tickets that Sandro annually picks up. It's not that funny, to be honest. Periodically, his licence is suspended and he gets one of the guys at Fort Batros to serve as his full-time driver. Even if there's no rush whatsoever, he yells at the driver to speed up, with the consequence that this unlucky individual soon has *his* licence suspended, which of course is a calamity for him. This has been the subject of much real and imaginary mail to Sandro, who, I know for a fact, makes no provision for the loss suffered by his drivers on his behalf. I have had to take it upon myself to make unofficial hardship payments to these unfortunates (out of the Family Office operational budget).

Using my corporate card, I pay Sandro's fines.

His son's writing assignment is on my desk. To get rid of it, I read it.

### My Summer Holiday

This year I spent my summer holiday in Dubai because I had to get a job and work. Usually I spend my summer holidays in Beirut. My grandfather lives there and we hang out on his yacht. Dubai is a lot of fun though. But its very hot. There are lots of malls to go to. I had a lot of fun. I swam a lot and listened to a lot of music. I like waterskiing and we did a lot of that. Usually I drove the motorboat and my friends skiied. I have a lot of friends here. My job was really boring though I have to say. I got pretty good at Sudoko though. I'm a brown belt. I'm going to make sure I get a better job when I leave my education. I don't want to loose my time on this earth.

Not too bad, I guess, given the limitations of the genre and the author. He really is not super-mature. (It would be nice if he'd use some of the high-value words I've taught him, but I don't want to get dragged into an editorial or pedagogic or hands-on role here.) Next paragraph:

194

I got into trouble with my Dad because I tried to take money out of the cashpoint that my family has. He caught me out, aaa! I was not trying to steal though. My Mum asked me to get it out for her. Its complicated!

Well, well, well. The kid took the fall for the mother. This essay is a cry for help. My duty is clear. I send Sandro a text advising him to read my e-mail ASAP. The e-mail reads:

> Hi Sandro – please see the attachment. This is a scan of Alain's summer essay assignment, which I've just read. You'll see that Alain suggests that Mireille played a role in his attempt to withdraw cash from the ATM.
>
> If Alain is being truthful – I have no opinion about that – it might explain another matter I need to raise with you. It seems that Alain has been attempting to pressure my assistant, Ali, into giving him (Alain) money. Young people can act uncharacteristically when they are in difficulty, and I would guess that Alain may be 'acting out' because of the ATM incident.

I feel a lot better. Everything is out in the open. I've done what was needed, and done it in a way that is, I believe, sensitive to all parties. Now it's up to the parents and their child to figure things out. My work here is done.

Meanwhile there's the problem of what to do with the kid for the rest of the day. We can't just sit around fuming and licking our wounds. In any case, my wounds have healed.

I go into his part of the room. 'OK,' I say. 'Let's go. Field trip.' I jingle the keys to the Autobiography.

'Where we gøing?'

We are going to the Al Fahidi Fort, which I've always wanted to visit. It has stood for two centuries and is the real deal, if by realness we mean oldness. These days the fortress is hemmed in by car traffic and by dense, dishevelled Bur Dubai, and the old magnificence – towers looming on white sands, warriors approaching on horseback – must be fantasized. For me, that's not a problem: I can't look up at those pale stone battlements without catching a glimpse of Beau Geste and, on the inland horizon, the gangsters of the sands. The fort now houses the Dubai Museum and, we are promised, artifacts from the bygone days. With luck, the kid and I will learn something. I've taken the precaution to not utter the word 'museum'. At his age, just hearing the word knocked me into the stupor I associate with being clubbed on the head.

And with stepping into the Dubai heat. Our summer sun is a goon. We cannot linger in the fort's large courtyard. We dash past cannons, a dhow, and a hut with walls made of dried palm fronds. We make it indoors.

What can I say about what happens next? We go down a staircase and are confronted with stuffed flamingos hanging mid-air on strings. There is a soundtrack of waves and bleating birds, and there's a panoramic maquette of the desert featuring the Creek and some trees, all on a ridiculously minuscule scale that presumably replicates the flying flamingo viewpoint. The kid gives me a WTF look. I start to explain that the museum dates back to 1971 and even think about bullshitting him about the interestingness of the technological gap that separates the now from the then. I can't keep a straight face, however. I say, 'OK, you're right. This place is weird.' From that moment on, we're in a comedy. We have a chuckle at a wood platform used as an outdoor bed, we feign awe at a goatskin drum, we stand in actual awe before a waxwork of life-sized Arab men drinking tea and puffing on shisha pipes. 'It's so bad it's good,' Alain says, and I can see he's proud of this comment. When he watches some film footage of long-gone fishermen dancing and chanting, the youngster, who let's not forget is as sizeable as John Candy, if a little shorter, does a funny shimmy. We're having a great time – and, I must insist, not at the expense of the good people who worked hard on these exhibits forty years ago, or out of disrespect for the local traditions honoured here. There's room in the world for a bit of innocuous, good-natured irony. It's not anybody's fault that, until very recently, this has always been an uneventful, materially poor, culturally static corner of the world, with inhabitants who did not prioritize their own future prestige or devote themselves to producing deathless *objets* for their museological self-representation in posterity. I find this refreshing. One detects, in the as it were whiteness of the pages of the history of Arabia Deserta, a conformity with ideals of modesty that contrasts favourably, in my book, with the vainglorious agendas of certain other nations. (Ted Wilson (I recall from my YouTubing of a conference talk he gave) thought that Dubai's blank past was a great 'storytelling' opportunity. This shocked me a little. I hadn't understood that it's no longer officially denied that history is cooked up. I'm fully aware that country branding is as old as Genesis, but have we become so despairing that we openly boast of our frauds on the facts? Jeepers creepers, whatever happened to lip service and the ceremony of innocence? Do we no longer require of our governors that at the very least they dissemble their motives and spare us, if nothing else, shame? Evidently not. Evidently we live in a world in which deep thinkers or investigative journalists are no longer required to bring to light the mechanisms by which our world, and our sense of it, is controlled. The controllers, like those buildings that wallow in their pipes and ducts, now jubilantly disclose their inner workings. (In this sense, the Ruler is behind the times. He'll learn soon enough, I'll bet. It won't be long before we'll be deafened by the screeches of whistles being blown by whistle-blowers blowing the whistle on themselves.))

The most striking exhibit is the diorama of the pearl diver in action. He wears an ancient diving suit and a makeshift breathing apparatus, and reaches down to the seabed he will never reach. The display commemorates Dubai's claim to notability as a former pearl-diving centre. I don't doubt that there used to be some pearl-related activity, but it's odd that I haven't heard a whisper about pearls since I got here. (Where are these famous pearl beds that were once so important? How come I've never seen an oyster?) I'm not sure, in any case, that it's such a terrific idea to lay claim, in memory, to the courage of these swimmers and the supposed glamour of underwater treasure-hunting. I may of course have been misinformed, but I think I remember reading that the divers were essentially in the ownership of the pearl merchants/boat owners and needless to say didn't get to keep the pearls they defied death to find. (I'm not saying they were blood pearls, counterparts of today's blood diamonds. I don't have the evidence to support this grave charge. (We should be wary of applying the noun adjunct 'blood' to everything and anything that comes to us with the taint of exploited labour. It would devalue the usefulness of the term; there would be no end to it. One cannot live in a world of blood pants, blood bread, blood spoons, blood saltshakers, blood water, and blood air.))

I'm minded to say something to the kid about the historic context of this diver. It's a lost cause, however, because one doesn't know what the cause is. Who can really know what actually happened and what one is to make of it all?

We drive back to the office in silence. The good cheer fades. How could it not?

It's back to business. Alain hits the number puzzles, I hit the stamps and bosses. Very little is said, either in the office or afterwards, when I drive the kid home. I make no mention of weighing him. I will have nothing more to do with this boy's body.

Notwithstanding the occasional comment posted on Ted Wilson's Wall, interest in the Ted Wilsons passed quickly enough. Other scandals occupied us. Let's see: there was the English couple from Emirates Hills, the W—s, whose Sudanese help, hours after she was fired, was found dead on the golf course. There was the saga of the marriage of B. and M. C—, whose union survived revelations of B.'s cross-dressing, M.'s prescription-drug abuse, and certain colourful claims made by their neighbours. And there was that sad story of the Dubai-based American, a gentle soul by all accounts, who bred falcons in Kazakhstan for sale in Saudi Arabia and was fatally stabbed with a screwdriver out there, in the Chu Valley, and presumably died a lonely death. The Wilsons were no longer talked about because they were no longer around. In Dubai, like anywhere else, we focus on our own.

(I don't want to attempt a taxonomy of expat chatter, but some distinctions should be made. Scandalized gossip is not to be confused with other modes of chitchat or outraged discussion:

- *Stories of drunken antics*: doing dumb, dangerous things *while intoxicated* is considered amusing, not scandalous.
- Nobody has much to say about *Western tourists getting into official trouble* (for making out in public, wearing too-skimpy clothes, being caught at the airport with microscopic traces of drugs on their shoes, etc.). People overseas may be interested; we're not. The view here is that visitors should respect and inform themselves about Emirati laws and customs. If they don't, that's their lookout.
- Although a person's *financial failure/employment termination* is always carefully analyzed, very few take talkative pleasure from it. There but for the grace of God goes one.
- *Official injustices done to high-net-worth expats* are discussed with sobriety. Take the story of Karl V—, who was arrested, imprisoned for a year, then deported – all because of alleged

homosexual acts in a parked car. That got the attention even of straight people. Why? Because all of our heads are on one kind of chopping block or another. (This isn't to diminish the special and inexcusable perils faced by the LGBT community here.)

- *Misfortunes or injustices suffered by low-net-worth expats* are simultaneously in our field of awareness and not on our conversational radar. (For example, Karl V—'s lover was a workman from India. He wasn't talked about, even though his unjust punishment was indistinguishable from Karl's.)
- *Tragedies.* We remain sensitive to death, serious illness, the suffering of children, etc., within the expat community.
- We don't talk about *injustices done to Emiratis by Emiratis.* We don't care.
- When it comes to the *judicial mistreatment of raped women,* we are affronted; and our affront has no communal limitation. Take the story of the young Emirati teenager who was abducted from her home and driven out into the desert, where she was raped, beaten, and left for dead. No asterisk of nationality is placed next to our sympathy for her experience or our horror at the fact that, after she somehow made it home, the rapists were exonerated and their victim, on account of her alleged failure to wear sufficiently modest attire in her own garden (into which the two rapists had furtively peeped), was officially blamed and disgraced for her alleged provocation of the rapists. This is no less appalling to us than (for example) the story of the French woman who was raped by three men (Christian foreigners, note well) and was charged with adultery after she reported the facts to the police. (The overseas press picked up both these stories, and there was a furore without borders. International outrage has no effect on our domestic outrage, except maybe to reduce it, because we disidentify with the fingering holier-than-thou crowd

who look down their noses on Dubaians of every stripe, always unaware, in their anxiety to piss on us from a great height, that they have forgotten to wipe the shit from their shoes. (That's not to question anyone's freedom of speech or opinion. I'm just saying.)))

Nor should it be forgotten that, of the people who might have been interested in the Wilsons' miseries, at least half left Dubai within a year. Yes – we have had a lot to brood over, starting with the near-bankruptcy of the emirate and the great economic paralysis that befell the land. (This development, so ruinous to so many, prompted a lot of gloating in the foreign media (British, in particular), where opinionators delightedly recognized a case of 'hubris', an intensely annoying word only used, in my opinion, by a nose-in-the-air jerk who is about to stride into a manhole. (These criticizers – who denounce our carbon footprint from their own catastrophically deforested, coal-built countries – not satisfied with character-izing the Emiratis as until-recently-illiterate camel-jockeying upstarts who have finally been taught a good lesson; not content with repeating unverified scare stories (the taps at the Atlantis give forth cockroaches; The Palm is sinking; The World is dissolving); and not sufficiently gratified by their 'exposés' of the 'dark side' of the 'desert playground', also attacked us, the expats. Apparently we were fleeing the 'sheikhdom' in 'droves' (i.e., mindlessly, like driven cattle) or in 'a Gadarene rush' (i.e., like the demoniac pigs who ran into the sea). I don't let this stuff get to me. I do, however, look forward to the day Dubai has bounced back and the hubris experts, down in their manholes, are begging for a helping hand.))
So I've had a lot on my mind; a thousand and one troubles have kept me awake at night; and yet for some reason I have continued to think about the Wilsons.

Initially my thoughts followed Mrs Ted Wilson; that is, in my mind's eye I travelled to Chicago and omnisciently followed her into her own home, and into her bedroom, and into the shower, and watched her doing all the things associated with those places. These crimes of fantasy were of course perpetrated in secret, and with impunity. One's thoughts are not yet searchable, thank God. Let me say, if I'm allowed to, that it's not as if in these scenarios I was interacting with Mrs Ted Wilson or doing gross stuff that would be wrong; and it's interesting that increasingly I have watched her doing everyday, out-in-the-open stuff – shopping, driving around, drinking coffee. I think what I've wanted, most of all, is someone nice and safe to hang out with. Evenings in The Situation can get awfully long.

I have not Googled Mrs Ted Wilson. The Jenn Rule applies.

(The Jenn Rule provides: It is wrong to Google a person who does not want to be Googled by you. As its name implies, the Rule was promulgated by me to me, in response to my incessant Googling of Jenn, an exhausting but irrepressible habit that did nothing to advance my understanding of how she was doing, if that was in fact my purpose. It dawned on me, after about a year of banging my head against a rigid superficies of data, that Jenn would not want me peering into and sniffing around her life; and it followed that I shouldn't. I would not want her to shadow me online, that's for sure. Once I had established, or discovered, the Jenn Rule, I saw no valid reason to limit its scope to Jenn. Thus, it applied to Mrs Wilson because she would likewise not want me to Google her. (Note, however, that the Rule does not apply to cases where A, the searcher, is unknown to B, the searchee, who by definition cannot want to not be Googled by A. (Confession: my observation of the Jenn Rule is not really attributable to any uprightness in my character. I broke the Rule many times. It was only when a 'Jennifer Horschel' search consistently yielded only third-party Jennifer Horschels (a few do exist) and it came to me that my Jenn had become unsearchable by me – it was only then that I stopped Googling her and found myself in compliance with the Rule. (I was of course terrified by Jenn's sudden virtual absence, but I calmed down when I saw that nothing online or anywhere else pointed to her death. I could and can only conclude that she broke her own rule against getting married and in the process completely shed her maiden name, for which she also had no great fondness, I suspect, especially after some prick at the office thought it would be smart to dub her J-Ho. Although the tag didn't stick and Jen came to see a funny side, I have to think that her feelings were hurt. (I did briefly re-break the Rule in order to track her down under her new identity, and I found out, by viewing the relevant photographs, that none of the Jennifers still working at my old firm was Jenn. Clearly, she had also made a professional move. (I stopped my prying there, which again was hardly laudable. To refrain from making investigative phone calls is not exactly a triumph of abnegation. (Is Jenn a mother now? I hope so. Is she happy? I hope so.))))))

While as it were haunting Mrs Wilson, I'd 'see' her raging and weeping about her ex-husband, and it was this, I suppose, that eventually turned my own thoughts to the *disparu*. What happened to him? Where is he now? There was and is no information to be had, not even by way of a rumour. Ted Wilson has never been sighted again in Dubai or, as far as I know, anywhere else. Nowadays it's he, rather than his beautiful first ex-wife, who loiters most often in my thoughts. I locate him fantastically. He is always somewhere in the East. At first I saw him in Bangkok and in Hong Kong, in Kuala Lumpur and Jakarta, and then, as I considered his position more carefully and understood that these places would be too exposed, that he would be able to survive there only by surfacing into identification, I saw him in smaller, still more remote places such as Balikpapan and Makassar and Davao City. I came up with these last-named ports by drifting always eastward on the online atlas, whereupon I'd image-search these dots on the map and understand that they were large, roaring, self-involved cities with refineries and airports and mature economies that probably would not make special deferential provision for the random incoming white man, and I – I mean Ted Wilson, of course – would have to move on still farther, in search of somewhere still smaller and more receptive to a stranger of dislocated competence who must remain incognito and yet keep his head above water. Is such a destiny still possible? It must be; there must be countless Lord Jims out there, bearded beyond recognition, every once in a while glimpsing with horror a face they know. And it may even be possible, I dream out of sympathy with Ted Wilson, that somewhere out there in the isles of the East, in the Sulu Sea or the Banda Sea or the Timor Sea, there is a neglected little port where honorary consuls drink sundowners on verandas, and ceiling fans whir almost in vain, and sinecures are not extinct, and the long call of the orangutan may yet be heard, a green and placid little harbour where an older white man of indefinite occupation may yet, without further inquiry, be received as a gentleman. This is what I imagine, in relation to Ted Wilson.

But here's the thing: the fate of Mrs Ted Wilson II went undiscussed. It was beyond our pale. It became known, or said, that she had avoided deportation and continued to work as a singer at the Arabian Courtyard, in Bur Dubai. No more was offered, and I made no inquiries. There wasn't anything I could single-handedly do about the general neglect of Mrs Ted Wilson II, if 'neglect' is even the right word. Yet I came to be bothered by the disparity in the attention paid to the Wilson wives, not least by me. I felt ashamed – specifically ashamed, that is, which is to say, filled with a shame additional to the general ignominy that is the corollary of insight, i.e., the ignominy of having thus far lived in error, of having failed, until the moment of so-called insight, to understand what could have been understood earlier, an ignominy only deepened by prospective shame, because the moment of insight serves as a reminder that more such moments lie ahead, and that one always goes forward in error.

Some months ago, I was startled by a phone call from the past. Don Sanchez, the vertical athlete, was in town, and staying at the Arabian Courtyard. I had no memory of giving Don my contact details and had no wish to see him again, decent man though he is, and I really, really didn't want to paint the town red with the guy. It was only because I couldn't resist the possibility of laying eyes on Mrs Ted Wilson II that I agreed to meet him at the Arabian Courtyard's Sherlock Holmes English Pub. Don wanted to meet 'somewhere more adventurous', but I twisted his arm. That wasn't very nice of me, I know, but those were my terms.

The Sherlock Holmes is like so many of the British-themed pubs that have spread all over the planet, a gloomy, friendly, wood-everywhere bar with dark Victorian-style wallpaper and a scattering of TV monitors showing 'live' broadcasts of defunct soccer matches. It's a fine establishment, in other words. Don and I ate hamburgers and French fries and drank pints of Foster's. Don explained that this was his 'one drinking night': the inaugural Burj Khalifa tower race, which was the reason he'd flown over, was four days away, and his 'hydration schedule' allowed for the consumption of his 'four last pre-race units' of alcohol that evening. Don needed no prompting to tell me about the physical preparations he'd made for the race, which he said was the 'most severe challenge' he'd ever 'accepted'. He told me he had left the Lincoln Tunnel luxury rental ('I felt I'd gone as far as I could with the set-up there') and moved into a fortieth-floor abode on the Upper East Side ('which was lucky timing, because I had no way of knowing that I'd be running the Burj, and frankly the forty-floor track is a superb amenity').

I was hearing all about his nutrition goals and training routine and run plan when the entertainers – two female singers and a male keyboardist – appeared, to the loud clapping of a bunch of Indian dudes who occupied the table next to the little stage.

I was excited myself. While Don shared his recent performance stats and detailed the changes he was making to his stride pattern, I studied the two singers. I'm not an ethnicities expert, but they looked like Filipinas to me – small, brown-skinned, dark-eyed young women with glossy black hair that fell straight to their shoulders. Which one, then, was Mrs TW2? Reproductive logic suggested that it had to be the older of the two – I assessed her to be in her early thirties – who wore a tight-fitting but entirely respectable very short black dress and high heels, and not the younger one, who looked to be in her early twenties and wore a short, sexy red dress and even higher heels and was the prettier of the two ladies, I guess most people would say, though personally I'm not one to start pitting women against each other in a competition of beauty.

The keyboardist hit the keys, and, before an audience of nine men and a woman, Mrs TW2 began to sing 'Jolene'. What a sweet voice! The nightingale of Dubai! She sang the song exactly and effortlessly in Dolly Parton's voice, which is saying something, in my opinion. I further tuned out poor old Don, who was so to speak verbally ascending a tower of data of concern only to himself, ordered another drink, and fell into an ecstatic, inebriated appreciation of Mrs TW2's artistic abilities. The young singer may have been the object of the Indian dudes' admiration, but I was rooting for the single mother and maritally wronged lead vocalist, who sang with great spirit at a venue whose league she was way out of. When Don suggested we go elsewhere, I bought him another drink and stayed right where I was. When Mrs TW2 sang 'Islands in the Stream', my cup overflowed.

Except that I'd developed a dislike of the keyboardist, a

– what, fifty-five-year-old? – white guy in a black shirt and a pair of John Lennon shades. His very long grey hair occasionally fell in front of his gaunt face, and as he played he would pull the hair back into place with a cruel-looking little finger. From time to time, Mrs TW2 gave him a frightened glance and received in return an indecipherable signal. The more I studied the on-stage dynamic, the stronger grew my conviction that this repellent individual was a Svengali under whose invisible rule these two women, Mrs TW2 especially, found themselves. You could be sure that he controlled the ensemble's finances and kept for himself the vast bulk of its earnings, a regime he certainly enforced by the malign use of his physical and/or mental powers. What a douche. I felt like going over there and pushing him off his little stool.

There was a break in the music. The Indians confidently called over the younger singer, and she went to join them as if she knew them well – which may have been the case. Acting under the inspiration of their example, and ignoring another request by Don to 'make tracks', I waved an inviting hand at Mrs TW2. She beamed at me but didn't move, ostensibly preferring to drink a glass of Coke with Svengali.

I got to my feet and went to her.

'Hi,' I said to her. 'Me and my friend' – I gestured towards Don, who appeared to be taking his own pulse – 'we were wondering if we could buy you a drink. You're a wonderful singer.'

Mrs TW2 beamed again. 'I'm glad you're enjoying the show.'

I smiled right back, making sure to blank Svengali, who was right there next to her, in order to demonstrate to Mrs TW2 that he wasn't all-powerful. Very amiable and harmless, I said, 'Where are you from? The Philippines?'

She beamed.

'I'm from the USA,' I said. I said something about 'my buddy over there' being in town for the Burj race. 'Is that a Coke?' I said.

Now Svengali leaned over to her, and they exchanged words. 'I have to sing now,' Mrs TW2 said very happily.

'OK, great,' I said, I think. That's when I gave her my card and said something innocuous, along the lines of, 'If you ever want to get in touch.'

Svengali spoke up. 'My friend,' he said. 'This is my wife. Please be respecting.'

That got under my skin – the ironic 'my friend'. I was going to say something about it, when the 'wife' assertion registered. Mrs Ted Wilson II was now Mrs Svengali.

'Hey, sorry, man, whatever,' I said.

Don Sanchez said, 'Well, I'm hitting the hay. It's past my bedtime.'

'Me too,' I said. A week or two later, Don e-mailed me a picture of himself in running apparel, arms raised skyward. He'd made it to the top.

Naturally, the incident in the Sherlock Holmes is mortifying to recall. I had too much to drink. I misread the situation. I embarrassed everyone concerned.

Ollie was of the opinion that my blundering was even greater than I thought. When I told him about meeting Mrs TW2, he said, 'How do you even know it was her?'

'I can't be sure,' I admitted.

We were having a sundowner at the Code of Hammurabi, which is one of the Unique's six bars/eateries.

Ollie said, 'Well, let's hope you're right. Good to know she's landed on her feet.'

He was trying to be kind to me, which made me feel a little foolish. I decided to drop the subject, which was, as I've said, by that point regarded as ancient history. Nor was it the occasion to mention that Mrs TW2, or the person I'd believed, rightly or wrongly, to be Mrs TW2, was now a Mrs Svengali, outwardly smiling and singing and inwardly robotic. (I believe that the conjecture retains its validity even if the woman I met was someone other than Mrs TW2. I saw what I saw.) Ollie doesn't go in for that kind of thinking.

'I might be leaving town,' he said.

'Oh? Where to this time?'

'I mean leaving for good. There's this opportunity opening up in Shanghai.'

'Oh,' I said.

'Yeah, we'll know a bit more in a few months. It depends on a few things falling into place.'

'Shanghai,' I said. 'Cool.'

'Yeah. Lynn is pretty psyched. I think she's ready for something new.'

'Cool,' I said.

Ollie went on to say that although Dubai was a 'great market', China was a 'truly exceptional market', even allowing for widely expected drops in its GDP growth rates. Ollie said it would be a super place to 'headquarter' going forward, although he would of course retain a 'strong presence' in the Gulf.

'That makes a lot of sense,' I said.

'It'll be an adventure,' Ollie said.

This was some months ago. I've heard nothing more about it. Don't go, Ollie. Don't leave me stranded.

Hello, here's the cavalry – Mila. I should get a special bugle tone for her texts.

You want two friends tonight? You can handle???

The threesome. The trio with brio. I'm well aware of the appeal. I've done the porn.

It's not for me. A sexual encounter should retain at least

the structure of the real thing, i.e., the one-on-one. The two-on-one, or the one-on-two, or the one-on-one-on-one – these are in formal contradiction, in my opinion, of the raison d'être of the coming together in closeness of persons. The problem of the third person is not the problem of the third wheel, which was solved once and for all, one would think, by the invention of the tricycle. It is the problem of the third as the third. His/her presence abolishes the bilateral relation of the first and the second – already fraught with difficulty – and installs in its place a trilaterality that, by its very multiplication of the possibilities for pleasurable physical interaction, by its generation of a beast with three backs and six arms and six legs and eight holes and one cock, involves the sexual participants in a metamorphosis in which they are turned into organs of an organism seeking only its sensual organization. Gone is the great promise of mutual caring enabled by one special other, whereby the carers together eliminate the terrible problem of space. (By 'space', I don't just mean the isolating sea of interpersonal separation. I also mean the cosmic sea.) Even a fiction of this caring (of the kind I happily settle for in my semi-pro pairings) is impossible. In its place comes a nonfiction of meat and bones, of blowjobs and handjobs and you-name-it-jobs, of stick-that-in-here and my-turn-your-turn-her-turn, of you-do-this-while-he-does-that-and-I-do-this. The falcon cannot hear the falconer. Everything turns to crap.

   One friend please

is my reply to Mila.

I've showered, shaved, and shat, and am all set to head out, when a doorman calls: Mr Ali is here.

I meet the great man in the lobby. 'Well, Ali, how are you keeping? Everything OK?' We shake hands. I tell him, 'One more day. Then Alain will be gone.'

Ali smiles. 'I have information for you, boss,' he says. During his brief sabbatical, this most diligent of assistants has made it his business to repeatedly visit the Project X site. 'Today, I speak to a man there,' he says. 'He is American. I ask him, "What is this building?" He tells me, it is a "mah-kp".'

I ask Ali to repeat that last word.

'Mah-kp,' Ali repeats. 'This is what he says. They are building a very big tower somewhere else. This is the mah-kp.'

'A mah-kp? What does that mean?'

Ali cannot tell me. He is relaying what the man told him.

'OK,' I say. 'That's very helpful. Thank you very much.' I'll get to the bottom of this later. 'Anything else?'

Ali shakes his head. I give him taxi money and send him on his merry way. I/Godfrey Pardew also go on our merry way, to the Unique Luxury Resort and Hotel.

I valet-park the Autobiography and brace for the Nubians. They're nowhere to be seen. I breeze unseen past the front desk: a first. It's exhilarating. The childhood dream of invisibility has come to pass.

My hostess is Oksana. She has an amazingly high forehead, very black hair in a ponytail, and small, decidedly elliptical eyes. (Where is she from? I'm guessing Novosibirsk.) The good-time girls I've had dealings with are usually dressed up, and made-up, semi-formally and semi-glamorously, as if en route to the commercial attaché's reception. Some even look as though they're about to ice-dance. Oksana looks like she's come back from the gym. She *has* come back from the gym: her discarded gym shoes are over there by the TV.

Good for her, I say.

She lights a cigarette. 'You want to fuck?' she says. 'You want to drink something?'

'Maybe a drink,' I say.

Oksana responds with an eye-roll towards the minibar.

I'm getting disdain? I'm being put in touch with

211

my unworthiness? Here? By her? I don't want to sink to the contractual level, but submitting to a personal assessment by Oksana isn't part of the deal. I insist only on niceness, and this isn't being nice. If she doesn't want to be in this room, neither do I.

I'm about to say something when I see, on the bedside table, something extraordinary: a Martial Arts Sudoku book, Black Belt.

I ask her, 'May I look?'

She sucks on her cigarette. We'll call that a yes.

My God, over half of the puzzles have been solved. The numbers are written down in a flawless, invariable hand. There isn't a correction or marginal notation in sight. These solutions are totally clean.

Oksana is a Black Belt?

'Bravo,' I say. 'These are very difficult. You must be very intelligent,' I say. (Clumsy, I know, but it's incumbent on me to speak to Oksana as if English were a foreign language for me, too.)

All I get out of her is more smoke.

Very shy, I hold out the book. 'Can you teach me? How you do it?'

Oksana is beautiful, I realize. How wonderful it would be to lie on this bed with her doing Sudoku puzzles, laughing and sharing and solving. And then a breakfast of fava beans, and then a car journey on sand flats and corniches, and then a trip by speedboat to an island, and there a small cabin build of clay and wattles made.

Oksana terminates her cigarette. Sitting on the edge of the bed, she begins to remove her clothing, starting with the white socks. Then it's off with the leggings and the T-shirt. In her underwear – sports bra and regular panties – she goes into the bathroom. She locks the door.

Oh, woe is me. Oh, woe is she.

She comes out a few minutes later, wearing a towel-turban

and a hotel bathrobe. 'OK,' she says, lighting up again. 'First, money. Then we fuck.'

Clearly, Oksana isn't aware of the protocol. I explain to her that I pay Mila and Mila pays her.

'Mila will not pay me,' Oksana says. 'My friends tell me this.'

I didn't come here to argue and bargain and transact.

'How much?' I say. The evening has now been spoiled.

'Two hundred American,' she says. 'This is what Mila promise.'

Two hundred? Out of five hundred? Mila gets to keep three hundred bucks plus tip? I've never heard of a booking agent taking 60 per cent plus. It's unconscionable. I cannot be party to such an arrangement. The Mila connection can no longer be.

I'm carrying cash. I pay two hundred dollars and make an announcement. 'I'm sorry, but I have a headache. I will go home now.'

Her eyes narrow even more; one glimpses the steppe, wild horses, the Great Khan. 'You are angry? You make problem for me?'

'No problem,' I say. 'I'm happy, really. I just have a headache.' I smile. 'It was nice meeting you.'

I see myself to the door. It's bye-bye, my Black Belt, and it's farewell and adieu, Godfrey Pardew.

Another solo celibate night in The Situation it is.

I get in, or on, the Pasha for a twenty-minute session. After three hundred seconds, I can't take one more rub of the roller. Off, or out, I get.

Night has fallen, and it's safe for me to approach the windows and look out. When I try this in daylight, I keep re-seeing that shadow, or bird, or dropping thing, out of the corner of my eye, and I find myself jerking my head leftwards time and again, always too late to catch sight of it. It's uncontrollable.

It does no good to remind myself that in all probability I saw nothing in the first place and my post-traumatic flashbacks, if that's what we're talking about, are founded on a trauma that never occurred. The falling shadow nonetheless appears; my head nonetheless jerks over my shoulder. This has been going on for a few days, and it's not getting any better, i.e., it's getting worse. It's got to the point where I can't take in the view from my apartment until the sun has set and all is dark. Is this what I've come to? Nocturnality? I have to keep a vampire's hours?

What with the moonlight and the lunar/man-made glow of the Marina, I have no problem discerning the pale X of Project X – the 'mah-kp'.

I permutate the vowels: 'make-up'; 'muck-up'; 'mock-up'.

Mockup. Let's consult the sum of all human knowledge. Let's Wiki it.

> In manufacturing and design, a mockup, or mock-up, is a scale or full-size model of a design or device, used for teaching, demonstration, design evaluation, promotion, and other purposes.

No mention of the construction of buildings. I Google 'mockup + building'. Here we go: a 'pre-construction mockup' is not uncommon, it seems. It seems that 'scale representations' of 'exterior wall systems' and 'other structures' may be useful to builders, engineers and architects, for a variety of purposes.

It follows that Project X is a scale representation of part of another building. It is, if I correctly recall what Ali told me, a representation of part of the 'very big tower' they're building 'somewhere else'.

So Project X isn't a project at all. It's a dummy run. It's a mockup. There's no actual residential proposition going up down there. The action has moved somewhere else. Privilege

Bay is toast and The Situation is fucked. The Uncompromising Few and the Pioneers of Luxury™ and the Dreamers of New Dreams must be re-named.

I'm going to bed.

And in the morning, immediately on waking up, I am jolted by gladness as I see blue sky through the window, and spontaneously I get out of bed and empty my bladder. The joy of this routine – invariably, the happiest time of my day – is, unfortunately, a simple matter of oblivious recurrence: in the drowsiness of renewed consciousness, the current blue morning is indistinguishable from the blue mornings of yore. I forget where I am and where things stand and what lies ahead. Then I remember.

It's the kid's last day. I'll get through it. Then Ali and I will regroup.

There's no sign of Alain at the office, though. His driver usually deposits him at 11 a.m. sharp. It's not till an hour later that a Batros shows – and it's Sandro. He makes straight for my chair.

'OK, so who is this guy – Ali,' he says.

'What do you mean, who is he?'

'That's what I mean: who is he? Why's he here?'

'He's my assistant. He's worked in this office for a long time. You've seen him a million times.'

Sandro says, 'What are his qualifications? Where'd he go to college? Where're his references?'

What is he talking about? 'Sandro, he's an office boy. He gets paid peanuts. I don't need references. He's a superb worker. I trust him totally.'

Sandro nods. 'You trust him. Right.'

'Yeah, I do. He's one hundred per cent honest.'

'More honest than my son?'

'What?'

'You're saying he's more honest than my son?'

215

'I don't understand the question,' I say, even though I do understand that this is big trouble.

He smiles at me like a mafioso. 'Alain says he didn't shake your guy down. He says your guy is making it up.'

'Why would he make it up?'

'You tell me,' Sandro says. Oh no – he's spotted my rubber stamps. He takes one and bangs it on my blotter. 'Why would my son lie?'

I say, 'Alain's a terrific kid, but he's a kid. Kids are always making stuff up, saying stuff that's not accurate, denying stuff. They're kids. They screw up.'

'These things are really great,' Sandro says. He's trying out another stamp, pressing it into the wrong inkpad. *Bang.* 'You made Alain go with this guy to the bathroom?' *Bang.*

Very carefully, like a lawyer, I say, 'You requested that Alain be weighed. Alain wished to be weighed in the bathroom, which was entirely appropriate. I asked Ali to accompany Alain to the bathroom to take note of the weight readings. He did not accompany Alain into the stall. Alain was in the stall by himself. When Alain stood on the scale, Ali could see the reading through the gap at the bottom of the stall. All he ever saw of Alain was his feet. If you recall, you oversaw the procedure the first day it happened.'

'Don't tell me what I recall and what I don't recall,' Sandro says. *Bang.* 'You let this guy, this stranger, take my son to the bathroom and be alone with him there.'

I'm trained for these situations. You have to push back, firmly and calmly. 'I put in place, with your approval, an appropriate procedure for carrying out your instructions.'

He grabs another stamp. *Bang. Bang.* 'I asked Alain if he was comfortable with the arrangement. He told me he wasn't. I said, Why not? No answer. I asked him did this guy, Ali, did this guy try anything funny. You know what he said? Nothing. I'm like, Did he or didn't he? He didn't want to talk about it.'

He's building a case out of a non-answer to a leading question? Has he gone mad?

'He told me something else,' Sandro says. Now he's handling one of my embossers. 'Your friend is an illegal. That right?'

'He's a bidoon. I e-mailed you about it a long time ago. What about it?'

'You know what? I'll be the judge of what you e-mailed me, OK?'

'I'll send you a copy, to refresh your memory,' I say.

'Don't worry about it, he's fired,' Sandro says. 'I don't want to see his face again.' He says, 'How does this thing work?' He's put a sheet of paper in the embosser's jaws. 'Do I just . . . ?' *Crump*. 'That's neat.'

'If you fire Ali, I'm quitting.' I say this serenely, because I've thought through and fantasized this scenario many times. I am ninety-nine per cent sure Eddie will be in my corner. He's not going to lose a high-value asset (me) on account of his crazy brother's whims.

Sandro says, '*If* I fire him? I just did.'

'In that case, I quit.'

'In that case, I'm calling security.'

Another line borrowed from TV. Or maybe Sandro, too, has often dreamed of this moment and knows his script backwards.

I get the cardboard box I've set aside for just this eventuality, and I rapidly box my personal embossers and stamps and the other possessions I keep here, which are very few. 'Here,' I say, and with great satisfaction I toss Sandro my Batros employee's ID card and credit card.

'The car keys,' Sandro says, wiggling his fingers. I almost forgot. The Autobiography is his, not mine. I hand over the keys.

Back at The Situation, the first thing I do is e-mail Eddie.

I'm sorry to inform you that, with effect from 12.36 p.m. today, I am no longer serving as the Batros Family Officer and related positions. Earlier this morning, Sandro capriciously and in bad faith terminated the employment of Ali, my assistant. This action, along with various actions taken and statements made by Sandro on this and other occasions, makes it impossible for me to discharge my responsibilities and/or remain in my job. I will happily provide you with more details, if you wish. Please note that I have not resigned. I have accepted the unlawful repudiation of my contract of service and am entitled to compensation on that basis.

I look forward to receiving your proposal of financial settlement.

Eddie responds within the hour:

Your resignation is not accepted old amigo. I'm in New York. Why don't you fly over tonight and we'll talk it over.

I knew it. When backs are against the wall, Eddie will come out shooting.

From the Belt Parkway, the city looks ragged. Manhattan shows in distant dribs and drabs. The three-quarters-built Freedom Tower, if that's still its name, looks – I'm afraid there is no other word for it – unintelligent. I saw the Burj Khalifa at a comparable stage of completion. The Arabian spire had the natural inwit of a blade of grass. Its American counterpart, for all its massiveness, looks like a stump – a gargantuan remnant. From my inspection through the taxi window, I actually find it hard to accept that this protrusion is indeed the so-called Freedom Tower. The building seems, as I say, not without nationalistic embarrassment, dumb – a meathead tower. It's not even that tall. Mistrustful as I am of the first impression; conscious as I am of my limitations as a critic of architecture; wary though I may be of the personal ruling: I cannot hold back a thumbs-down.

This is my first time back in New York since I left, four years ago/yesterday; it's the first time I've set foot in the land of President Obama. My basic reaction is one of unaccountable infuriation. It gets under my skin that the Belt is as worn-down as ever, with the same potholes and, I'm almost prepared to swear, the very same orange-striped traffic cones marking off the same dormant roadworks. The same battered NYPD saloons lurk roadside with the same lethargic and dangerous cops inside them; and the proud, industrious *Volk* still drives around as if the Rockaways mark the end of the factual world. I'm being irrational, I recognize. To interpret is to misinterpret, never more so than when one is gripped by the prejudicial dismay that's typical, so I've gathered, of the expatriate on his or her return home from brand-new Dubai, who must acclimatize to the older, stick-in-the-mud society of origin, and must be careful neither to overprize nor to overestimate her new knowledge, and of course must reconcile himself to the subtle pigheaded-ness of his native country, which will withhold from her any interest in, let alone understanding of or esteem for, her overseas experience and the value-adding perspective it has granted, and will not give an inch, and will force the returner from Dubai into one more contemplation of his inefficiency. So it's not surprising that I'm exasperated as my taxi edges towards down-town Brooklyn and its Marriott hotel, and offended by every-thing, even the poor old sun, modestly falling into New Jersey. It holds itself out as a bright cloud, and does nothing wrong.

The psychologizer will say that something is afoot, and the

psychologizer will be correct. This is J-Town, and I'm having Jenn-jitters. Even though I have no information as to her current whereabouts, I'm very afraid of running into her. I'm well aware that, in terms of probabilities, this is like worrying about being waylaid by Jerry Seinfeld – but guess what, I once walked right by Jerry Seinfeld, on Broadway at Seventy-Seventh Street. That's why I'm spending the night in a Brooklyn hotel, because Brooklyn, in Jenn's mind, is another extension of the Lehigh Valley, and a borough of shame. And it's not only to avoid road traffic that I travel by subway to my meeting with Eddie: in Jenn's mind, the subway is a zone of shame.

I don't want to make her out to be a snob. She isn't, or wasn't; she was prepared to live in a rent-stabilized one-bedroom, after all. It's just that she was involved in a quest for metropolitan dignity. This plucky, meritorious girl from ABE was trying to make good, and my job was to cheer her on and, when the going got tough, as it will, to cheer her up, i.e., to run out into the rain for DVDs, and open a bottle of wine, and lay me down like a bridge over troubled water. Talk about cluelessness. Talk about underestimating the loneliness of the viaduct. But what was the clued-in alternative? One still has no idea. One's heart goes out to this young couple on the A train who drowsily lean on each other as they hurtle towards Manhattan and who knows what else.

He rudely shoves her: she has accidentally drooled on his shoulder. He's very upset. He likes his jacket, and now his jacket has drool on it. He calls her a name. The train stops, and he gets up. She sort of screams at him to stay, and follows him. She's pregnant, I see, this nineteen- or twenty-year-old Hispanic girl who wears very high platforms. The train lurches into motion, and she loses her balance and begins to topple over. Instinctively, I move to one side and catch her.

She shouts at me – Get the fuck away from me, asshole.

I've got my hands up as if it's a stickup. I'm looking around the carriage for confirmation that this criticism is outrageous and I'm without blame and in point of fact saved the day. I get nothing but blank faces. Now here comes the knight in shining armour, the boyfriend, all fuck this and fuck that, and getting in my face, pointing and gesturing and threatening, and bitch this and cracker that.

'What did you call me?' I say. 'Cracker?' Now my face is right up against his. 'Say it one more time. Call me that one more time.'

The girl is still shouting at me and making accusations.

I call you what I like, bitch cracker, the boy says.

Everyone's watching now. Everyone's waiting to see what I'm going to do next.

I've made a mistake. I'm looking at a lose-lose-lose-lose-lose-lose.

The train brakes: West Fourth Street. I get out, as if it's my stop. The boy is yelling and laughing at me from the door of the train. His girlfriend is next to him, screaming with laughter and pride, hanging out of the door, standing by her man. I have brought them together. As they are pulled away, they mouth more insults at me and bang on the train windows. This will be one of the great stories of their romance.

I walk towards the station exit, sweating and shaking. I have to take care to not mutter audibly, because I'm thinking of things to say to the kid. Then another A train roars into the station. I can board it and be in the clear. Nobody on this train knows me: a new train is a new beginning and a clean slate.

Not quite. I'm still in New York, where I am ignominious.

I remember all too well how it began.

This was during the awful period when Jenn and I were co-workers but no longer involved. My office interactions were getting stranger. Colleagues had started to act with the weirdly chirpy and compliant standoffishness that is usually reserved for crazy neighbours, bores, people with halitosis, etc. When I engaged them in conversation, they'd say, 'Got it,' or 'Absolutely,' or 'You bet, X.,' and then they'd be out of there.

(Almost immediately after its aggressive introduction by Human Resources, my first initial became my office handle: everybody called me 'X.', even clients. (Even Jenn, even after I told her I didn't like it. 'Please,' I eventually insisted, 'can you not call me that?' 'It's alluring,' she said. 'It makes you kind of mysterious. How many other X.s do you know?' 'I don't like it,' I said. 'It's not my name. It's not me.' (To her credit, she did as I asked. But she was right: that goddamned X. made my name unique and that much easier to drag through the mud. If I state that John Smith is a coward, no John Smith will lose sleep. John Smiths have safety in numbers, like the gnus of the savannah. If I state that Q. John Smith is a coward, a gnu is separated from the herd. The predators are in business.)))

I was in my Lincoln Tunnel luxury rental, drinking and Googling my evenings away, when I decided, maybe guided by some sixth sense, to search an unusual person – me; that is, I Googled the professional name that was, as I say, thanks to the accursed X., distinctively mine. As I typed, the Autocomplete function spontaneously offered search suggestions. The following appeared in the search box next to my name:

    attorney
    sexual harassment
    embezzlement
    tiny cock

Naturally, I was horrified. Anyone who Googled me – as clients and professional colleagues did, all the time – would see this list. They would think less of me. It would make no difference if they followed the search suggestions and duly discovered that there was no actual web content connecting me to sexual harassment, or embezzlement, or a tiny cock, and/or if they understood that these Autocomplete suggestions were not the results of multiple arm's-length searches by disinterested parties but had been generated by a malicious person or persons Googling me again and again and again in conjunction with the words suggested by Autocomplete in order to create the defamatory and false impression that I was somehow infamously involved in scandals of money-related dishonesty and inappropriate workplace behaviour towards subordinates, and on top of it all was notorious for being meagrely endowed. Even if the Googler understood all of this – understood that I was the victim of a fiendish new form of defamatory publishing that one might term 'search libel' – I would still be lowered in his/her estimation for the simple, unfair reason that whoever is (whether rightly or wrongly or inaccurately or correctly) publicly ridiculed or embarrassed automatically suffers a loss of reputation and respect. Nor would it change anything if I were to make some sort of public announcement making clear that I was not, and had never been, implicated in any kind of financial or sexual wrongdoing. That would only aggravate the publicity. A fortiori if I were to post online a photograph that would quash beyond peradventure the nonsense about my not being well hung.

There was nothing to be done. I consulted, in the strictest confidence and professional privilege, an attorney who specialized in verbal torts. She expressed the opinion that this was a very interesting case. She advised that the absence of any express statement, whether defamatory or otherwise, made problematic even a defamation claim based on innuendo, since an innuendo was an unstated secondary meaning contingent on the existence of a stated primary meaning. She pointed out that the text originated algorithmically from a computer program, Autocomplete, rendering complex even the basic issue of authorship. She stated that, as a practical matter, there was no reliable way to identify the responsible spiteful human searcher or searchers. She told me, as if in admiration, that whoever had done this was possessed of low legalistic cunning.

'Do you know who it is?' she asked.

I said, 'I have no idea.'

The lawyer looked curious. 'Really? We could always send her a cease-and-desist.'

I felt that conclusions were being jumped to about the gender of the person injuring me. I couldn't say for sure that it was Jenn or some other female in the office or elsewhere. And the world was filled with male malice. Without making any claim to moral rarity, I wasn't about to go down the road of unfairness. 'I'm sorry,' I said. 'I wish I could tell you, but I can't.'

'In that case, I'd try not to worry about it,' the specialist in speech wrongs said. 'It'll go away. Enmity is a lot of work. People get tired. They move on.'

I was alarmed by how she'd put it: enmity. The Earth contained a person, or persons, with the will to cause me harm. It was hard to grasp. I could understand hatred and rage and pain. I could understand ruthlessness – one person falling under the wheels of another's advance – and I could understand tsunamis and bolts of lightning. What I couldn't understand was acting with a calculated and methodical intent to damage a fellow human for the sake of making that human suffer damage. I still cannot understand it.

In one respect, my adviser was wrong. My enemy did not tire or move on. The search libel did not go away. When Sandro Batros flew into town to talk to me about Donald Trump, I received him as a saviour.

And now I'm meeting Eddie to save me from Sandro.

We're having dinner at Per Se. The maître d' leads me to the best table, by the famous big window, with views of sparkling traffic and the wonderful night-time blackness of Central Park. Eddie is waiting for me, and embraces me. I'm still rattled by the subway altercation and pretty rattled generally, so it feels unusually good to get a big hug out of someone who knows me from way back and, now that I think of it, in Dublin once had lunch with my parents, at the Stag's Head. He may be the only person I'm still in touch with who knew me when I was not yet orphaned. This fills me with emotion.

'Let's get a drink in you,' he says.

And we drink, and we eat, and we talk about student days. Over Irish coffees, I say, 'Maeve MacMahon – remember her?'

'Maeve MacMahon,' Eddie says. He shakes his head, amazed. 'Maeve MacMahon.' The words make a dark, beautiful sorrow. Eddie says, 'Where is she now, I wonder? Maeve MacMahon.'

Where, indeed? Where has everyone gone? Where is everybody?

It's time, I feel, to get to the point. 'Eddie, about Sandro –'

He stops me with a signal of the hand. '*Ne parlons pas de cette bêtise, mon vieux,*' he states. 'Forget it. It never happened. There's something else we need to talk about.'

He asks me if I've recently heard from the authorities in Dubai. I'm about to say no, when I remember (because I'm bureaucratically competent) the Joint Notice from the Dubai Financial Services Authority and the International Humanitarian City Authority. I was supposed to meet these jokers the day after tomorrow, Tuesday. I mention this to Eddie, and he says, 'Yes, that's what I'm talking about. Now, listen carefully.'

I listen carefully, and I really don't like what I'm hearing.

In executive summary: the Dubai authorities are about to formally launch an investigation into possible malfeasance by the Batros Foundation. It is suspected that certain charitable activities of the Foundation – specifically, the provision and operation of health clinics for the African poor – have been used as a vehicle for laundering monies ('Many millions of dollars,' Eddie says, when I press him) debited without authority (i.e., stolen) from Libyan banks and transferred, via a series of offshore intermediaries, to the Foundation in Dubai, which has accepted these monies as donations. ('I don't know the details,'

225

Eddie claims. 'I've got nothing to do with Africa. But what I'd like to know is, how are our people in Dubai supposed to know if a donation is legit or not?') Apparently there are further questions about the redistribution of these donations to African sub-charities, i.e., whether the money in question was devoted to the Foundation's charitable purposes or whether, in fact, it made its way back to the thieves/donors/money launderers. 'It's all very probably a big nothing,' Eddie says, 'but that's not the point. Apparently the Libyans are pretty steamed up about their missing cash, and Dubai feels it has to do something. This needs careful handling.'

'I can see that,' I say.

Eddie says, 'The problem, from your point of view, is that, as the Foundation Treasurer, your name is all over these transfers to Africa.'

I say, 'I think you'll find that my role has always been pro forma. I have disclaimers stamped all over the recent transfers. My position is very clear.'

Eddie is sympathetic. 'I'm sure it is, but they're going to look for accountability. You know that. They're not going to let technicalities get in their way.'

Accountability? What's going on?

Eddie says, 'What we're hearing from Mahmud, and I can tell you he's reliable, is they're going to go after you. To make an example of you.'

'But I've done nothing wrong.'

'I know that. Everybody knows that. But that's not what this is about.'

I'm stunned.

'Listen,' Eddie says, leaning forward. 'You're not going back there. That's what I'm telling you. You're staying right here. You do not go back to Dubai.'

'Wait a minute. I've done nothing wrong – and *my* head rolls?'

Eddie makes a dismissive gesture. 'We don't know that. We

don't know how it's going to pan out. We're getting our lawyers all over it. We've got Mahmud on the case. They're going to raise hell. You're going to come out of this just fine.'

I'm spluttering. 'It's monstrous. I have to fight this. What's it going to look like if I stay here? I'm going to be a fugitive from justice? Eddie, I'm an attorney. If they do me for money laundering, I'm finished. I'm on the street.'

Eddie says, 'We'll figure something out. We'll take care of you.'

'How are you going to do that? This is my good name we're talking about.'

'Your name?' He laughs. 'What name? Nobody has a name.' He leans forward once more. 'Look,' he says, 'you don't have a job to go back to. As of now. I hereby terminate your employment. Do you understand? There's nothing to go back to.'

I'm fired? Again? 'Why am I fired? What are the grounds?'

'Come on, now,' Eddie says. 'Don't be like that. Here,' he says, filling my wine glass. He raises his glass, and I'm in such a daze, I do the same. 'Land without rent and death in old Ireland,' Eddie says, as if this were a toast from the old days, which it isn't.

It's not just because I'm half-asleep, blinking stars, and maybe not entirely sober – Eddie and I wound up singing 'Dirty Old Town' in a bar near Times Square at three in the morning, and I returned to the Marriott only so as to pick up my suitcase en route to Heathrow – that, when I arrive at Dubai International Airport, Terminal 3, it's as if I'm a dreamer. From the gate, one passes on a moving walkway through an unprecedented forest of silver-coloured pillars and then, by the paranormal merger of escalator and floor, one is delivered to the border-control stations, an archipelago of kiosks between which coasting border controllers, their all-white apparel copied in the sheen of the floor, make oneiric white shadows. I sail through their attentions. The dream intensifies. I am in a vast white palace filled with rows of the grandest white columns in the world. These fluted, mysteriously twinkling, enormous uprights, maybe ten feet in diameter, point to a civilization, wiser and more advanced than ours, elsewhere in the cosmos and elsewhere in time, and the sensation of otherworldly transportation – not expected by the air traveller, who has the idea that she has completed her journey – is reinforced by the decorative metal band on the white ceiling above the central concourse, an airy argentine river containing lights and the images of the same lights, reflected from the marble floor, and the images of those images: this overhead reflection of reflections, a pluperfect constellation, is repeated underfoot, where the dots of light on the ceiling, an infinity, are optically doubled; and so there are heavens above and heavens below. This is the realm of the luggage carousels. Gigantic circling coelacanths, their scaly black belts carry suitcases from Manchester and Trivandrum and the Seychelles. It almost feels like an option to hop aboard and go around like a bag for ten minutes and be picked up and towed away on one's little wheels and, in the fullness of time, be taken wherever – Dar es Salaam, Rio de Janeiro, Ho Chi Minh City. A taxi and an elevator move me from the airport to my bed, and I wake up in a Tuesday morning refreshed and clear-eyed – and still it seems as if I'm dreaming.

There is no awaking from the facts. I have no job, no car, and (a futile attempt at online banking confirms) no access to my dirhams: my bank has frozen my accounts, presumably upon being notified, by the Batros Group, that my contract of service has been terminated. I have no right to be here. Unless I promptly find employment – very difficult for anyone, in this economy; very, very difficult, for the tainted jobseeker – I will be forced to pack my bags: a foreigner is permitted to live in this country only if, and for so long as, she or he is a worker sponsored by an employer. ('Employer', in this sense, cannot include oneself: the sole contractor or freelancer is a juridical nonentity in Dubai. One cannot be one's own boss.)

And I have no Ali. I'm assuming he, too, has been formally canned. I cannot be sure, because he is not responding to my messages. That isn't illogical. I am no longer his manager; he is free to ignore me. And why wouldn't he? I put him in the way of harm. I failed him.

Yet from a different tributary of feeling come strength and excitement. I'm pumped up as I head off to the DIFC for my encounter with the regulators. They want a piece of me? I'll give them a piece of me.

When I arrive at the FSA office, high up in The Gate, I'm told the rendezvous has been cancelled. After waiting around and pushing for answers, I'm informed that the regulators have been made aware that I'm no longer a Batros employee and that consequently they lack jurisdiction to meet with me. It does no good to explain that I offer myself as a volunteer, in order to be of assistance. There will be no encounter.

So be it. My day will come. I will have my say. This will not stand.

'This will not stand,' I repeat to Ollie, very importantly. We have convened for an emergency drink, in the afternoon, at Calabar. Our table overlooks the artificial lake that serves as a waterfront for Dubai Mall. I well remember the huge cavity that was here before, and I regret not having witnessed the record-breaking inundation that produced this body of water.

Ollie says, 'What won't stand?' When I start to reply, he interrupts with, 'Yeah, I know all that. I'm just saying, there's nothing to take a stand against. I know they've sacked you, but what you're talking about hasn't happened. Nobody's coming after you – yet.'

'You think they won't?'

Ollie says, 'I wouldn't stick around to find out. I'd be gone.

There's nothing for you here except a shitstorm. Mate, get out while the going's good.'

I don't answer him. What Ollie doesn't understand is that I will not be bounced from country to country. I can be pushed only so far and no farther. There comes a point when I draw a line in the sand.

Ollie says, 'Are you all right for money? Just say the word.'

I'm OK, I tell him. (Although my Dubai cash is inaccessible, I have funds in my New York account – 26,455.70 USD – and I have my old New York credit cards. I'm not completely illiquid.) To be honest, I'm a little disappointed with my old buddy of the depths. When I told him about Sandro's despicable conduct, he didn't really react. I'm not expecting Ollie to tell Sandro Batros to go fuck himself and find someone else to take care of his fungal feet; but I think I detect, in his demeanour, evidence of a self-interested computation: he has his commercial interests to consider. This unspoken reckoning of utilities may not be inconsistent with mateship, but neither is it pretty.

'Look, I can't skip town,' I tell him. 'It's a question of principle.'

Ollie takes a swig of pineapple juice and clatters his glass on the table. 'Fair enough,' he says. 'I won't be around to see it all go down, unfortunately.'

A cold, cold chill. 'Shanghai?' Why is this word, Shanghai, in my life?

'Yeah,' Ollie says. He tells me that they've found a great pre-school for Charlie, and an apartment that's 'smallish, but fantastic. We're even shipping out Walda, the nanny.' Ollie says that he's started to get excited, and I believe him. He's already calling it 'Shangers'.

'Sweet,' I say.

A little while later, we part company. The world goes on. It doesn't care – unless it has you in its sights.

I have long had my suspicions about the escape to figuration

– the flight to metamorphic representation of which I'm so often guilty. How can A be turned into B? Doesn't A = A? Isn't B really a way to hide A? Yet I'm also aware that the great personages of the history of thinking, to whom I owe my small measure of liberty from ignorance, have seen fit to deploy apparent misrepresentations in order to progress into the unknown. It's in the spirit of the doomed, last-ditch sortie that I embrace the idea of the submarine to attempt to account for the deep element of illusion into which, it feels like, I have been hurled, as if – and here one definitively leaves behind the stockade of the literal – as if at some point in one's past one was thrown unconscious overboard, and one has only now gained an awareness of one's situation, which is that of the human person going downward in water, and one is in a fix, to put it mildly, and heedless fish-people swim by, and a terrible bathyal reality prevails, and one can only go down, and cannot breathe, and one's humanness has no medium. The perils of such a fantasia are evident – what about people who have actually been thrown overboard, for example? Is their experience to be frivolously appropriated? Nonetheless, once I'm restored from my aquatic delirium, I'm left with a new, possibly valuable, clue-like question: when was I tossed into the sea? Because, as I review my history of living without a feeling of insight, I cannot say that it all started yesterday, at Dubai International Airport. I have trouble identifying a moment, if I may flip the question, about which I can say, At that moment, I certainly had not yet gone under; at that moment, I was on the good ship. Indeed it seems to me that every epoch of my life has involved a snorkeller of sorts, a gasper . . . O brightening glance! There must be a way to Wiki this. There must be an answer.

I go to sleep. When I stir, at dawn in The Situation, nothing has changed. The facts are all still there. Tomorrow is not a new day.

Except that sometimes the details are new. Today's new detail is Watson. Watson is the most trusted and put-upon Batros lawyer in Dubai, and all of our dealings have been pleasant and successful. I would not go so far as to call him a friend, but I will say that I like and respect him and have reason to hope he feels the same way about me. 'Good morning,' he says on the intercom, 'I was wondering if I might come up. I've got some paperwork here, I'm afraid.'

'Of course,' I say.

Watson accepts coffee. He asks for permission to sit at the table, and he waits for me to join him before he reaches for his briefcase, and he asks for permission to place the briefcase on the table. Again, I grant permission. I must say that I warm to this man. He is a compact, reticent Scot. 'Please accept this by way of personal service,' he says, handing me a document titled 'Terms of Settlement'.

I read the document. The 'Reason for Termination' is stated to be 'Gross Misconduct'. My 'End of Service Benefits' are stated to be 'None'.

I say, 'Right, well of course I take issue with all of that.'

Watson bows his head. 'Your countersignature isn't necessary,' he says, 'but it would make life easier. And I'm going to need your passport,' he says. He explains that the company will cancel my employment visa, which will be followed by the cancellation of my residence visa. I will then have thirty days to leave. 'In the circumstances,' Watson says, the company 'declines' to make the customary payment of repatriation expenses.

I say to him, 'Tell me about the gross misconduct. I have no idea what I'm supposed to have done.'

Watson says, 'I'm not able to help you with that today, I'm afraid.'

'I'm very, very unhappy about this,' I say. 'They're making me the fall guy. It's completely unacceptable.'

Watson says, 'You're aware the Dubai police are taking an interest in this matter?'

'Let them. I've done nothing wrong.'

Watson bows. 'May I speak unofficially – collegially?' I tell him he may. Wearing the hat of the colleague, Watson says, 'My guess is that the authorities will not confine their investigations to your role at the Foundation.' He says, 'I apprehend there are some question marks about your dealings with Alain Batros. Privately tutoring children is against the law here. For the protection of minors.'

'That's ridiculous. He was an intern, for God's sake.'

'If you gave him academic help,' Watson says, 'there may be a perception that you unlawfully acted as his tutor in the privacy of your office. And there's the question' – Watson raises a finger to cut me off – 'there's the concern about Mr Ali's dealings with Alain, and your role in those dealings.'

'You've got to be joking,' I say.

Watson says, 'Your corporate computer would appear to have been put to illegal use. The technicians have found an unauthorized virtual network, and somebody has used your computer to make visits to pornographic websites. That's a problem, obviously.'

I deem it best to say nothing.

Watson says, 'Does the name Godfrey Pardew mean anything to you?'

So that's how it's going to play out. I'm a fiend. I'm a round-the-clock criminal.

*Really, Eddie? You would do this?*

'Collegially,' I say, 'how do you think it would pan out?'

Watson says, 'In my experience, someone in your position should have at the forefront of his mind the real possibility of a criminal conviction and a lengthy custodial sentence – five to ten years is by no means out of the question. In any event, you're looking at hostile, complex, expensive, drawn-out legal proceedings: best-case scenario, a lengthy investigation coupled with house arrest. The house arrest could go on for years, as I'm sure you're aware.'

Watson is only telling me what everybody here already knows. A handful of men have famously chosen to fight for their honour in Dubai rather than be convicted in absentia of crimes (relating to financial failures, almost invariably) of which they claim to be innocent. By and large, it seems to have not worked out for them, insofar as one receives continuing reports about their suffering and/or mistreatment in prison and/or in the court system and/or while under house arrest for the duration of indefinite 'investigations' (i.e., in a halfway house between guilt and innocence in which the compulsorily domesticated party is denied the creditable adversity of being in jail and, simultaneously, the good standing associated with so-called freedom).

I ask Watson straight out: 'What do you suggest?'

He gets up, takes his first and only sip of coffee. 'I'll come back in a couple of hours to collect your passport. If I were you, I'd think very carefully about whether you want to be here. I understand that I may not be the only visitor you receive this afternoon.'

'I see,' I say, quite literally, because I'm envisioning Dubai policemen charging in and taking me away.

We shake hands. 'Thank you for your hospitality,' he says.

No sooner have I closed the door behind Watson than I start packing. Mysteriously, I find myself moving with the efficiency of an assembly-line worker, i.e., someone who has performed my actions thousands of times. I limit myself to that quantity of belongings capable of fitting into one laptop bag and one carry-on case. The decision is easily made, because I have nothing physical I'm attached to, and because to eliminate stuff is a dark, strong joy. There is the temptation to keep going – to eliminate even one's only bag. The temptation must be resisted, arising as it does from a mistaking of actual luggage for that which is dragged around psychically. Ridding oneself of a perfectly wearable pair of underpants solves nothing.

I must not, in my haste, forget my passport. Very good: it's still valid. Mine is the new, so-called biometric edition. A huge bald-eagle head dominates the page above my photograph. The bald eagle would only have to lean over to gobble up my head. These days, the US passport looks like a picture book for children. To flip through it is to contemplate, beneath festive clusters of exit and entry stamps, renderings in pen-and-ink of an alleged American quintessence: a farmer and two oxen ploughing the prairie; cowboys riding with cattle; a grizzly bear devouring a salmon; a Mississippi steamboat; a sailing ship off the New England shore; and so on. This folksy, somewhat ominous little graphic paperback ends with an image of North America viewed from space, as if through the eyes of an awed celestial being. The moon is in the picture, too, perhaps to indicate our nation's extraterrestrial reach.

The blue pages put me in mind of the carpets of Zurich, pale-blue fields on which I daily spent hours playing and massacring with the plastic little cowboys and soldiers and Indian braves that served as dolls for small boys of my generation. These battles – GIs firing bazookas at the redskins behind the table leg, flamethrowers clearing gladiators out of the deep-pile carpet – connected the young me to his rumoured fatherland, for which I felt a homesickness that strangely only deepened when I moved there. It is from this era that I retain one of my few ineliminable memories of my mother. She is standing at the sink, washing up in Switzerland.

There are quotations above the pictures, I see:

> Let every nation know, whether it wishes us well or ill,
> that we shall pay any price, bear any burden, meet any

hardship, support any friend, oppose any foe, to assure
the survival and the success of liberty.

*John F. Kennedy*

Let us raise a standard to which the wise and honest
can repair.

*George Washington*

The cause of freedom is not the cause of a race or a
sect, a party or a class – it is the cause of humankind,
the very birthright of humanity.

*Anna Julia Cooper*

My country is now in the sixth grade?

I bear in mind that expatriation is distortive. I accept the
proposition that I wrongly see the USA as a Jenn-land and my
feelings about it are accordingly twisted. I quash my rebel's excitement. I factor into my thinking the panic of the fugitive. I reject
as unreliable and extraneous to the decision I must make the
jolt of abhorrence caused by my passport and my sudden insight
that American nationhood is part of an outdated worldwide
protection racket and that it should be possible, surely, to live
without a state's say-so. I set to one side all theories and systems.
Bailiffs, clear the room: Jenn, Don Sanchez, the Batroses, the
three Ted Wilsons, the contemptible couple from the A train – I
want all of them out. I must be left alone. I must deliberate.

I will deliberate in the Pasha. When I take a seat, I shift a
little in order to remove my passport from a buttock pocket.
The egg-shaped blue marks of the Department of Homeland
Security declare ADMITTED and ADMITTED and ADMITTED.

The phone. Ali!

'Ali!' I say, clambering out of the Pasha. 'How are you? Are
you OK?'

'I am at the airport, boss,' Ali says.

He's one step ahead of me, as always. He has foreseen my departure and is in position to wave goodbye.

From what he next tells me, I gather that Ali is about to board a plane. I gather that his application for Emirati citizenship somehow resulted in an unrefusable offer of citizenship of the Union of the Comoros. I gather that he has a wife and two children. I gather he is now about to leave for the Comoro Islands in the company of his wife and two children. I gather he has no option. I gather that, as a Comorian national, he can no longer be in Dubai because he now has another place where he can be.

'I want to say thank you, boss,' Ali says. 'You have helped me.'

'No, I thank you, Ali' is all I can think to say to him. 'Good luck to you and your family. Stay in contact,' I say, very stupidly, because there is no way that Ali and I will be able to stay in contact. 'OK,' he says, and he disconnects. My friend is gone.

But gone how? To what effect? Not to devalue Ali's subjectivity, but for me his fate lacks depth. The Comoros?

Surely there's time for one last search.

The top search suggestion is 'Comoros crash': the Comoros are notable, in the first place, as a site of aviation accidents. They constitute a sovereign state and comprise a chain of volcanic islands in the Mozambique Channel, northwest of Madagascar. Since independence from France was achieved in 1975, the islands have seen twenty coups/attempted coups. Comorian and French are the main languages; Arabic is also spoken. The main economic activity is agriculture: vanilla is cultivated there, and the islands are the world's largest producer of ylang-ylang, the oil of which is an ingredient of Chanel No. 5 perfume. Photographs of the Comoros show a lake in a crater, a mongoose lemur perched on the rusted tin roof of a one-roomed residential proposition, and a very rundown little port, Moroni, the capital. Its old colonial warehouses give prettily on to forested uplands; its fishing boats lie prettily at anchor; there is no sign of activity.

Hold the airplane door, Ali, I'm coming.

Let's not be rash. Let's take a closer look.

Unemployment is very high in the Comoros. About half the population lives on less than 1.25 USD a day. People regularly try to 'escape' to the nearby island of Mayotte, a French overseas department, and a good number drown in the attempt. As for Moroni, it sits at the foot of a highly active volcano. 'Moroni' is Comorian for 'in the heart of the fire'.

I will not be joining Ali.

I'm shutting the laptop when, for old times' sake, and for the first time in a long time, and for the last time, I swear, I search myself, X. and all. Autocomplete suggests:

> dubai
> attorney
> forcible touching
> gay

The defamation continues. It's shocking. It's enough to make me want to lie down.

It's back into the Pasha. And it's back, on recollection's ice, to Mar-A-Lago.

The wedding of Melania Knauss and Donald Trump was an unusual event, but I think it may have been especially out of the ordinary for Jenn and me, who in the context of that gathering qualified as so-called 'real people' or 'civilians'. This was in January 2005, in the very early, very successful days of *The Apprentice*, and many well-known NBC 'personalities' and stars of reality television were wedding guests, and of course there were celebrities from other walks of life and reality. Jenn and I knew nobody there and yet, by an enchanting paradox, we were able to identify many of those present. These individuals had the charisma and suddenness of fauna. Here was Barbara Walters, startling as a secretary bird; there, like a small upstanding crocodile, was Paul Anka. It was especially outlandish to sight them in the church. The fellow next to me on the pew had a familiar TV-face – Pat O'Brien, I later figured out, the *Access Hollywood* host who afterwards had a brush or two with disrepute, poor devil – and I remember that I could not help feeling it odd that he and his ilk should have to squeeze into the hard pews and humble themselves on the kneelers like everybody else. Jenn and I of course were known to nobody, but by virtue of our mere occurrence were understood to possess imperceptible power or renown, and certainly wealth. Almost every net-worth present at the wedding was very high, I would say. At dinner, I was seated near two likeable, non-famous, not-loaded-looking guys who said they were connected to the bridegroom by business. It was a relief to locate people on my own level, and we were able to talk about this and that. I kind of dried up when they began to exchange details of the résumés of their pilots. This isn't in any way to pooh-pooh them or the occasion.

As the dinner drew to an end, my attention veered to a neighbouring table, where a man was eating almost in solitude: save for a woman who was clearly his wife, the seats around him were vacant. Looking more closely at this forlorn diner, I recognized him from the newspapers: Conrad Black, the newspaper publisher who had given up his Canadian citizenship in order to accept a British peerage. Now Lord Black was an alleged embezzler. The SEC proceedings against him were only several months old and nothing had been proven, yet already a distinct cloud of downfall hung over this man, and apparently one or two of those seated near him had decided to eat somewhere else. I observed all of this unreflectively. I did not feel, stirring within, the organizing of moral faculties. I looked at Black like a boy looking at a duck. In the years since, I've kept half an eye on the Conrad Black story, though not out of any special sympathy for its protagonist, who seems unaccountably to have a Napoleonic idea of himself and, to be honest, rubs me the wrong way with his scornful pronouncements from on high, and absolutely doesn't strike me as the kind of dude I'd like to chill with, not that that's a valid measure of anything. No, I've followed his fate out of the same childish, selfish strain of curiosity that led me to gawk at him in the first place – that yearning to enter the territory where, deep in a forest, a dragon breathes heavily on a hoard of knowledge.

After dinner, there was dancing around the swimming pool. Jenn and I spectated. 'The richer you are, the worse you dance,' she said. I wanted to dance but I didn't ask her to, because she didn't like to dance, I think because it made her afraid. At a certain point, the Conrad Blacks took to the floor. The wife had eyes only for the husband, and vice versa, and as they swayed and shuffled on the spot, always smiling, they took turns to murmur confidences into the other's ear. For the duration of a song, they were the only ones on the dance floor, and Jenn said, 'Who are those two?' I said, 'He's Conrad Black. I can't remember her name. Mrs Conrad Black.' 'Huh,' Jenn said. I imagine that, like me, she was wondering what to make of this performance of amorousness, which I suspect left many feeling by comparison romantically wan. The uncharitable observer – is there another kind? – would say that the flaunting of a supposed connubial superiority was an important part of the fun the Conrad Blacks were having. I say, Maybe so; but subsequent events have shown that, whatever else they may be accused of, they are not guilty of making an insubstantial marriage. It is reported that Mrs Conrad Black – a personage of independent notoriety, it would seem – has moved full-time to the couple's Palm Beach residence in order to be near her husband in his correctional facility, this even though she suffers from a skin condition that responds poorly to tropical sunlight, and even though she owns a pair of huge guard dogs, of

Hungarian provenance, whose thick white fur makes them, too, ill-suited to Florida living.

As is well known, Lord Black's relations with the forces of justice only deteriorated after the Trump wedding, and I haven't kept up with the various convictions, judgments, suits, appeals and proceedings (including moves to 'strip' him of membership of the Order of Canada, to bar him from holding US company directorships, and to discourage him from sitting in the House of Lords) that have engulfed him. I take no sides. I will only say that, if the moves against Black show no sign of ending, neither does Black's strangely joyful struggling. For the time being he remains in prison in Florida. Here, I find myself moved to a certain respect and sympathy – and, is it possible, envy: he has, as it were, surfaced from illusion. He is purely disgraced. He is behind bars. He wears a jumpsuit. His enemies have revealed themselves – as have, I feel sure, his friends. Also, obscurely, he is in the clear. Maybe I'm perverse, but I connect imprisonment to a limit of culpability. It's certainly true that, so long as he's inside, Black can hardly be punished more.

The Swedish frictions came to an end some while ago. I have no wish to move. Because of my new phobia or new PTSD, the Pasha now faces away from the windows, and to open my eyes is to see a white wall. In its way, it is a magnificent vista. I could stay where I am, looking at that wall, for a long time – and in fact this is what I do, quite without foreboding. On the contrary: any minute now, Watson, followed soon after by the others, will as it were rat-a-tat-tat on the door.

I am grateful for assistance received from the Dorothy and Lewis B. Cullman Center for Scholars and Writers; the John Simon Guggenheim Memorial Foundation; the National Endowment for the Arts; and the Corporation of Yaddo.